WV 270 GRA

AC

Dedication

This seventh edition of *Ballantyne's Deafness* is dedicated to the memory of John Ballantyne and to his family.

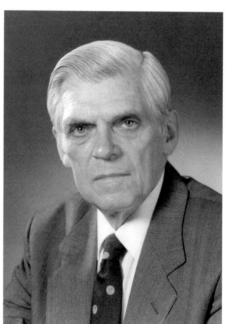

Ballantyne's Deafness

Seventh Edition

Edited by

John M Graham MA BM BCh FRCS

Consultant Otolaryngologist
Royal National Throat, Nose and Ear Hospital
London, UK

and

David M Baguley BSc MSc MBA PhD

Consultant Clinical Scientist and Director of Audiology
Cambridge University Hospitals NHS Foundation Trust
Cambridge, UK

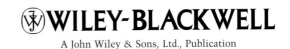

WILEY-BLACKWELL

A John Wiley & Sons, Ltd., Publication

This edition first published 2009
© 2009 John Wiley & Sons
Sixth edition first published 2001
© 2001 Whurr Publication

Wiley-Blackwell is an imprint of John Wiley & Sons, formed by the merger of Wiley's global Scientific, Technical and Medical business with Blackwell Publishing.

Registered office
John Wiley & Sons Ltd, The Atrium, Southern Gate, Chichester, West Sussex, PO19 8SQ, United Kingdom

Editorial office
John Wiley & Sons Ltd, The Atrium, Southern Gate, Chichester, West Sussex, PO19 8SQ, United Kingdom

For details of our global editorial offices, for customer services and for information about how to apply for permission to reuse the copyright material in this book please see our website at www.wiley.com/wiley-blackwell.

Library of Congress Cataloging-in-Publication Data
Ballantyne's deafness / edited by John M. Graham and David M. Baguley. – 7th ed.
    p. ; cm.
Includes bibliographical references and index.
ISBN 978-0-470-77311-6 (pbk. : alk. paper) 1. Deafness. I. Ballantyne, John C. (John Chalmers) II. Graham, J. M. (John Malcolm) III. Baguley, David (David M.) IV. Title: Deafness.
[DNLM: 1. Hearing Loss–diagnosis. 2. Hearing Loss–therapy. 3. Audiometry–methods. 4. Hearing Aids. WV 270 B188 2009]
RF290.B17 2009
617.8–dc22
2008049890

A catalogue record for this book is available from the British Library.

Set in 10 on 12 pt Sabon by SNP Best-set Typesetter Ltd., Hong Kong
Printed in Singapore by Markono Print Media Pte Ltd

1 2009

Contents

Contributors

Sally Austen BA(Hons) MSc CPsychol AfBPsS
Consultant Clinical Psychologist, National
Deaf Mental Health Services (Birmingham),
Birmingham and Solihull Mental Health
Foundation Trust, Birmingham, UK

Patrick R Axon MD FRCS(ORL-HNS)
Consultant Otolaryngologist, Cambridge
University Hospitals NHS Foundation Trust,
Cambridge, UK

David M Baguley BSc MSc MBA PhD
Consultant Clinical Scientist and Director of
Audiology, Cambridge University Hospitals
NHS Foundation Trust, Cambridge, UK

Doris-Eva Bamiou MD MSc PhD
DoH HEFCE Clinical Senior Lecturer,
UCL Ear Institute. Consultant in
Neuro-otology, Neuro-otology Department,
National Hospital for Neurology and
Neurosurgery, London, UK

Judith C Bird MSc
Clinical Scientist (Audiology), Cambridge
University Hospitals NHS Foundation Trust,
Cambridge, UK

Rachel L Booth MSc PhD
Principal Clinical Scientist (Audiology),
Manchester Royal Infirmary, Manchester, UK

Martin J Burton MA DM FRCS
Consultant Otolaryngologist, Oxford Radcliffe
NHS Trust. Senior Clinical Lecturer, University
of Oxford, Oxford, UK

Huw Cooper BSc MSC PhD
Consultant Clinical Scientist (Audiology),
University Hospital Birmingham NHS
Foundation Trust, Birmingham, UK

Adrian Davis OBE FFPH FSS FRSA MSc PhD
Director, NHS Newborn Hearing Screening
Programme. Director, MRC Hearing and
Communication Group, University of
Manchester, Manchester, UK

Katrina Davis BA (Cantab) MB BChir
ST2 Post in Psychiatry, Institute of Psychiatry,
South London and Maudsley NHS Foundation
Trust, London, UK

Neil Donnelly MSc(Hons) FRCS(ORL-HNS)
Fellow in Neurotology and Skull Base Surgery,
Cambridge University Hospitals NHS
Foundation Trust, Cambridge, UK

Graham P Frost BSc(Hons) MSc RHAD
Technical Director, PC Werth Ltd, London, UK

William PR Gibson MD FRCS FRACS
Professor of Otolaryngology, University of
Sydney. Director, Sydney Cochlear Implant
Centre, New South Wales, Australia

John M Graham MA BM BCh FRCS
Consultant Otolaryngologist, Royal National
Throat, Nose and Ear Hospital, London, UK

Roger F Gray LRCP MRCS MB BS MA
FRCS(ORL-HNS)
Consultant Otolaryngologist, Cambridge
University Hospitals NHS Foundation Trust,
Cambridge, UK

Lucy Handscomb MA
Hearing Therapist, St Mary's Hospital,
London. Lecturer in Audiology, Centre for
Hearing and Balance Studies, University of
Bristol, Bristol, UK

Sarah Healy MB ChB MRCSEd DOHNS
ST2, Ear, Nose and Throat Surgery, Leicester
Royal Infirmary, Leicester, UK

William PL Hellier MB ChB FRCS(ORL-HNS)
Consultant ENT Surgeon, Southampton
University Hospital and Royal Hampshire
County Hospital, Winchester, Hampshire, UK

Penny R Hill MSc DPhil
Clinical Scientist (Audiology), Manchester
Royal Infirmary, Manchester, UK

Rachel Humphriss MSc CS
Lecturer, University of Bristol, Bristol, UK

Richard M Irving MD FRCS
Consultant in Otology, Neurotology and Skull
Base Surgery, University Hospital Birmingham
and Birmingham Children's Hospital. Honorary
Senior Lecturer, University of Birmingham,
Birmingham, UK

Richard D Knight PhD MSc CS
Clinical Scientist (Audiology), Audiology
Department, Cambridge University Hospitals
NHS Foundation Trust, Cambridge, UK

Simon KW Lloyd BSc FRCS(ORL-HNS)
Locum Consultant Otolaryngologist, Royal
National Throat, Nose and Ear Hospital and
Royal Free Hospitals NHS Trust, London, UK

Mark E Lutman BSc MSc PhD
Professor of Audiology and Head of Hearing
and Balance Centre, Institute of Sound and
Vibration Research, University of Southampton,
Southampton, UK

Catherine A Lynch BSc MSc
Clinical Scientist (Audiology), The Emmeline
Centre for Hearing Implants, Cambridge
University Hospitals NHS Foundation Trust,
Cambridge, UK

Josephine Marriage BSc MSc PhD RHAD
Paediatric and Research Audiologist.
Director, Chear Ltd, Royston, Hertfordshire,
UK

David McAlpine BSc DPhil(Oxon)
Professor of Auditory Neuroscience. Director,
UCL Ear Institute, London, UK

Don J McFerran MA FRCS
ENT Consultant, Colchester Hospital
University NHS Foundation Trust, Colchester,
Essex, UK

Laurence McKenna MClinPsychol DG Dip Cog
Ther PhD
Consultant Clinical Psychologist, Royal
National Throat, Nose and Ear Hospital,
London, UK

Anne O'Sullivan BSc MSc ACS
Consultant Speech and Language Therapist,
Royal National Throat, Nose and Ear Hospital,
London, UK

Henry Pau MD MBChB FRCSEd
FRCSEd(ORL-HNS) FRCS
Consultant Ear, Nose and Throat Surgeon and
Honorary Senior Lecturer, University of
Leicester, Leicester, UK

Peter A Rea BM BCh MA FRCS
Consultant Otolaryngologist and Lead
Clinician, The Leicester Balance Centre,
Leicester Royal Infirmary and The London
Road Clinic, Leicester, UK

Shakeel R Saeed MBBS(Lon) FRCS(Ed)
FRCS(Eng) FRCS(Orl) MD(Man)
Professor of Otology/Neuro-otology, UCL Ear
Institute. Consultant ENT and Skullbase
Surgeon, The Royal National Throat, Nose and
Ear Hospital and Royal Free Hospital, London,
UK

Pauline Smith BSc MSc
Clinical Scientist, MRC Hearing and
Communication Group, University of
Manchester, Manchester. Clinical Scientist,
Hearing Services, Leicester Royal Infirmary,
Leicester, UK

Neil Weir MA FRCS
Honorary ENT Surgeon, Royal Surrey County
Hospital, Guildford, Surrey, UK

Tony Wright LLM DM FRCS TechRMS
Emeritus Professor of Otolaryngology, UCL
Ear Institute. Consultant ENT Surgeon, Royal
National Throat, Nose and Ear Hospital,
London, UK

Foreword 1

John Ballantyne CBE FRCS DLO HonFRCSI HonFRCPS(Glas) HonFCS (SA) 1917–2008

John Ballantyne was a champion of deaf people of all ages, a skilful and versatile surgeon, author, editor, teacher, mentor, musician and above all friend to otolaryngologists, patients and many others throughout the world.

Deafness, originally written to help parents of deaf children and the adult deaf, and later used by generations of audiologists in training, was published while John Ballantyne was Assistant Director to the Audiology Unit at the Royal National Throat, Nose and Ear Hospital, London (1953–58).

When he moved on to the Royal Free Hospital in 1958 he collaborated with his senior colleague WG 'Bill' Scott-Brown in editing and contributing to the second edition of his legendary textbook *Diseases of the Ear Nose and Throat*, and later with John Groves produced the third and fourth editions. These editions and other books, together with the editorship of *The Journal of Laryngology and Otology* (1978–88), benefited hundreds of readers and authors and gave John Ballantyne global prominence.

The first *Journal of Laryngology and Otology* supplement, published in 1978, was co-authored by John Ballantyne, Professor Ted Evans and the late Andrew Morrison (Ballantyne *et al.*, 1978). It concerned the state of the art of cochlear implantation and paved the way for further work by the Medical Research Council and later adoption of the technique by the Department of Health and Social Security (DHSS). As Chairman of the DHSS Advisory Committee on Services for Hearing Impaired People (ACSHIP), John Ballantyne introduced hearing therapists, drew attention to the needs of the adult deaf, and contributed to the establishment of audiological physicians.

He received recognition for his endeavours on behalf of deaf people in the form of eponymous lectureships, prizes, high offices in British otolaryngology, and honorary fellowships of the surgical colleges of Ireland, Glasgow and South Africa. He was awarded the CBE in 1984.

John Ballantyne died in June 2008 in his 91st year.

Reference

Ballantyne JC, Evans EF, Morrison AW (1978) Electrical auditory stimulation in the management of profound hearing loss. *Journal of Laryngology and Otology* 92(suppl 1).

Neil Weir

Foreword 2

Ballantyne's Deafness

Ballantyne's Deafness is a classic resource for audiologists, specialist teachers, audiological physicians, ENT surgeons, and psychologists interested in perception. I am delighted to see it revived in the competent hands of John Graham and David Baguley, who have themselves pushed back the frontiers. John Graham has been at the forefront of cochlear implantion and David Baguley has contributed to many aspects of audiology.

John Ballantyne anticipated cochlear implantation in the UK, leading a fact-finding trip to California. The subsequent report to the Department of Health in 1978 was pivotal in obtaining funding for the first implant centres a few years later. Such was his enthusiasm for better lives for deaf people that he would have been sure to welcome the glittering array of advances displayed on these pages.

I had the privilege of being John Ballantyne's last registrar at the Royal Free Hospital London in the late 1970s. It was an experience I treasure because it was a time when every condition had a diagnosis and a treatment to be utilised fearlessly. In theatre, John was a decisive and skilled operator who just got on and solved the problem. I tiptoed along behind, ready with the adrenaline and cocaine crystals, which JB mixed to such good effect for his nasal cases. A stapedectomy took 40 minutes. In clinic it was a different story, with care to see each patient's symptoms in the light of their work and experience, often leading to different management for patients with identical symptoms (absolute voice rest for a teacher with vocal strain and a local anaesthetic throat spray for a talented professional singer nearing the end of a concert tour in London – we got free tickets to the performance). John's teaching was always clear and to the point, starting with the fundamentals, especially of the scientific basis of our specialty. This was the style in the early editions written with his daughter Deborah, herself an audiologist. By the sixth and now the seventh edition there was too much in this important field for a single author, so we now have contributions from the leaders in the field. These are the new developments in that rich seam that runs between audiology and surgery. The editors have done their best to make the text as accessible as possible, so that we can enjoy a common language. This is important because, provided each can understand the other, the interface between different disciplines is the area where advances are made. Microelectronics and microsurgery are but the latest examples. I have every expectation that the techniques that will be used by the next generation of specialists will be put forward in this seventh edition, making it a fine tribute to John Ballantyne's long and enduring vision for the relief of deafness.

Roger F Gray

Comment by the editors: This tribute to John Ballantyne was written in February 2008, while John Ballantyne was still alive, and we have included it with the minimum of changes.

Preface

John Ballantyne died in June 2008, in his 91st year, not long before the publication of this, the seventh edition of the book he originally wrote in 1960. Generations of parents of deaf children, audiologists, surgeons and physicians, speech and language therapists, teachers, psychologists, paediatricians, public health audiologists, audiological scientists and engineers in the field of hearing have every reason to be grateful to John Ballantyne for his continuing influence, through this book, in explaining in simple and clear terms what it means to be deaf or to care for a deaf child, and how we may all contribute to this most fascinating of fields of endeavour.

We hope that this edition will continue on the path created by John Ballantyne. Although some technical aspects of our field have changed and developed in ways our predecessors may not have predicted in the 1960s, the fundamental principles of multidisciplinary clinical care, with the patient at the focal centre of this care, have not changed, and should never do so.

Some of the authors who have contributed to this seventh edition are new; some have updated their contributions to previous editions, to incorporate fresh information and new techniques. All contributors are busy professionals and have given generously of their time and skills. As editors we express our gratitude to them all for their hard work and for helping us to produce this book within a relatively short period of gestation.

For this edition of *Ballantyne's Deafness*, we have tried to continue John Ballantyne's original and successful concept of a book designed to serve as an introduction to the field of hearing and deafness and an inspiration to those entering the field to develop their expertise and insight.

As a tribute to John Ballantyne, we have included two forewords, written by surgeons who worked closely with John and were inspired by his example. Neil Weir has provided a foreword based on his address at the memorial celebration of John's life. Roger Gray has provided a vignette, written early in the preparation of this edition while John was very much alive, although rather frail. We are grateful to both for providing insights into the life and work of a truly remarkable man. We are also very much indebted to Kate Lay and Vicki Holmes, in the medical illustration departments of the Ear Institute and the Royal National Throat, Nose and Ear Hospital, London, for their skill and enthusiastic help, usually at very short notice and beyond the normal call of duty, in preparing and adapting many of the figures in a number of the chapters.

Lastly, the editors dedicate this book to our wives. It is far from easy to share one's marriage with a large number of authors, publishing editors, passing deadlines and the hypnotic glare of the computer screen, in the knowledge that most of the time spent on such a project is taken from evenings and weekends at home and on holiday. We are truly grateful to Sandy Graham and Bridget Baguley, for their constant support, forbearance and understanding.

John Graham and David Baguley

Abbreviations

A1	primary auditory cortex
AABR	automated auditory brainstem response
AAF	anterior auditory field
AAOHNS	American Academy of Otolaryngology – Head and Neck Surgery
ABI	auditory brainstem implant
ABR	auditory brainstem response
AC	air conduction
ACE	advanced combination encoder
ACSHIP	Advisory Committee on Services for Hearing Impaired People
ADHD	attention deficit hyperactivity disorder
AEP	auditory evoked potential
AHL	acquired hearing loss
AIED	auto-immune inner ear disease
ALD	assistive listening device
AM	amplitude modulation
AMTAS	Automated Method for Testing Auditory Sensitivity
ANF	auditory nerve fibre
AOAE	automated otoacoustic emissions
AOM	acute otitis media
AP	action potential
APD	auditory processing disorder
APHAB	Abbreviated Profile of Hearing Aid Benefit
APHL	acquired profound hearing loss
AR	acoustic reflex
ARHL	age-related hearing loss
ART	acoustic reflex threshold
ART	auditory nerve response telemetry
ASD	autistic spectrum disorder
ASHA	American Speech-Language-Hearing Association
ASSR	auditory steady-state response
ATT	automated toy test
AVCN	anterior ventral cochlear nucleus
BAHA	bone-anchored hearing aid
BAHOH	British Association for the Hard Of Hearing
BC	bone conduction
BDA	British Deaf Association
BDI	Beck Depression Inventory
BEA	better ear average
BiCROS	bilateral contralateral routing of signal
BKB	Bamford–Kowal–Bench (sentence test)
BOA	behavioural observation audiometry
BPPV	benign positional paroxysmal vertigo

BSA	British Society of Audiology		DIC	inferior colliculus dorsal shell
BSER	brainstem electric response		DNA	deoxyribonucleic acid
BTA	British Tinnitus Association		DNLL	dorsal nucleus of the lateral lemniscus
BTE	behind the ear (hearing aid)			
CAEP	cortical auditory evoked potential		DP	distortion product
CAM	complementary and alternative medicine		DPOAE	distortion product otoacoustic emissions
CANS	central auditory nervous system		DSL	desired sensation level
CAP	compound action potential		DSM	*Diagnostic and Statistical Manual of Mental Disorders*
CAPD	central auditory processing disorder			
CB	cognitive behaviour		DSP	digital signal processing (hearing aid)
CBT	cognitive behavioural therapy		EABR	electrically evoked auditory brainstem response
CERA	cortical electric response audiometry			
CF	characteristic frequency		ECAP	electrically evoked compound action potential
CHAPS	Children's Auditory Processing Performance Scale		ECNL	equivalent continuous 8-hour noise level
CHARGE	coloboma, heart defects, atresia of the choanae, retardation of development, genital abnormalities, ear abnormalities		ECochG	electrocochleography
			EHL	estimated hearing level
			ELLAEP	electrically evoked long-latency auditory electric potential
CHL	conductive hearing loss		ENG	electro nystagmography
CI	cochlear implant		ENT	ear, nose and throat
CIC	completely in the canal (hearing aid)		ENU	*N*-ethyl-*N*-nitrosourea
			EP	evoked potential
CIS	continuous interleaved sampling		EPI	echo planar imaging
CM	cochlear microphonic		ESP	early support protocol
CMV	cytomegalovirus		ESR	erythrocyte sedimentation rate
CN	cochlear nucleus		ESRT	electrically evoked stapedial reflex threshold
CNS	central nervous system			
COCB	crossed olivocochlear bundle		FDA	Food and Drug Administration
CPA	cerebellopontine angle		FM	frequency modulation
CROS	contralateral routing of signal		fMRI	functional magnetic resonance imaging
CSF	cerebrospinal fluid			
CSOM	chronic suppurative otitis media		FMT	floating mass transducer
CT	computerised tomography		FTC	frequency-tuning curve
CTA	computed tomographic angiography		GBC	globular bushy cell
			GCSE	General Certificate of Secondary Education
CTSIB	clinical test of sensory interaction and balance			
			GHABP	Glasgow Hearing Aid Benefit Profile
CUNY	City University of New York (sentence test)			
			GP	general practitioner
3D	three-dimensional		HADS	Hospital Anxiety Depression Scale
DAI	direct audio input			
DAS	dorsal acoustic stria		HIE	hypoxic ischaemic encephalopathy
dB	decibel		HL	hearing level
DC	direct current		HQ	Hyperacusis Questionnaire
DCN	dorsal cochlear nucleus		HRT	hormone replacement therapy

HST	hearing support teacher/therapist	MGB	medial geniculate body
HTA	Health Technology Assessment	MHAS	Modernising Hearing Aid Services (programme)
HVDT	Health Visitor Distraction Test		
Hz	Hertz	MIDD	maternally inherited diabetes and deafness
IAC	internal auditory canal		
IAM	internal auditory meatus	MLAEP	middle-latency auditory evoked potential
IC	inferior colliculus		
ICC	inferior colliculus central nucleus	mMGB	medial medial geniculate body
ICD-10	International Classification of Diseases and Related Health Problems, 10th edition	MMN	mismatch negativity
		MMR	measles, mumps and rubella
		MNTB	medial nucleus of the trapezoid body
ICF	International Classification of Functioning, Disability and Health		
		MOC	medial olivocochlear (pathway)
		MPO	maximum power output
ICX	inferior colliculus external nucleus	MRA	magnetic resonance angiography
IEC	International Electrotechnical Commission	MRC	Medical Research Council
		MRI	magnetic resonance imaging
IHC	inner hair cell	MSO	medial superior olive
IHR	Institute of Hearing Research	MTT	McCormick Toy Test
IID	interaural intensity difference	NAB	Newcastle Auditory Battery
IMAP	Institute of Hearing Research Multicentre Auditory Processing (testing battery)	NADP	National Association of Deafened People
		NAL	National Acoustics Laboratory (Australia)
IQ	intelligence quotient		
ISI	Insomnia Severity Index	NART	National Adult Reading Test
ISO	International Standardization Organization	NDCS	National Deaf Children's Society
ISSNHL	idiopathic sudden sensorineural hearing loss	NFl	neurofibromatosis type 1
		NF2	neurofibromatosis type 2
ITD	interaural time difference	nHL	normal hearing level
ITE	in the ear (hearing aid)	NHS	National Health Service (UK)
JCIH	Joint Committee on Infant Hearing	NHSP	Newborn Hearing Screening Programme
KKS	King–Kopetzky syndrome	NICE	National Institute for Health and Clinical Excellence
KSS	Kearns–Sayre syndrome		
LDL	loudness discomfort level	NICU	neonatal intensive care unit
LLAEP	long-latency auditory evoked potential	NIHL	noise-induced hearing loss
		NIL	noise immission level
LOC	lateral olivocochlear (pathway)	NOHL	non-organic hearing loss
LSO	lateral superior olive	NRI	neural response imaging
LSP	language service professional	NRT	neural response telemetry
MDT	multidisciplinary team	NSH	National Study of Hearing
MEG	magneto-encephalography	NSHL	non-syndromic hearing loss
MEI	middle ear implant	OAD	obscure auditory dysfunction
MELAS	mitochondrial encephalopathy lactic acidosis and stroke-like episodes	OAE	otoacoustic emissions
		OHC	outer hair cell
		OME	otitis media with effusion
MERRF	myoclonic epilepsy and ragged red fibres	PATHS	Promoting Alternative Thinking Strategies

PCHI	permanent childhood hearing impairment	SSCD	superior semicircular canal dehiscence syndrome
PET	positron emission tomography	SSEP	steady-state evoked potentials (test)
PMP	personal music player		
PMS	patient management system	STIR	short tau inversion recovery
PORP	partial ossicular replacement prosthesis	TARGET	Trial of Alternative Regimes for Glue Ear Treatment
pps	pulses per second	TE	transient evoked
PSQI	Pittsburgh Sleep Quality Index	TEN	threshold equalising noise (test)
PST	prolonged spontaneous tinnitus	TEOAE	transient evoked otoacoustic emission
PSTH	peri-stimulus time histogram	THI	Tinnitus Handicap Inventory
PTA	pure tone audiometry/audiogram	THQ	Tinnitus Handicap Questionnaire
PTSD	post-traumatic stress disorder	THI-S	Tinnitus Handicap Inventory: Screening Version
PVCN	posterior ventral cochlear nucleus		
QALY	quality-adjusted life-year	TOAE	transient otoacoustic emission
REIR	real ear-insertion response	ToM	theory of mind
REM	real ear measurement	TORCH	toxoplasmosis, rubella, CMV or herpes
RETFL	reference equivalent threshold force level		
		TORP	total ossicular replacement prosthesis
RETSPL	reference equivalent threshold sound pressure level		
		TRQ	Tinnitus Reaction Questionnaire
RIC	receiver in the canal (hearing aid)	TQ	Tinnitus Questionnaire
RITE	receiver in the ear (hearing aid)	TRT	tinnitus retraining therapy
RNID	Royal National Institute for Deaf People	ULL	uncomfortable loudness level
		UNHS	universal neonatal hearing screening
rTMS	repetitive transcranial magnetic stimulation		
		VAS	ventral acoustic stria
SBC	spherical bushy cell	VBI	vertebrobasilar insufficiency
SCENIHR	Scientific Committee on Emerging and Newly Identified Health Risks	VCN	ventral cochlear nucleus
		VEMP	vestibular evoked myogenic potential
SFOAE	stimulus frequency otoacoustic emission	vMGB	ventral medial geniculate body
		VNG	video nystagmography
SLI	specific language impairment	VNLL	ventral nucleus of the lateral lemniscus
SHL	syndromic hearing loss		
SNHL	sensorineural hearing loss	VOR	vestibulo-ocular reflex
SOC	superior olivary complex	VORP	vibrating ossicular prosthesis
SP	summating potential	VRA	visual reinforcement audiometry
SPL	sound pressure level	WDRC	wide dynamic range compression
SRT	speech recognition threshold or stapedius reflex threshold	WHO	World Health Organization

Introduction

David Baguley and John Graham

Human hearing is a wonderful sense, giving access to environmental sound to keep us safe and secure, to spoken language to involve us in the lives of our companions, and to song and music to enthral and enrich us. While people with hearing loss can of course live fulfilling lives, access to all these experiences can be a challenge. With this book we seek to draw the reader into an understanding of hearing impairment and its remediation, introducing a topic that has fascinated us personally and professionally.

The title of the first five editions of this book was simply *Deafness*. John Ballantyne wrote it as an introductory guide for those working with deaf adults and children and their families. In order to discuss deafness and loss of hearing you must first have some understanding of hearing itself.

Taste, smell, sight and hearing are traditionally known as our 'special senses'. Hearing allows us to be aware of sounds in our environment; it allows us to develop language and communicate; it enables us to enjoy what we hear, whether this is music, the information contained in language or the sounds around us. Hearing allows us to be emotionally moved by music, by the content of the spoken language of a poet, by the voice of an actor, by the sounds of nature. Emotions can also be negative: the anger generated by the content of what we hear someone say, the fear generated by an unexplained sound in a dark room. Without hearing, we risk losing these components of our daily life.

Deafness is not simply a reduction in the amplitude of the sounds we perceive. Our sense of hearing involves many different elements: the external and middle ear structures; the cochlea, with its inner and outer hair cells; the transfer of molecules within the cochlea; the encoding of the electrochemical signals travelling in the afferent and efferent nerves connecting the cochlea with the brain; the hearing pathway along which these signals travel through the brainstem and midbrain to the primary hearing areas of the cerebral cortex, with feedback and interaction at all levels of this pathway, and with onward links across the whole brain from the primary auditory cortex. This hugely complex network of systems interacts with most of our conscious and unconscious functions, from emotions to balance, the ability to stand and walk and dance, our vision and the control of our eye movements, and a myriad of others.

As more and more is understood about hearing, the concept of deafness as a simple attenuation of hearing, easily corrected with an ear trumpet, hearing aids or a cochlear implant can be seen to be highly simplistic. We hope that this book, in providing a broad overview of hearing and deafness, will also give insight into this wonderfully complex system. It is hardly surprising, for instance, that no two cases of hearing loss, whether acquired or congenital, can be exactly the same, either in their cause and site of origin, or in their impact on the individual who suffers the hearing loss, or in the most effective method of correcting or compensating for this hearing loss. In a clinical setting, constraints of time will reduce the amount of useful analysis that can take place. We can usefully separate sensorineural deafness, caused by lesions in the cochlea and cochlear nerve, from conductive deafness; this allows us to decide whether the cause of the deafness can be actively treated, perhaps with surgery, or simply compensated for by hearing aids. Potentially life-threatening lesions such as acoustic neuromas can be identified. For the rest, it is still hard or impossible to identify the precise causes or even the sites of the lesions that produce deafness, and of the disorders that affect our hearing. Clinicians working in the field of hearing and deafness need constantly to make appraisals and decisions based on practical and often empirical judgement. With time, we would expect our work to become better and better informed, allowing deeper and wider skills to be applied for the benefit of those who turn to us for help.

Terminology

In this chapter we introduce terminology and concepts that underpin both the scientific understanding of hearing loss and associated symptoms, and the clinical interventions that are available.

The vocabulary used to describe hearing impairment is wide and varied. The word *deafness* can be used in a general sense. If, however, the word *Deaf* is used, especially with a capital D, then a specific meaning is now conveyed, referring to the Deaf community that communicate with sign language and for whom the onset of reduced hearing has usually been *congenital* or before spoken language has been learned (*prelingual*). Within this community, language that describes deafness as an impairment is problematic: rather, it is seen as a difference, not a disability. For those born with good hearing but in whom reduced hearing abilities are acquired, the terms *hearing loss* or *hearing impairment* are commonly used, and the onset is *post-lingual*. *Presbycusis* (*presbyacusis* in the United States of America) is a term used to describe hearing loss acquired with age.

Some people are troubled by sound of internal origin, without an external source, and this is called *tinnitus*. This symptom can derive from bodily sounds, which are not usually perceived, and this is described as *somatic tinnitus*: more commonly it is a *subjective tinnitus* ignited within the auditory system. A commonly associated symptom is *hyperacusis*, in which sounds in the external environment are perceived as intrusive and distressingly loud, even when of moderate intensity.

A biopsychosocial perspective

The term *biopsychosocial* was introduced in 1977 by Engel, and has some important applications to hearing impairment (Engel, 1977). To break it down into component parts: the *bio* element refers to the biological aspects of a situation, and the physiological dimension of hearing impairment is of major significance, both for understanding the situation, and for future treatments that may regenerate elements of the cochlea (see Chapter 11). The *psycho* element includes the psychological aspects to hearing loss, which may include a vulnerability to anxiety, depression and other mental health issues (see Chapters 17 and 18). Less dramatically, an adult with presbycusis may experience difficulties with concentration, and may also feel less confident. *Social* refers not only to the individual's ability to function in society, but also to the way that society views a particular condition. In the case of hearing loss, there are ways that society views the symptom that may be burdensome. The hearing-impaired person can be a figure of fun, or worse, perceived as one of limited intelligence, as a result of their inability to hear.

Underpinning these thoughts is the fact that hearing impairment is not experienced in isolation. It impacts upon one's partner, one's family, and the entire social and professional context in which a person exists.

Impairment, handicap and disability

These terms are not synonymous, and each refers to a different aspect of a situation. These terms have been defined by the World Health Organization (WHO) in 1980 (WHO, 1980).

> An impairment is any loss or abnormality of psychological, physiological or anatomical structure or function; a disability is any restriction or lack (resulting from an impairment) of ability to perform an activity in the manner or within the range considered normal for a human being; a handicap is a disadvantage for a given individual, resulting from an impairment or a disability, that prevents the fulfillment of a role that is considered normal (depending on age, sex and social and cultural factors) for that individual.

In terms of deafness, the *impairment* is the reduction in auditory function, the *disability* is the restriction in activity consequent upon that, and the *handicap* then is the extent to which the individual cannot achieve their potential. The WHO framework was revised in 2000, and now refers to

- losses or abnormalities of bodily function and structure (previously impairments)
- limitations of activities (previously disabilities)
- restriction in participation (previously handicaps)
- contextual factors (WHO, 2000).

As previously, the physical situation, the limitations that places on an individual, and the outworking of that in their context are all considered. This is discussed further in Chapter 17.

Deaf culture and the deaf community

As mentioned above, there are those who believe that to be born deaf is not a disability or a handicap, but an entry into the world of deaf culture. For those who have been born with a degree of deafness that prevents them from acquiring spoken language, the acquisition of sign language has been essential to allow them to communicate. The various national sign languages have become an integral part of the education of profoundly deaf people across the world. Sign languages have a long and rich heritage. Within the Deaf world there are poets, comedians, playwrights, and spiritual leaders, all indications of a thriving and rich culture. However, the deaf community of any country will inevitably be small in relation to the general population and will rely either on written communication or the help of interpreters to communicate fully with the hearing population. It is estimated that in the UK, among a population of 60 million, the number of those who rely on signing to communicate is approximately 50,000 (Adrian Davis, personal communication), although it will touch the lives of many others.

Before the advent of cochlear implants, and their application to congenitally deaf children, it was widely accepted that education through Sign was imperative for the congenitally profoundly deaf. The advent of cochlear implants has changed this. The majority of congenitally deaf, signing couples who have a profoundly deaf child will prefer their child to be brought up as part of the deaf community, and will not consider the provision of a cochlear implant to be either necessary or desirable. This view is rightly respected by professionals working in the field of hearing. However, most congenitally deaf children are born to hearing parents, who are likely to consider that cochlear implantation is desirable if it enables their child to learn speech and spoken language and to experience the world of sound in a way that approximates to their own experience.

Auditory dysfunction

Another dimension to be considered is the type of auditory dysfunction experienced by an individual. This might be thresholds that are reduced from normal values, but also difficulty with discrimination, which may affect the ability to detect small differences in the timing, intensity or frequency of sound. Hearing loss that is unilateral may involve problems with localising sound. In some individuals with hearing loss, the ability to tolerate loud sound may be reduced, which may both trouble and perplex them. Additionally, some people are able to detect the presence of sound, but are unable to understand it, especially in the presence of background noise. This situation has been given the descriptor *auditory processing disorder*, and can almost be considered as the auditory equivalent of dyslexia.

Each of these auditory dysfunctions is a representation of the biological element of the biopsychosocial perspective, and it should be borne in mind that psychological and social consequences will follow accordingly, appropriate to the type of dysfunction. An example would be a person with problems discriminating speech in noise, who may find their social scope limited, and become isolated and ultimately depressed.

Professionals associated with deafness

Deafness requires a multidisciplinary approach and involves a wide range of professionals. The titles of the professions involved varies from country to country, but it is usual for a multidisciplinary team to involve clinical audiologists (with university training in audiology), otolaryngologists with surgical training, physicians with specialist audiology training, speech and language therapists, and teachers of the deaf. In specialist units, clinical psychologists may also be involved, and in some countries engineers will perform many tasks.

Clinical model

While mindful of the cultural issues and sensitivities described above, the perspective of this book is essentially clinical: that is, seeking how the impairment, disability and handicap associated with deafness (in all its forms) can be reduced. For some, with acquired hearing loss, this will mean a process of intervention (such as hearing aid fitting or surgery) and then *rehabilitation*; for others with a congenital hearing impairment this will mean childhood interventions of education and hearing aid use, and a process of *habilitation*.

This clinical perspective is underpinned by a number of concepts. Firstly, it is cautiously optimistic that, in many situations of hearing impairment, benefit can be conferred and the situation improved for the individual, friends and family. Further, it is based upon the idea that not only can *coping strategies* be introduced in the lives of people affected by hearing impairment, but also that the human central nervous system (CNS) can change such that new abilities can be acquired.

The traditional view of the human CNS was that in adulthood it became fixed, with limited scope for learning or recovery from injury. This is now believed not to be the case: rather that the human CNS exhibits remarkable *plasticity* that allows learning, which is represented by physiological changes in the brain, and reorganisation following injury which can lead to the recovery ability. These phenomena were predicted by Ramon y Cajal (1852–1934), a pioneering Spanish neuro-anatomist, and have entered the mainstream of clinical neuroscience within the last decade. What is interesting within the present topic is that the *central auditory system* exhibits plasticity and the ability to reorganise to a very significant degree. Change in cochlear thresholds (usually a reduction in sensitivity) results in reorganisation in central auditory processing, exhibited as change in the tonotopic frequency maps within the auditory cortex, where frequency areas where good hearing remains are more substantially represented that those where hearing loss is severe. Also, fitting a hearing aid or cochlear implant in an individual with a long-standing cochlear hearing loss appears to instigate a process of acclimatisation and reorganisation in central auditory processing so that the new auditory experiences can be consolidated and used without effort. These new findings urge us to intervene in a timely fashion in people with hearing impairment, as there is evidence in adults of a 'use it, or lose it' principle regarding hearing function within the human brain, and in children of *critical periods* when language skills can be acquired.

Within this book we hope to have laid out the wide scope of knowledge regarding deafness (and balance impairment and tinnitus), such that the reader will be inspired to look further into this fascinating and rewarding area.

References

Engel GL (1977) The need for a new medical model: a challenge for biomedicine. *Science* 196:129–136.

World Health Organization (1980) *International Classification of Impairments, Disabilities and Handicaps*. Geneva: World Health Organization.

World Health Organization (2000) *International Classification of Functioning, Disability and Health*. Geneva: World Health Organization.

The prevalence of deafness and hearing impairment

Adrian Davis, Katrina Davis and Pauline Smith

2

Introduction

Prevalence information about the numbers of people in the population who are deaf is important in planning and delivering services. The scale of deafness and hearing impairment is a key public health issue in developed economies for the coming decades of the new millennium. Not only will there be a premium on communication in the coming years, but people will live longer and healthier lives. These longer lives need communication through sound as a basis for a high quality of life and an independence that is a right of all. The level and design of service provision in any country will depend on a number of interacting factors as well as the structure and financing of health services: public opinion, lobbying by pressure groups, market factors, local and national politics, as well as financial limitations.

The major influence on the prioritisation of provision should be good prevalence data about people affected by deafness. With good prevalence data we can then estimate the cost-effectiveness and benefits of screening and treatment, and measure improvements over time. We need to consider the questions: 'Do those that need a service get it?'; 'Do they get a good-quality service?'; 'Do those that get the service benefit from it?'.

This chapter looks primarily at the prevalence of deafness and the ways in which prevalence data are relevant to the work of clinicians and planners of health services. The two terms 'prevalence' and 'deafness' both give potential for confusion. The term 'prevalence' is used here to refer to the number of people in a defined population, with a stated characteristic at a particular time (e.g. the number of people who had a hearing problem in 2009). Sometimes the prevalence is stated as a percentage of the population. A term related to prevalence is 'incidence', which is defined as the number of new cases in a defined population with a stated characteristic over a particular time period (e.g. the number of people with a new hearing problem arising between 1 January 2007 and 31 December 2007).

The term 'deafness' has many dimensions, some of which are explored elsewhere in this book. Unfortunately, 'deaf' or 'deafness' has a number of unwanted connotations. From a practical point of view, it is often difficult to decide how and where to draw the line between who is 'deaf' and who isn't, particularly when carrying out a survey to determine the prevalence of 'deafness'. To overcome this problem of terminology, in the rest of this chapter the more easily quantifiable term 'hearing impairment' is used.

The prevalence of hearing impairments by gender, socioeconomic group and, most importantly, age, is an essential ingredient in the planning of audiological and ear, nose and throat (ENT) services. At the broadest level, the purchasers of healthcare can estimate the needs of the population from the prevalence of hearing impairment. In the system in use in England, commissioning is devolved to the local level, e.g. primary care groups, except where prevalence for particular conditions is low. Other methods of purchasing hearing healthcare will apply in other health economies, e.g. managed healthcare in the USA. Within many healthcare systems, there is a role for wider policy decisions to be made, e.g. in negotiating contracts for hearing aids. Individuals can pay for their own healthcare, and in some healthcare systems co-payments, insurance and re-imbursement systems will also operate. Obviously these needs will vary according to the age groups and severity (and type, as explained in other chapters in this book) of hearing impairment. Audiological healthcare providers share this interest in the overall levels of need. They have an interest in (1) the extent to which the public seek out their services, (2) whether the mix of services is appropriate for the population served (both now and in the future), (3) the extent to which the services supplied meet the demand and (4) the quality of the service offered (and how it is perceived by consumers of the healthcare).

External factors and the prevalence of hearing impairment

Knowledge of the extent to which external factors influence the prevalence of hearing impairment (e.g. meningitis in children, noise exposure in adults, genetic susceptibility to noise and ageing) at particular ages may help in defining what scope there is for primary prevention of hearing

pathology. Legislation is effectively reducing exposure to noise at work: a European directive, 'Noise at Work Regulations', took effect in February 2006, and established the minimal security level at the equivalent noise exposure limit to 80 dB(A) for an 8-hour working day (or 40-hour working week). However, a recent European Commission study (2008) highlights a newer source of exposure:

> Besides noise at workplaces, which may contribute to 16% of the disabling hearing loss in adults, loud sounds at leisure times may reach excessive levels for instance in discos and personal music players (PMPs). It is estimated that over two decades the numbers of young people with social noise exposure has tripled (to around 19%) since the early 1980s, whilst occupational noise has decreased. The increase in unit sales of portable audio devices including MP3 has been phenomenal in the EU over the last four years. Estimated units sales ranged between 184–246 million for all portable audio devices and between 124–165 million for MP3 players . . .
>
> Published data indicate that excessive acute exposures to PMPs music at maximal or near maximal output volume can produce temporary and reversible hearing impairment (tinnitus and slight deafness) . . . there is a lack of data concerning . . . whether excessive voluntary PMP-listening leads to lasting and irreversible cognitive and attention deficits after the cessation of the noise (European Commission, Health and Consumer Protection DG: Scientific Committee on Emerging and Newly Identified Health Risks (SCENIHR), 2008).

Until we have further longitudinal data on these newer at-risk groups, it appears that external factors seem to play a small (but sometimes critical) part in the population prevalence of hearing impairment. Consequently, the main public health emphasis should be on screening and early intervention to limit longstanding forms of hearing disability that can have severe disabling effects on individuals.

Current users of prevalence data

Information concerning the prevalence of hearing impairment has been used by a wide variety of professional bodies and individuals for a variety of purposes: educators, in planning educational opportunities for the hearing-impaired child and adult; social workers and nurses who have responsibility for the elderly; physicians planning their practice approach and targets; and market researchers ascertaining the number of potential clients for new products.

Another large set of individuals who ask for prevalence information are those who are either hearing impaired themselves, are closely related to someone with a hearing disability, or are working for a hearing-related organisation (e.g. Royal National Institute for Deaf People (RNID), National Deaf Children's Society (NDCS), British Association for the Hard of Hearing (BAHOH), National Association of Deafened People (NADP), British Deaf Association (BDA) in the United Kingdom). Knowledge of the extent to which the prevalence of hearing impairments changes with age, the natural history of hearing impairments and the relative contribution of aetiological factors, such as noise exposure, can be important factors in the counselling of many hearing-impaired people; in addition it could help determine priorities within an organisation.

Prevalence measures: population studies

The prevalence of hearing impairment as an indicator of population need for hearing services should not and cannot be estimated by performance indicators, such as the number of hearing aids fitted last year, due to the hidden nature of hearing impairments and the substantial size of the existing unmet need. Prevalence estimates can only be ascertained by population measures, usually through survey of the appropriate population. For prevalences in excess of 2%, this is feasible, although a large study would be required for an accurate assessment of prevalences in the

region of 2–5%. In order to evaluate the approximate prevalences for rare conditions (e.g. the number of people who might benefit from a cochlear implant), reliance on other survey techniques is necessary.

Most of the data quoted in this chapter come from UK studies; large-scale prevalence studies are costly and complicated; there are not many of them and they are more likely to be carried out in managed public health economies. There are no data to indicate that the prevalence of hearing impairment will vary significantly from one country to another. It is reasonable to assume that prevalence data from recent well-managed large surveys in the UK will be applicable to populations in other developed health economies. We have quoted prevalence figures in terms of percentages of the population, or incidence, to help with translation to non-UK populations.

The following section briefly discusses some pertinent aspects of method in prevalence studies. The chapter will then concentrate on the prevalence of hearing impairment in adults, and its variation with age, and the prevalence of hearing impairment in children, and will give an example of the use of prevalence data in the UK, in planning and delivering screening programmes and services for the hearing impaired.

Methods for collecting prevalence data on hearing impairment

Postal questionnaires: self-reported data

The UK prevalence data on hearing impairment in adults have been taken predominantly from the National Study of Hearing (NSH), which was conducted by the Medical Research Council (MRC) Institute of Hearing Research (Davis, 1989, 1995). The fieldwork for the four individual studies comprising the NSH was conducted between 1980 and 1986. Four of the five main samples taken for the survey (more than 50,000 people were contacted by a postal questionnaire) were concentrated in Cardiff, Glasgow, Nottingham and Southampton; the fifth sample was taken from Great Britain as a whole.

These surveys gave self-reported information on the population's hearing, tinnitus and use of the public health system. This information has limited value for planning purposes, due to the extent to which the young have a tendency to overrate their disability for a given level of hearing impairment and the old consistently to underrate their disability. Jerger and colleagues (1995) state what many authors report: 'many old persons and their relatives are reluctant to confront the reality of hearing handicap and try to hide the fact that they need sound amplification.'.

Prevalence studies which overcame this tendency to distort hearing disability in self-report studies were needed to supplement self-reported data from the NSH.

Case studies as a supplement to self-reported data

The NSH estimated that 20% have a bilateral hearing impairment at 25+ dB hearing level (HL), and at least 10% of the adult population would substantially benefit from a hearing aid. Less than 4% used a hearing aid in the 1980s.

A recent Health Technology Assessment (HTA) (Davis *et al.*, 2007) updated the NSH data and estimated how many adults would benefit from modern, well-fitted hearing aids. It also examined strategies by which people might be either case-found or screened for benefit from amplification and provision of a hearing aid. The research took place between 1998 and 2007. It consisted of (1) a population study, (2) a clinical effectiveness study to examine the acceptability, benefits and performance of different screening programmes and (3) retrospective case-control studies with patients fitted with hearing aids after screening several years previously, to assess long-term compliance.

As part of the HTA population study, a postal questionnaire to gather data on the prevalence of all major ENT symptoms was sent out to 26,160 households selected at random in various parts

of England, Wales and Scotland. This consisted of questions on all ENT symptoms and use of services. The complete dataset consists of 34,362 respondents in Great Britain, giving 31,793 cases for whom good data were available. To supplement the postal self-reported data, 506 respondents were then interviewed, 351 were assessed for benefit from amplification and 87 were fitted with a hearing aid.

The prevalence of hearing impairment in adults

Measures

There are many measures of hearing impairment, the most general being the hearing threshold levels obtained for pure tones at different frequencies. In order to simplify the information available from the pattern of these thresholds over frequency (the audiogram), the NSH study used an index of impairment for the average hearing threshold level over the frequencies 0.5, 1, 2 and 4 kHz, in the better ear. This measure (better ear average, BEA) tends to underrate the problems that a person with asymmetrical hearing might have, but is probably one of the better predictors of overall hearing disability, and includes the ability to hear speech in a background of noise, and the ability to use environmental sound cues appropriately.

Prevalence: the results of the 1995 study

The prevalence of hearing impairment is shown in Figure 2.1. About 30% of the adult population has an impairment in at least one ear, with two-thirds of these having an impairment in the better ear at 25 dB HL or greater. Between 20% and 30% of adults also have great difficulty hearing speech in a background of noise. This is not surprising, as most people find this task difficult. However, Davis (1995) showed that this degree of reported difficulty was associated with a hearing threshold that was considerably raised

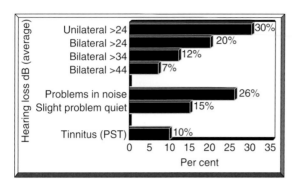

Figure 2.1 The overall prevalence of impairment and reported disability in those aged 18 years and over in Great Britain. PST, prolonged spontaneous tinnitus. (Source: NSH data reproduced from Davis A (1995) *Hearing in Adults.* London: Whurr Publishers Ltd.)

compared to the thresholds of those who did not complain. Tinnitus, which is highly associated with hearing impairment, is reported to occur spontaneously in about 10% of people (i.e. not only after loud sounds), and to last for more than five minutes.

Prevalence: the results from the 2007 HTA update study

The HTA report (Davis *et al.*, 2007) updated the prevalence data from the NSH reported in 1995 (Davis, 1995). Researchers from the MRC Hearing and Communication Group at the University of Manchester collected data from the UK on the prevalence of reported hearing problems, the uptake of primary care and specialist hearing services, and the acceptability, benefits and performance of different screening programmes. They also conducted case-control studies with patients who had been fitted with hearing aids after screening several years previously, to assess long-term compliance, and undertook an evaluation of the cost-effectiveness of potential screening programmes.

Out of the complete dataset available for analysis, a total of 31,793 cases, almost one-fifth of the sample, answered 'yes' to the question 'Do you have any difficulty with your hearing?', and this rose to almost one-third of the sample in the age range 55–74 years. Other ENT symptoms

were near to this prevalence: dizziness, which encompasses a range of pathologies as well as vestibular ones; sore throat, the prevalence of which decreases with age; and nasal problems. Voice problems were less prevalent. There was a high prevalence of co-morbidity of the following ENT symptoms: hearing, balance and tinnitus.

The same prevalence data broken down for manual and non-manual occupations show that people in manual occupations reported more ENT symptoms of all types. This is more evident in males than in females, and in the older age groups; 31% of the whole sample reported some degree of hearing difficulty on at least one of the questions in the postal questionnaire.

The HTA study focused on the specific age range 55–74 years of age because the main focus of the study was on the pros and cons of early screening for hearing disability. It found that 12% of people aged 55–74 years have a hearing problem that causes them moderate or severe worry, annoyance or upset. It also found that, although 14% have a bilateral hearing impairment of at least 35 dB HL, only 3% currently receive intervention through use of hearing aids. These hearing problems, which mainly affect ability to hear speech in noise, had a mean reported duration of about 10 years. People under 75 years who reported concerns were less likely than those over 75 years to have sought and obtained help or intervention for this problem in the form of a referral or hearing aids.

Prevalence of degree of hearing impairment by age group

Twenty-six per cent of people have a 35 dB HL hearing impairment in the worse ear, of whom 23% do not have a hearing aid. On the better ear criterion, there are 14%, of whom 11% do not have a hearing aid. The percentages are greater in men and in the older age group, those aged 65 years or more. In the younger age group, 6% of the 60–64 year olds have this degree of impairment, of whom five out of six who are

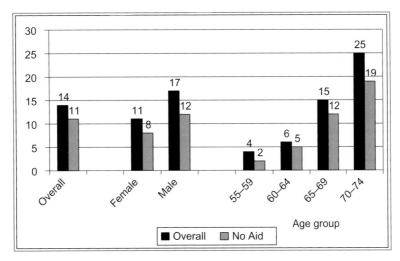

Figure 2.2   Percentage of population with a significant hearing impairment at 0.5, 1, 2 and 4 kHz on any ear using a criterion of 35 dB HL or greater as a function of gender, age and aided status (aid or no aid), projected from the Strand 1 population study. (Figure 4.1 reproduced with permission from Davis *et al.* (2007) Acceptability, benefit and costs of early screening for hearing disability: a study of potential screening tests and models. *Health Technology Assessment* 11(42), Crown Copyright.)

hearing impaired at the 35 dB HL level do not use hearing aids.

In terms of prevalence of hearing impairment (at 25 dB HL and greater) with age: until the age of about 45 years mild hearing problems are rare, so that the prevalence estimates are small; beyond the age of 50 years the prevalence estimates are well over 10%, approaching 50% by 70–74 years of age. There are gradual changes with age: the median BEA increases by about 2.5 dB per decade in people aged 20–40 years, but increases by up to 10 dB per decade in those aged 60–80 years (Figure 2.2).

Prevalence of hearing aid use and self-reported effectiveness of hearing aid use

In the 55–74-year-old age group, almost *one-third* of the sample in the HTA study answered 'yes' to the question 'Do you have any difficulty with your hearing?'. *This is in contrast to the 5.7% of people in the sample who were using a hearing aid at that time.* There is potentially considerable unmet need in the population and potential benefit from amplification from using

hearing aids. The 55–74-year-old age group would be appropriately targeted with hearing screening, to try to avoid the rise in the prevalence of severe hearing handicap (those who are severely annoyed, worried or upset about their hearing); at age 75+ years, this prevalence is about 60%. Only 50% of those with such handicap use amplification at age 55–64 years, reducing to about 40% at 54–74 years and about 20% at age 75+ years.

Prevalence of tinnitus and balance problems

Tinnitus, noises in the ears or in the head, correlates highly with the individual's hearing impairment. The best predictor of tinnitus is the severity of hearing impairment in the worse ear at high frequencies. The HTA study results show that hearing difficulties and tinnitus increase steadily with age, the prevalence being higher in males than in females, and there is a clear increase in uptake of aids with age.

The NSH also asked questions about tinnitus and balance problems. Over one in three adults report some tinnitus, mainly transient, but this section concentrates on the 10% who report tinnitus that lasts for more than 5 minutes and is not only present after very loud sounds. About half of this tinnitus group report that their tinnitus is moderately or severely annoying. Bilateral tinnitus is reported in about 3% of those with better hearing thresholds than 25 dB HL in the worse ear at high frequencies, with unilateral tinnitus reported in about 2%. These tinnitus prevalences increase in line with severity of impairment to 10% (bilateral) and 15% (unilateral) for those with 85 dB HL or more in the worse ear, averaged over the high frequencies (5% of the population). The prevalence of tinnitus is very susceptible to small changes in the protocol that define the precise condition of concern, and in any tinnitus study this has to be well controlled. However, there is no doubt from two UK studies (Coles *et al.*, 1990; Sancho-Aldridge and Davis, 1993) that the quality of life for 2% of the population may be moderately affected by tinnitus, and that for perhaps as many as 5 per 1000, or about 0.3 million in the UK, the quality of life is greatly affected by their tinnitus.

Nearly 7% of the population have consulted a doctor about their tinnitus. The main statistical factors predicting consultation are the severity of the tinnitus annoyance and the degree of hearing impairment. However, socioeconomic group and age are the best predictors of the one-third who were seen by the family doctor and who were subsequently referred to a hospital department.

Prevalence of co-morbidity of hearing problems, balance and tinnitus in the HTA study

Table 2.1 (Table 1.11 from the HTA study from Davis *et al.*, 2007) shows the high prevalence of co-morbidity of ENT symptoms: hearing, balance and tinnitus.

Earlier referral could reduce this handicap and deal with co-morbidity, leading to treatment of other ENT symptoms; in particular there is a high proportion of hearing-impaired people who also report tinnitus and dizziness. This indicates that the 55–74-year-old age group would be appropriately targeted with hearing screening, to try to avoid the rise in the prevalence of severe handicap at age 75+ years.

Prevalence of self-reported severe annoyance due to hearing, tinnitus or balance problems

Figure 2.3 shows the numbers of people reporting that they are severely worried, annoyed or

Table 2.1 Reported prevalence of hearing problems, tinnitus and balance problems and their co-existence. (Table 1.11 reproduced with permission from Davis *et al.* (2007) Acceptability, benefit and costs of early screening for hearing disability: a study of potential screening tests and models. *Health Technology Assessment* 11(42), Crown Copyright.)

	Overall crude prevalence			Overall weighted prevalence
All sample	%	*n*	95% CI[a]	%
Hearing	31.0	10,386	(30.5, 31.5)	30.5
Hearing & tinnitus	11.7	3901	(11.4, 12.1)	11.4
Hearing & balance	15.4	4864	(15.0, 15.8)	14.9
Tinnitus & balance	11.0	3491	(10.7, 11.3)	10.7
Hearing & tinnitus & balance	7.4	2328	(7.1, 7.7)	7.2

[a]NB confidence intervals (CIs) calculated using Wilson's method.

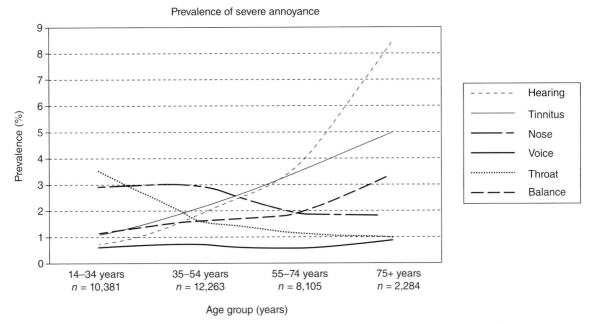

Figure 2.3   The prevalence of severe annoyance caused by major ENT symptoms plotted in 20-year age bands. (Figure 1.2 reproduced with permission from Davis *et al.* (2007) Acceptability, benefit and costs of early screening for hearing disability: a study of potential screening tests and models. *Health Technology Assessment* 11(42), Crown Copyright.)

upset by each of the ENT symptoms that they report.

These results show that hearing problems are a significant public health problem with a substantial number of adults aged 55–74 years reporting severe problems with their hearing and considerable co-morbidity. A substantial proportion of these adults fail to access hearing services (Department of Health, 2007).

Prevalence and severity of hearing loss

The prevalence for a range of severity of hearing impairment from the NSH data showed that 16.1% of the adult population in the UK, aged 18–80 years, have BEAs of 25 dB HL and greater. As the severity of hearing impairment increases, the prevalence decreases. At a severity of 65 dB HL and greater, the best estimate is about 11 people per 1000, at 95 dB HL and greater about 2 per 1000, and at 105 dB HL and greater about 1 per 1000. For the worse ear, however, there are about 6 per 1000 at 105 dB HL and greater.

Generally at degrees of severity of 45 dB HL and greater, there are no substantial differences between men and women in the percentage with hearing impairments. Below 45 dB HL, men have a substantially higher chance of having a mild-to-moderate hearing impairment. At 25 dB HL and greater, the prevalence estimate is 18.1% (confidence interval (CI) 16.4–19.7%) for men and 14.4% (CI 12.8–16.0%) for women. This difference is almost certainly due to the greater degree and duration of noise exposure experienced by men aged 40 years and older compared with women. As noise affects thresholds in the 4–6 kHz region more than at lower frequencies, this difference, which is slight for BEA, is greatly increased at high frequencies (3–8 kHz).

Prevalence of sensorineural and conductive hearing loss

The majority, 87%, of the hearing impairments at 25 dB HL and greater are of a sensorineural type rather than having a substantial conductive component (see Chapter 6 for an explanation of the difference between the types of hearing impairment). The criterion used here to qualify for a conductive component was an average difference of 15 dB between the air- and bone-conduction thresholds averaged over 0.5, 1 and 2 kHz. The proportion with no conductive component in the worse ear is less than in the better ear, at 69%. At greater severities than 25 dB, the proportion of people with no conductive component in the better ear decreases to 82% at 35 dB HL and greater, and to 69% at 45 dB HL and greater.

The prevalence of hearing impairment at all severities in the population is highly dependent on age. This is the case even for profound hearing impairments, indicating that most hearing impairments are acquired. At 95 dB HL and greater, the estimate in terms of numbers from the NSH data is about 100,000 people in the UK population, of whom probably about 15,000 were impaired pre-lingually. This can be scaled to other populations with similar age distributions, as a lower-bound estimate (the lowest that any estimate might be), as can the data in the following section.

Prevalence of pre-lingual deafness and visual impairment with deafness

For young age groups, the proportions of pre-lingually impaired individuals are much higher than the average figures suggest. The proportion of the profoundly impaired individuals who could be candidates for cochlear implants obviously depends on the actual audiometric and other selection criteria used by different health economies, and might be as low as a few per cent or as high as 50%.

The proportion of hearing impaired with visual impairments is high, as ageing is a common factor in the increasing prevalence of both these sensory impairments. The number of people with substantial visual disability and severe hearing impairment or worse is not currently known with any degree of statistical precision, but is unlikely to be more than 1 in 10,000.

Prevalence and demographic profile

The number of people in the UK with hearing impairments of different degrees of severity, taking gender into account, can be deduced from the prevalence of hearing impairment and the demographic profile. The estimated number of hearing-impaired people using the mid-1990s NSH estimates for the age and gender profile of Great Britain was that there were about 8.58 million people with BEA hearing impairments of 25 dB HL and greater. This decreases to about 2.94 million with moderate degrees of impairment. We know that there are substantially more women than men with hearing impairments, despite roughly equal prevalences, because more women survive into the seventh, eighth and ninth decades of life. Indeed at 45+ dB HL, about one-quarter of those disabled by this level of impairment are women of 80 years or older.

Over the next two decades, due to increasing survival, the number of hearing-impaired people will probably rise by 20%, in line with other chronic disabilities. Thus by the year 2016 there may be 700,000 people with severe hearing impairments (65 dB HL and greater) compared with an estimated 580,000 in 1988. The number of people with profound hearing impairment is of particular interest because they have very special needs. Those in younger age groups are possible candidates for cochlear implantation if it is acceptable to the individual and society, and meets agreed standards of quality and cost-effectiveness. The data suggest there are less than 200,000 people over 18 years with profound hearing impairment, of whom 20,000–30,000 are people with profound deafness from childhood. This means that around 80% of those with profound hearing impairment reached this level in adulthood – either through new hearing impairment or deterioration of an existing impairment. Not only is the prevalence of profound hearing impairment highest in the over-80-year-old group, but the incidence of new profound hearing impairment is greatest in this age range. Reducing the dependency brought about by deafness in this group will be a great challenge, since the risk-benefit of cochlear implants is likely to be unfavourable.

The prevalence of hearing impairment in children

When discussing the prevalence of hearing impairment in children, it is important to use and understand various definitions in order to estimate prevalence with accuracy, and match that prevalence with need. In this section, we shall refer to *congenital* hearing impairment, meaning that which is present and detectable using appropriate tests at or very soon after birth – the converse being *acquired* hearing impairment. Children may also experience *temporary* hearing impairment such as otitis media with effusion (OME or glue ear). This does not concern us here, because its individual consequences are not as severe as those with *permanent* childhood hearing impairment (PCHI). Where significant PCHI is present pre-lingually, this will obviously have great impact on the rest of the child's life.

The CEC report *Childhood Deafness in the European Community* (Martin *et al.*, 1981) puts the lower bound on hearing-impairment prevalence at around 1 per 1000 in children with a BEA of 50 dB HL born during 1969 and ascertained by 1977 (i.e. at 8 years of age). Despite the significant medical and social changes since that time, this remains a good benchmark. For example, while vaccination means that congenital rubella is much rarer in Europe, there has been a large increase in the number of pre-term babies surviving with hearing impairments.

Traditionally, studies have tended to be cross-sectional and based on retrospective ascertainment. One of the largest such studies, aiming at a calculation of prevalence of PCHI across the whole of the UK, was by Fortnum *et al.* (2001). After adjusting for estimated under-ascertainment, they suggested there were around 21,500 children aged 3 to 18 years in the UK with a BEA of 40 dB HL. The prevalence of a diagnosed hearing impairment at age 3 years was around 1.1 per 1000, rising to 2.1 per 1000 at age 9–16 years. Such studies have some validity in the context of planning diagnostic and rehabilitative facilities for hearing-impaired children.

In the 1990s, the technology of evoked oto-acoustic emissions (OAE) and auditory brainstem response (ABR), providing proxy measures of hearing, even in newborn babies, opened up the potential to screen for congenital hearing impairment. Evidence of the prevalence of congenital hearing loss led to the recommendation of programmes for screening. Universal neonatal hearing screening (UNHS) has been piloted in the UK since 2001, and became standard in England in 2006. Results from studies on UNHS express a 'rate' of hearing impairment detected per baby screened. Depending on the coverage (percentage of babies screened very soon after birth), the sensitivity of the test, and the confidence of the diagnosis, the prevalence of congenital hearing impairment can be measured with increasing confidence. Uus and Bamford (2006) gave the rates for the Newborn Hearing Screening Programme (NHSP) in England, based on the 21 pilot sites around the UK, between February 2002 and June 2004. The programme achieved 96% coverage, with 169,487 babies screened. Among the babies referred from the screen, 90% were followed up, and a confirmed permanent bilateral hearing loss of moderate or greater severity was found in 169. This leads to a rate of 1.00 (95% CI 0.78–1.22) per 1000 babies screened.

Prevalence is by no means even across the population. The most notable risk factors are a family history of permanent hearing impairment, present since childhood, or a lengthy stay in a neonatal intensive care unit (NICU) (Fortnum and Davis, 1997). The identification of some risk factors has come from understanding the aetiology of PCHI, and for others after observational studies. At least half of all cases of permanent childhood hearing impairment are known to have a genetic cause (Reardon, 1992a, 1992b; Morton and Nance, 2006). Mutations in around 120 genes have been identified as contributing to PCHI – around 80 causing syndromes that include hearing loss and over 40 responsible for 'non-syndromic' hearing loss. A targeted neonatal hearing screening programme in the Redbridge District of London for 10 years between 1990 and 2000 (Watkin *et al.*, 2005) demonstrated that newborn babies identified as high risk using appropriate guidelines (3.5% of total) made up 58% of children who would go on to be diagnosed with PCHI by the age of 5 years.

Risk factors remain important because the high risk may extend beyond the neonatal period, indicating the need for further observation of children as they develop. The NHS Newborn Hearing Screening Programme (NHSP) in the UK publishes their own guidelines on the management and surveillance of high-risk individuals (NHSP Clinical Group, 2006), which they identify as babies with a family history of PCHI, cranio-facial abnormality, Down's syndrome, congenital TORCH infection (toxoplasmosis, rubella, CMV (cytomegalovirus) or herpes) or neurological disorder, plus those with perinatal problems leading to assisted ventilation in the NICU for more than 5 days, exchange transfusion or high levels of ototoxic drugs. Weichbold *et al.* (2006) examined the histories for 23 9-year-old children who had developed bilateral PCHI after a clear newborn hearing screen. Eleven children had a risk factor (as defined by the Joint Committee on Infant Hearing (JCIH), 2000). Among these, three had a family history of hearing loss; two had recovered from meningitis; two had a craniofacial malformation. They also found that five children had received ototoxic therapy and two had been born before the 33rd gestational week (one child had a combination of the last two). Six children (26%) showed no risk indicators for postnatal hearing loss.

Using prevalence data: patient and population level

Explanations are important for all patients, but for patients with hearing impairment, where we know that not enough seek help early and not enough accept and use hearing aids, explanation has a particular value. We do not thrust hearing aids upon patients; we have to motivate them to seek help, go through the process of learning to use their aids and then continue to use them. Helping patients to see their hearing loss in context can be an important part of motivating them (see Chapter 23).

Where hearing loss is preventable, prevalence data can measure progress in prevention. Alberti (1996) estimated that half of all disabling hearing loss worldwide was preventable by primary means, from vaccination to better protection from noise exposure. This is already happening. For example, thanks to a successful vaccination programme, hearing losses related to congenital rubella syndrome, measles or mumps are now rare in the developed world. There has also been some progress in highlighting consanguinity as a potent risk factor for PCHI in some communities (Elahi *et al.*, 1998).

Prevalence data are clearly vital for planning, evaluating and improving screening and services for hearing-impaired people. In the UK, detailed information and evidence about services for the hearing impaired are only slowly becoming available in terms of (1) the coverage, timeliness and effectiveness of prevention programmes (e.g. paediatric/neonatal screening, vaccination, noise conservation, pre-retirement screening), (2) the extent to which those who might benefit from advice or a hearing aid have their needs met and (3) the extent to which the quality of the service provided meets the needs of the individual (e.g. failure rate of hearing aids, non-use rate, waiting times for initial consultation, quality of ear moulds, availability of rehabilitative support).

Prevalence data in the UK are being used to plan and improve services

Recent Health Technology Assessments (Davis *et al.*, 1997, 2007; Bamford *et al.*, 2007) are all attempts to collate information on need and current and ideal screening practices for newborn babies, young children and adults respectively.

The prevalence data and the results of the UK work indicate that screening in adults, if it is targeted on the younger age range (55–74 year olds), will identify more people who are currently not likely to self-refer: this is where the additional benefits (e.g. from identification 10 years earlier) are more likely to be found. Prevalence data, with costs of screening and intervention, have to be balanced against gains in quality of life and costs saved.

The HTA report (Davis *et al.*, 2007) explored the potential cost-effectiveness per quality-adjusted life-year (QALY) of different screening programmes for hearing impairment targeting 55–74 year olds. The most efficient and practicable method was to use two questions in primary care concerning hearing problems and a hearing screen using a pure tone of 35 dB HL at 3 kHz, which could be used in primary care if costs per device were appropriate. The average cost of the screening programme was £13 per person screened, or about £100 if treatment costs were included. Using the prevalence data indicated that this screening programme makes good economic sense in relation to a service costing £100–120 m per year.

Prevalence: consumer approach

Hearing services do not necessarily have a good image with other health professionals and members of the public; historically this may be due to long waiting times for assessment and provision of hearing aids as well as a poor perception of the hearing aids used in the NHS. The population study of the HTA report found that 72.4% of people who subsequently used audiology services reported that they were very satisfied with primary care services, with 89.4% of them being fairly or very satisfied with them. Those who became users of audiology services more frequently reported that they were very satisfied with primary care services; 60.2% reported that they were very satisfied with audiology services, with 89.4% being fairly or very satisfied. A greater percentage of people with hearing aids reported being very satisfied, compared with people without hearing aids.

In general, respondents were satisfied with the services, the users having higher opinions of the audiology service than the non-users. The main concerns expressed were (accurately) the waiting times and the size of the NHS hearing aids. For adults the dissatisfaction is a product of a number of issues, which can be summed up as accessibility of services, availability of good-quality hearing aids, provision of good rehabilitation services,

appropriate repair and advice services, and the time needed to access the services.

Service development: using prevalence data in the UK

The HTA prevalence data enabled an estimation of the numbers of people aged 55–74 years who would benefit from modern and well-fitted hearing aids. It also examined strategies by which people might be either case-found or screened for benefit from amplification and provision of a hearing aid. The research found that, although 12% of people aged 55–74 years have a hearing problem, only 3% of them have hearing aids. So the proportion of people with a hearing loss that is unmanaged by provision of hearing aids is very high.

Good amplification was shown to benefit about one in four of the 55–74-year-old population, and the degree of hearing loss was a good predictor of benefit. There was a strong correlation between benefit from amplification using headphones and benefit from using hearing aids. The offer of two hearing aids was accepted by about 70% of those who were offered an aid, which increased to 95% for those with 35+ dB HL.

There is now considerable interest in the UK in providing hearing aids as early as possible to the adult population. The Modernising Hearing Aid Services programme (MHAS) has been completed in England, with similar programmes in Wales, Northern Ireland and Scotland. This has provided audiology departments with new, digital signal processing (DSP) hearing aids, and with the infrastructure, patient management systems (PMS), IT and training to provide a quality service and deliver the national patient journey from referral to follow-up. As part of this initiative there is much work concerned with meeting need in the population and meeting a demand that appears to be increasing. The prevalence data we have are an essential part of this work.

The degree of unmet need, the late age of presentation of most patients, and the problems they have in adapting to hearing aids at an older age suggest that screening for hearing impairment in older people ought to be investigated as a priority. New technology, such as audiometric screeners and automated otoacoustic emissions (AOAE), is promising as a screen, but the primary care-based two-question screen is a low-cost way of identifying a high percentage of those people whose quality of life would benefit from hearing aids.

Summary and conclusion

Prevalence data give a clearer picture of the scale of the problem now and in the future. They are essential for service planning and delivery. Over the next 15 years, hearing impairment will be an increasing population problem, because of the ageing population profile. It is likely to increase by 10 to 15% in population terms – without any shift in the prevalence of hearing impairment.

The rate of change of hearing impairment at age 60–70 years is such that the increase in prevalence of the target group in the UK outweighs by 2:1 the change in provision of services. So the current services do not meet the known future needs, let alone the current prevalent needs – primarily due to lack of identification and referral to hearing services (Davis *et al.*, 2007). This is likely to be the case in other health economies. Hearing health services are not a high-profile or glamorous specialty, but they have the potential to improve the quality of life for the very large number of hearing-impaired people who would benefit from new technology, for example the DSP, open-fit and in-the-ear (ITE) hearing aids (see Chapter 17).

Hearing loss affects one in six of the European population and this is projected to increase to one in four by 2050. Hearing loss is age related and affects three out of four adults over the age of 70 years, thus constraining their autonomy and capacity to live independently. A recent Australian study reports that hearing loss ranks with asthma, diabetes and musculoskeletal diseases in terms of burden of disability, and should be considered as a national health priority (Access Economics, 2006).

The key points that emerge from this chapter are that:

1 prevalence data are important for service planning and delivery respectively. There are about 8.6, 5.1, 2.9 and 0.15 million adults in the UK with bilateral hearing impairments of at least 25, 35, 45 and 95 dB HL over the frequencies 0.5, 1, 2 and 4 kHz

2 prevalence of all severities of hearing impairment increases rapidly with age after 50 years, and up to one in three of the hearing impaired is over 80 years of age

3 there is substantial unmet need, in terms of people who would benefit from a hearing aid: only 19%, 33% and 55% of people with a bilateral impairment of at least 25, 35 and 45 dB HL respectively have tried a hearing aid

4 congenital hearing impairment is a substantial public health problem affecting more than 1 in 1000

5 fifty-eight per cent of children with hearing impairment at age 5 years have risk factors as babies, but up to 42% of them do not, which is important when planning screening and support services for deaf children

6 in order to meet this challenge we need innovative hearing health services that are evidence based and have the capacity in the longer term to begin to meet the need in a sustainable way.

References

Access Economics Pty Ltd (2006) *Listen Hear: the economic impact and cost of hearing loss in Australia.* www.audiology.asn.au/pdf/ListenHearFinal.pdf (accessed 7 November 2008).

Alberti PW (1996) The prevention of hearing loss worldwide. *Scandinavian Audiology* 25(suppl 42):15–19.

Bamford J, Fortnum H, Bristow K *et al.* (2007) Current practice, accuracy, effectiveness and cost-effectiveness of the school entry hearing screen. *Health Technology Assessment* 11(32).

Coles RRA, Davis A, Smith P (1990) Tinnitus: its epidemiology and management. In: Hartvig

Jensen J, ed. *Presbyacusis and Other Age-related Aspects*. Proceedings of the 14th Danavox symposium. Copenhagen: Danavox Jubilee Foundation.

Davis AC (1989) The prevalence of hearing impairment and reported hearing disability among adults in Great Britain. *International Journal of Epidemiology* 18:911–917.

Davis A (1995) *Hearing in Adults*. London: Whurr Publishers Ltd.

Davis A, Bamford J, Wilson I, Ramkalawan T, Forshaw M, Wright S (1997) A critical review of the role of neonatal hearing screening in the detection of congenital hearing impairment. *Health Technology Assessment* 1(10).

Davis A, Smith P, Ferguson M, Stephens D, Gianopoulos I (2007) Acceptability, benefit and costs of early screening for hearing disability: a study of potential screening tests and models. *Health Technology Assessment* 11(42).

Department of Health (2007) *Improving Access to Audiology Services in England*. Gateway reference 7837. London: Department of Health.

Elahi MM, Elahi F, Elahi A, Elahi SB (1998) Pediatrics. Hearing loss in rural Pakistan. *Journal of Otolaryngology* 27:348–353.

European Commission, Health and Consumer Protection DG: Scientific Committee on Emerging and Newly Identified Health Risks (SCENIHR) (2008) *Potential Health Risks of Exposure to Noise from Personal Music Players and Mobile Phones Including a Music Playing Function. Preliminary Report*. Brussels: SCENIHR.

Fortnum H, Davis A (1997) Epidemiology of permanent childhood hearing impairment in Trent region, 1985–1993. *British Journal of Audiology* 31:409–446.

Fortnum H, Summerfield Q, Marshall DH, Davis AC, Bamford JM (2001) Prevalence of permanent childhood hearing impairment in the United Kingdom and implications for universal neonatal hearing screening: questionnaire based ascertainment study. *British Medical Journal* 323(7312):536–540.

Jerger J, Chmiel R, Wilson N, Luchi R (1995) Hearing impairment in older adults: new concepts. *Journal of the American Geriatric Society* 43:928–935.

Joint Committee on Infant Hearing (2000) Year 2000 Position Statement: principles and guidelines for early hearing detection and intervention programs. *Pediatrics* 106:798–817. www.jcih.org/jcih2000.pdf (accessed 7 November 2008).

Martin JA, Bentzen O, Colley JR *et al*. (1981) Childhood deafness in the European community. *Scandinavian Audiology* 10:165–174.

Morton CC, Nance WE (2006) Newborn hearing screening – a silent revolution. *New England Journal of Medicine* 354:2151–2164.

NHSP Clinical Group, edited by Sutton G; contributors Green R, Parker G, Robertson C *et al*. (2006) *Guidelines for Surveillance and Audiological Monitoring of Infants and Children Following the Newborn Hearing Screen*. Version 3.1. Manchester: University of Manchester. http://hearing.screening.nhs.uk/surveillance (accessed 7 November 2008).

Reardon W (1992a) Genetic deafness. *Journal of Medical Genetics* 29:521–526.

Reardon W (1992b) Genetics of deafness: clinical aspects. *British Journal of Hospital Medicine* 47:507–511.

Sancho-Aldridge J, Davis A (1993) The impact of hearing impairment on television viewing in the UK. *British Journal of Audiology* 27:163–173.

Uus K, Bamford J (2006). Effectiveness of population-based newborn hearing screening in England: ages of interventions and profile of cases. *Pediatrics* 117:e887–e893.

Watkin P, Hasan J, Baldwin M, Ahmed M (2005) Neonatal hearing screening: have we taken the right road? Results from a 10-year targeted screen longitudinally followed up in a single district. *Audiological Medicine* 3:175–184.

Weichbold V, Nekahm-Heis D, Welzl-Mueller K (2006) Universal newborn hearing screening and postnatal hearing loss. *Pediatrics* 117: e631–e636.

The structure and function of the ear

Tony Wright

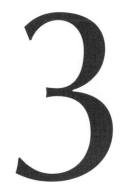

Introduction

Over the years, both convention and convenience have separated the ear into its three parts – outer, middle and inner – for descriptive purposes (Figure 3.1). This convention has served well but now must be integrated into advances in the knowledge of how the ear works as an essential component in survival. The ear has two major and separate functions – hearing and balance. Hearing is needed as an early warning system for detecting and locating potentially threatening environmental sounds. In addition, in many animals, and especially in humans, the ears form a major part of a communication system. As far as balance is concerned, the inner ear is crucial for survival, not only by accurately and rapidly detecting head movement so that the eyes can stay fixed on prey or predator but also by giving important information about sudden changes in the environment, both external and within the person's self, to avoid falls and injury. This chapter concentrates on the hearing.

The external ear

The auricle (pinna)

The body of the auricle is formed from elastic fibrocartilage and is a continuous sheet except for a narrow gap between the tragus and the anterior crus of the helix, where it is replaced by a dense fibrous tissue band. This gap is the site for an endaural incision which, properly performed, should not damage cartilage or its perichondrium, and which, by splitting the soft-tissue ring surrounding the bony ear canal, allows wide exposure of the deeper parts. The endaural incision is one of the possible approaches to the middle ear used for ossiculoplasty and stapedectomy (see Chapter 9).

The cartilage extends about 8 mm down the ear canal to form the outer third of the canal. The cartilage of the auricle is covered with perichondrium, from which it derives its supply of nutrients, as cartilage itself has no direct blood supply. Stripping the perichondrium from the cartilage, as occurs following injuries which result in collec-

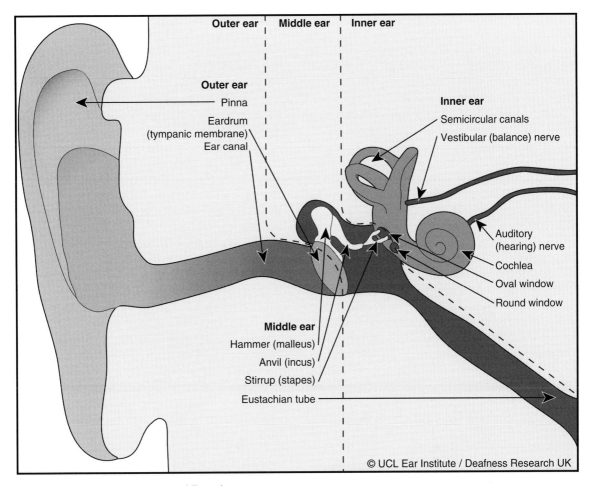

Figure 3.1 Diagram of the outer, middle and inner ears.

tions of blood between perichondrium and carti-lage, can lead to cartilage necrosis with a crumpled up, 'boxer's' ear. The skin of the auricle is thin and closely attached to the perichondrium on the outer, front surface. On the back surface, between the mastoid process and the auricle, there is a definite subdermal layer which allows dissection during surgery for bat-ears. The skin of the auricle is covered with fine hairs and, most noticeably, in the concha and the scaphoid fossa, there are sebaceous glands opening into the root canals of these hairs. The cartilage of the auricle is con-nected to the skull by ligaments and by muscles which are supplied by branches of the facial nerve.

The external ear canal and tympanic membrane

The external ear canal in adults is approximately 2.4 cm long with the outer third having cartilagi-nous walls and the deeper two-thirds bony walls. At the deep end of the canal, and stretched across it, is the eardrum or tympanic membrane. The diameter of the canal varies greatly between indi-viduals and between different races. Starting from the outside, the canal curves forwards and slightly downwards so that in adults a direct view of the tympanic membrane usually requires the auricle to be gently pulled upwards and backwards to straighten out the cartilaginous canal.

The continuing curve of the deep bony canal results in the tympanic membrane lying at a slant across the bony canal, with an acute angle between the drum and the anterior canal wall. This anterior recess is a difficult area for access at surgery and can be hard to see in the clinic.

The eardrum (Figure 3.2) is a circle of thin skin about 8–9 mm (one-third of an inch) in diameter. Despite its name, it is not flat like the skin of a drum but is slightly conical with the curved sides sloping inwards, like a traditional loudspeaker cone. The eardrum has three layers. The outer layer, in contact with the deep ear canal, is covered with a thin layer of skin. The inner layer, which is continuous with the lining of the middle ear, consists of rather flat cells that have the ability to transform into the type of cells that line the nose and sinuses and produce mucus. The middle layer of the eardrum is very important and consists of elastic fibres arranged both like the spokes of a wheel (radial fibres) and in circles (circumferential fibres), so that this layer is like a sprung trampoline net. The major portion of the eardrum is tense and absorbs sound (pars tensa). The small upper portion of the membrane is more floppy because the fibres of the middle

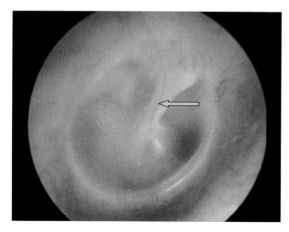

Figure 3.2 Endoscopic photograph of a right tympanic membrane. The arrow indicates the handle of the malleus with a small, normal blood vessel running down it. To the left of the malleus handle can be seen the long process of the incus, and just below and to the right of the tip of the malleus handle is a reflection of the light used to illuminate the membrane. This 'light reflex' usually indicates that the membrane is healthy and in the correct position.

layer are not organised in regular patterns, and this region is called the pars flaccida.

The external canal is lined with skin (epidermis). Body skin normally grows directly from the basal layers towards the surface, where it is shed into the surroundings. Excess proliferation in the scalp trapped by the hair is dandruff. If this pattern of growth were to occur in the external ear canal then the canal would soon become filled with dead skin (keratin). Instead of maturation taking place directly towards the surface, there is outward, oblique growth of the epidermis of the canal skin and pars flaccida, so that the surface layers effectively migrate towards the external opening of the canal. The normal rate of migration is about 0.05 mm/day, although this range is hugely variable and in some conditions there is complete failure of migration with a consequent build-up of shed keratin in the ear canal (Alberti, 1964).

The skin of the pars tensa has a different derivation from that of the deep canal, and cell divisions occur randomly within the layer of basal cells. The effect of this, in a circular sheet with the handle of the malleus forming a central boundary extending halfway down the membrane, is to create outward, mass migration of the skin of the pars tensa. Ink dots applied to the surface have an outward pattern of movement. However, if a hole is made in the tympanic membrane and a graft laid underneath the membrane (an underlay graft), then migration of the skin from the outer edge of the perforation is directed centrally to cover the graft. This occurs because the boundary conditions have altered, and fortunately provides the basis for the healing of grafts and for the re-epithelialisation of mastoid cavities. Even a small piece of pars tensa skin has this ability and so is a precious material and needs to be preserved during ear surgery if a bare area needs covering. The property of canal skin to migrate, however, can also bring problems with the formation of a cholesteatoma if the skin becomes displaced into the middle ear (see Chapter 9).

At the outer limits of the ear canal are some short hairs which project towards the opening of the canal. In this region are clusters of wax-forming ceruminous and sebaceous glands. The ceruminous glands are modified sweat glands that produce a watery, white secretion that slowly darkens turning semi-solid and sticky as it dries. Since these glands are sweat glands, they respond to many stimuli such as adrenergic drugs, fever and emotion, which, along with direct mechanical stimulation, can all produce an increased or altered secretion.

The sebaceous glands produce an oily material (sebum) which is usually excreted into the root canals of the hair follicles. The mixture of desquamated cells, cerumen and sebum forms wax. This is a good agent for inhibiting the growth of many fungi and bacteria and is strongly bactericidal for certain bacterial species (Stone and Fulghum 1984; Campos *et al.*, 2000).

Human ear wax consists of 'wet' or 'dry' forms and is inherited as a Mendelian trait (see Chapter 11). Dry wax, lacking cerumen, is yellowish or grey, and brittle, while wet wax is brownish and sticky. The wet phenotype is dominant over the dry type, and is frequently seen in populations of European and African origins. East Asians show the dry phenotype and there are intermediate distributions of these phenotypes among the Native North Americans and Inuits of Asian ancestry. A single-nucleotide polymorphism in the *ABCC11* gene is responsible for the determination of earwax type, with the AA genotype corresponding to dry wax and GA and GG to wet wax (Yoshiura *et al.*, 2006). However, the areas of skin that take part in cerumen production have all the components of an active local immune system and probably protect the canal by an antibody-mediated local immune response (Sirigu *et al.*, 1997).

Wax is not usually found in the deep ear canal, and a lump of 'wax' overlying the upper portion of the tympanic membrane (pars flaccida or attic region) is rarely true wax, but is nearly always associated with an underlying cholesteatoma as it is, in fact, dried-up, oxidised keratin. The sense of the old adage – 'beware the attic wax' – is still just as true today as it was in the past (see also Chapter 9).

Sound waves are partly collected by the pinna, which in humans has only a limited function. However, it is common experience that dogs prick up their ears as a response to an interesting sound, and this enables them not only to hear

better but also to localise the source of sound more accurately. In man the convolutions of the pinna do help a little in both respects, but complete loss of the pinna only reduces the hearing a few decibels, although sound localisation is impaired.

The ear canal not only protects the eardrum from direct damage but also has a role in hearing. The resonance properties of a tube that is open at one end and closed at the other, result in sounds being enhanced over a certain frequency range at the closed end of the tube, rather like the sound produced by blowing over the top of an empty bottle. For the dimensions of the human ear, this enhancement is most marked in the range 1500–6000 Hz, which includes most of the frequencies used for speech and for 'discriminating' one complex sound from another, for example speech in background noise.

The middle ear (tympanum)

The middle ear itself (mesotympanum) lies deep to the eardrum and is an air-filled space that holds three small bones (ossicles) that connect the eardrum to the inner ear (Figures 3.3 and 3.4).

These bones are called the malleus (hammer), incus (anvil) and stapes (stirrup), because of their resemblance to these objects. The malleus has a

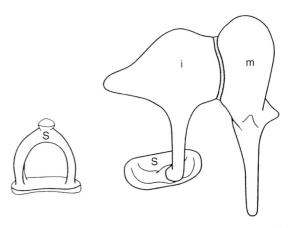

Figure 3.3 Drawing showing the malleus (m), incus (i) and stapes (s).

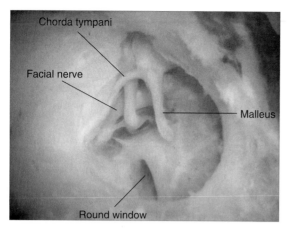

Figure 3.4 Image of a dissection of the right middle ear. The tympanic membrane has been removed. At the top of the figure a part of the wall of the deep ear canal has been drilled away to reveal part of the head of the malleus and body of the incus. To the left the long process of the incus descends to enter the middle ear, and the tip is attached to the stapes. Just above the stapes runs the facial nerve and just below is the round window niche. The chorda tympani, which carries taste from the front two-thirds of the tongue on each side, runs across the middle ear, from front to back, to join the facial nerve on its way to the brain.

handle and a head, and the handle lies within the layers of the eardrum. The head of the malleus sits in the upper part of the middle ear space called the attic (epitympanum) and is connected to the rather bulky body of the incus. From the incus, a long strut (the long process) descends back into the middle ear proper and is connected to the head of the stapes. The two arches (crura) of the stapes join the footplate, which sits in a small (3 mm × 2 mm) hole in the skull called the oval window (fenestra ovalis). This is the opening into the fluid-filled space of the inner ear. Just below the oval window is another small hole into the inner ear called the round window (fenestra rotunda). This is closed by a thin membrane, and when the footplate of the stapes moves 'in and out', then the round window membrane moves 'out and in' because the fluid in the inner ear transmits the pressure changes.

The malleus and incus are supported in the middle ear by several membranes and ligaments, which minimise their weight, allow them to move easily and bring them a blood supply. Unfortu-

nately, this leaves only a little space for the passage of air from the middle ear to the attic.

Running through the middle ear is the facial nerve (VII nerve; 7th nerve) that has left the brain and has to pass through the skull on its way to supply the muscles of facial expression, i.e. frowning, winking, smiling, scowling and so on. The nerve lies in a thin bony tube (Fallopian canal) and runs horizontally from the front to the back of the middle ear just above the oval window and stapes, before it turns downwards to leave the base of the skull. The nerve then turns forwards to reach the face. The facial nerve is therefore relatively vulnerable in diseases of the middle ear, and indeed in middle ear surgery itself.

Running through the eardrum is the nerve that carries taste from the front two-thirds of the tongue, the chorda tympani nerve. This nerve is on its way to join the facial nerve in the middle ear where it then 'hitch-hikes' a lift back to the brain.

Finally there are two small muscles in the middle ear. The one at the front (tensor tympani) is attached to the upper part of the medial surface of the handle of the malleus, and tenses up the eardrum when swallowing activates it. The muscle at the back of the middle ear (stapedius) arises near the facial nerve, is supplied by it, and attaches to the head of the stapes. It responds to loud sounds by contracting and stiffening the chain of small bones, and probably reduces transmission of prolonged loud sounds to the inner ear.

When sound waves enter the ear canal, the large area of the eardrum, which is not rigid but flexible and buckles slightly to help absorb the sound, collects the energy. The malleus, incus and stapes then transfer this energy to the relatively small area of the oval window (Figure 3.5).

This system, which comprises the large flexible eardrum linked by a chain of bones with a small lever action to the inner ear, is really quite efficient in converting airborne sound waves into sound waves in the fluids of the inner ear. Normally when sound hits the surface of a liquid, 99.5% or more is reflected. The middle ear mechanism results in about 50% of the sound reach-

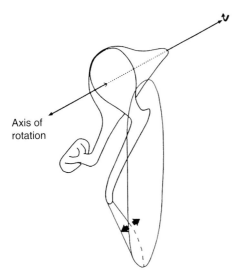

Axis of rotation

Figure 3.5 Diagrammatic representation of the middle ear transformer mechanism. The three contributors are: (1) the large surface area of the tympanic membrane to collect sound, which is transferred to the much smaller area of the stapes footplate, (2) the lever effect of the length of the malleus to the length of the incus and (3) the buckling effect of the elasticity of the tympanic membrane.

ing the eardrum being transferred to the inner ear. The middle ear mechanism therefore acts to match the very different impedances of air and fluid; all animals that live on land and can hear have a similar mechanism, although the details are different with birds only having one bone – the columella – between the eardrum and inner ear.

In mammals the middle ear is lined with a tissue which is rather like the lining of the nose with mucus-producing glands and with cells whose surface is covered with moving flexible microscopic hairs or cilia. The middle ear is therefore an air-filled space lined with living tissue capable of producing both debris from dead surface cells and mucus from the glands. This gives two possible problems: first, clearing the debris and mucus and second, a more subtle but potentially very important problem. Oxygen is absorbed from the air in the middle ear into the blood vessels running through its lining in much the same way that oxygen is absorbed in the lungs. Some carbon dioxide is given off into the air in the middle ear, but overall, and with

the passage of time, the effect of oxygen absorption would be a drop in middle ear pressure as the oxygen is removed. With higher atmospheric pressure outside the eardrum, something would have to give, and the only thing that can move is the eardrum. This would be pushed inwards by the external pressure and would stop normal function. Eventually the whole middle ear would collapse and a significant hearing loss would develop.

When working properly, the Eustachian tube (Figure 3.6) prevents both these problems. This tube runs forwards and inwards from the front wall of the middle ear to open into the back of the nasal cavity above the soft palate (the naso-pharynx). The end nearer the nose is soft and flexible and opens on swallowing or yawning. Although the precise mechanism is unclear, this tubal opening allows enough air to be drawn up into the middle ear by the negative pressure mentioned above to replenish it and keep the middle ear pressures close to atmospheric. It has been calculated that only one or two millilitres of air per ear per day – that is less than half a teaspoon of air – are necessary to maintain proper ventilation of the middle ear, but without this the middle ear fails.

The Eustachian tube is also the conduit along which the cilia move the normal mucus produced in the middle ear to the back of the nose, where, in turn, it is swallowed. This thin film of mucus,

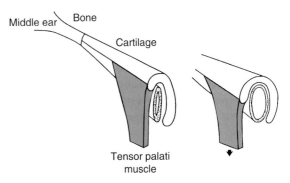

Middle ear   Bone

Cartilage

Tensor palati muscle

Figure 3.6 Diagram of the action of the Eustachian tube. The cartilage walls of the inner portion of the tube have the tensor palati muscle attached. When this muscle contracts as it does during swallowing, the cartilage buckles and the tube opens a little.

carrying the debris produced in the middle ear, is moved by the cilia along the floor of the Eustachian tube with air passing above it to reach the middle ear from the nose. Thus, the two functions of ventilation and self-cleansing are achieved when the system is working properly. Unfortunately in man, the mechanism is rather fragile and often fails to function adequately, possibly because of the shape of the skull needed to accommodate the large brain. The end result of this can be that an over-production of mucus – as frequently happens in children – fails to be cleared and this mucoid fluid accumulates in the middle ear and prevents the eardrum moving, which, in turn, reduces the hearing. When the fluid has been present for three months or more, the condition is called 'glue ear' or otitis media with effusion (OME) (see Chapter 9).

There is also an extension of the air-filled spaces of the middle ear backwards into the mastoid bone, which, if you put your hand onto the back of the skull just behind the ear, can be felt as a rounded bump. The mastoid bone should be hollow, with air-filled spaces broken up by small and incomplete bony partitions. The average mastoid has an air volume of about 15–20 ml, and this helps buffer pressure changes in the middle ear and reduce adverse effects on the tympanic membrane. Individuals with small mastoid air spaces seem to be at a much greater risk of developing middle ear and mastoid disease. Whether it is the middle ear and mastoid disease that causes the failure of the mastoid to develop, or whether the small size reduces the buffering power and therefore causes the development of disease, is yet to be fully answered. The likely answer, although, is that it will be a bit of both.

The inner ear

Anatomy of the cochlea (Figure 3.7)

The inner ear is probably the most remarkably intricate piece of the body. Not only does it perform hearing by converting sound into electrical impulses that then travel along the hearing

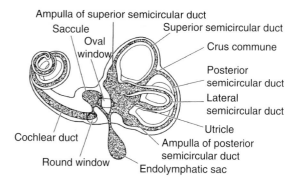

Figure 3.7 Schematic diagram of the inner ear. The solid lines represent the bony shell that houses the sensory structures of hearing and balance. This is the bony labyrinth which is filled with a fluid called perilymph and contains the membranous labyrinth which is stippled in the diagram. The different parts of the membranous labyrinth are labelled. The membranous labyrinth is filled with a very special fluid called endolymph.

nerve to the brain (the acoustic nerve; auditory nerve; VIII or 8th nerve), but it also plays a major role in balancing. The balance portions of the inner ear (vestibular labyrinth) can detect acceleration of the head in any direction, whether it be in a straight line (linear) or twisting and turning (angular). The electrical signals that arise in response to head movement pass along the balance nerve (vestibular nerve; stato-acoustic nerve; VIII or 8th nerve) to the brain (see also Chapter 24).

The portion of the inner ear that hears is the cochlea (Figures 3.7–3.10). This is a hollow coiled tube, called the bony labyrinth, set in the very dense petrous (rock-like) temporal bone. This tube is filled with fluid, which is much the same as general body fluid (lymph) and that which surrounds the brain (cerebrospinal fluid – CSF). This inner ear fluid is called perilymph. Inside the perilymph is another coiled tube which is triangular in cross-section and is called the cochlear duct (scala media).

It is the cochlear duct that contains the all-important 'hair cells' – which convert sound to electricity. These hair cells are arranged in two groups that follow the coils of the cochlear duct and spiral upwards from base to apex. There is

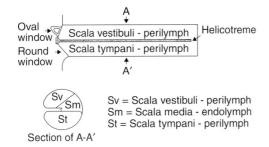

Section of A-A'

Figure 3.8 It is rather difficult to understand the workings of the cochlear portion of the inner ear and it is possibly easier to imagine it uncoiled. The upper diagram shows the uncoiled tube which is split into an upper portion – the scala vestibuli (sv), and a lower portion, the scala tympani (st), by a shelf of bone. This bony shelf does not extend all the way along the cochlea but stops short at the apex so that there is a connection between the two scalae called the helicotreme. These two scalae are filled with perilymph.

If we cut across the tube at AA' and look at it end on, we can see that the bony shelf does not stretch all the way across the tube but is replaced by a thin membrane going to the outer wall of the tube. There is also a sloping membrane running upwards from the edge of the bony shelf to the outer wall thereby creating a triangular space called the scala media (sm). The scala media or cochlear duct is filled with endolymph and contains the auditory sensory cells.

a single row of inner hair cells (IHCs), which lie closer to the core of the cochlea, and three or four rows of outer hair cells (OHCs), which are further away (Figure 3.9). In a healthy, young ear there are about 3500 IHCs and about 12,000 OHCs. Each hair cell has a cluster of small rigid hairs (stereocilia) that project from the thicker upper surface of the cell into the special fluid that fills the cochlear duct. This fluid is called endolymph and is remarkable in that it has a strongly positive electrical charge associated with it – about 80 mV – and is rich in potassium (K^+).

The hair cells in their rows are grouped together with their supporting cells in the organ of Corti. This is a small ridge which sits on a thin, very flexible membrane called the basilar membrane. The basilar membrane forms the floor of the triangular cochlear duct (Figure 3.10). The sloping roof is another very thin membrane (Reissner's membrane), and the side wall is a thickened region rich in blood vessels (the stria vascularis), which is responsible for maintaining the composition of the endolymph.

Adjacent to the base of the hair cells are the nerves that carry impulses to the brain (afferent nerves). At least 90% of these nerves come from the IHCs. Each IHC has about 10 nerve endings

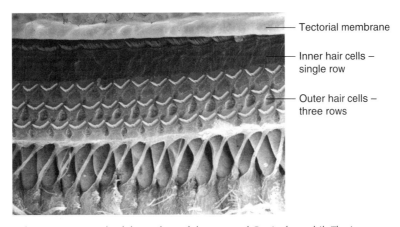

Figure 3.9 Scanning electron micrograph of the surface of the organ of Corti of a gerbil. The image was taken by Professor Andrew Forge of the UCL Ear Institute and I am grateful for his permission to use it. Projecting from the surface of the organ of Corti are clusters of fine hairs (stereocilia) that arise from the sensory hair cells. The hair cells are arranged in two groups called the inner and outer hair cells (IHC and OHC respectively). There are usually three rows of OHCs and one row of IHCs in rodents, although the pattern in humans is somewhat disorganised. The stereocilia that project from the OHCs are arranged in a V- or W-shaped array, while those from the IHCS are linear. The tectorial membrane, which normally covers the organ of Corti, has shrunk back during preparation of the specimen to reveal the hair cell stereociliary bundles.

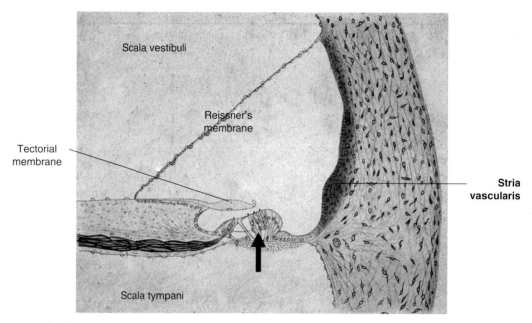

Figure 3.10 This drawing of a cross-section of the human cochlear duct (see also Figure 3.8) was made by Gustav Retzius and was part of an incredible study of the inner ears of a whole range of animals in 1881. The technical quality of his work was stunning. I have added the captions but did not want to obliterate the fine detail. The arrow indicates the Organ of Corti.

attached to it, and there are about 30,000 nerve fibres in the acoustic nerve.

The OHCs do have nerves attached to them but most are nerves coming from the brain (efferent nerves), whose function is probably to keep the cochlea 'in tune' and add sensitivity to the inner ear by way of an internal cochlear amplifier, which adds about 60 dB gain to enable quiet sounds to be detected.

The afferent hearing nerves travel inwards, along with the balance and facial nerves, through a canal in the inner part of the skull (internal auditory meatus (IAM); internal auditory canal (IAC)) to reach the brainstem. This part of the brain deals with many automatic functions such as pulse, blood pressure, general alertness, balance and so on.

How the cochlea works

As sound waves hit the perilymph beneath the footplate, they create a wave that travels along the length of the cochlea. This travelling wave builds up to a specific maximum for each particular pitch and then falls rapidly away to nothing. The location of the peak of the wave varies at different pitches: for high-pitched sounds the wave peaks near the base of the cochlea, whereas for low-pitched sounds this peak is near the apex (Figure 3.11).

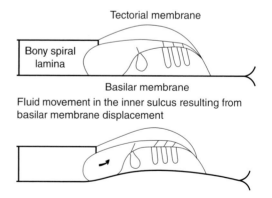

Figure 3.11 A diagram redrawn from von Bekesy, who discovered how sound travelled through the inner ear to stimulate the hair cells and was awarded the Nobel Prize for his work in 1961. As sound pressure waves pass through the cochlea, the flexible basilar membrane moves up and down in response to the sound. As the membrane moves 'up', the stereo cilia of the IHCs are deflected away from the bony spiral lamina and this is the stimulus that results in the IHCs generating a signal in the fibres of the acoustic nerve.

As this pressure wave passes through the cochlea, there is movement of the thin basilar membrane and with it the organ of Corti containing the hair cells. Overlying the hair cells is a gelatinous membrane called the tectorial membrane. One edge of this is attached to the bony core at the centre of the cochlea (the modiolus), while the other edge is loosely attached to the organ of Corti outside the outermost OHC. The tips of the hairs of the OHCs are lightly embedded in the under-surface of the tectorial membrane, while the tips of the IHCs, which you will remember connect with most of the nerve fibres,

do not reach the tectorial membrane and stand free in the endolymph. As the travelling wave reaches its peak, the OHCs near this peak give a small, physical 'kick' to enhance the movement of the basilar membrane. This internal amplifier causes the endolymph to squirt towards the hairs of the IHCs (Figure 3.12).

If the movement of fluid is great enough, then the hairs are deflected and very small channels open up somewhere near the tips of the hairs. The potassium (K^+) in the endolymph can now flood down through these small channels, being propelled by the very strong positive electrical

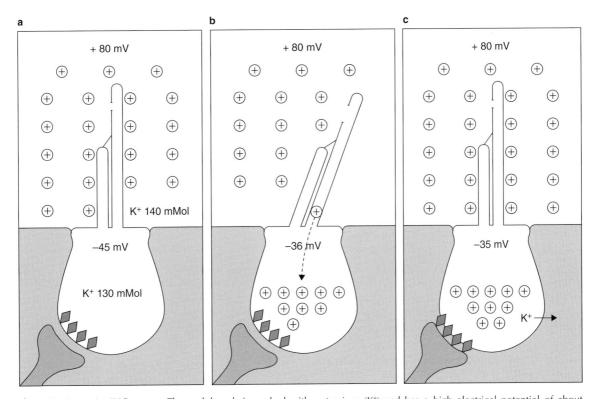

Figure 3.12 a, An IHC at rest. The endolymph is packed with potassium (K^+) and has a high electrical potential of about +80 mV. The inside of the IHC has a negative, resting potential of −45 mV. Near the tip of the longer stereocilium is a small gate, although it is too small for the K^+ to squeeze through. The shaded diamonds are neurotransmitters in the cell membrane waiting to be released. **b,** The stereocilia are being deflected by sound and the small link between the shorter and the longer stereocilia pulls on the membrane covering the stereocilium to widen the gate enough for the K^+ to be driven into the IHC body by the large voltage gradient. Consequently the negative voltage in the cell becomes less marked. **c,** Eventually the intracellular potential becomes much less negative and the cell is said to be depolarised. This alters the cell membrane and enables the release of packets of neurotransmitter (probably acetyl choline) that result in stimulation of the acoustic nerve. By now the stereocilia have returned to the upright position, no more potassium enters the cells, and the cell contents are returned to the resting state as K^+ is pumped out of the cell and the potential returns to its original state.

charge of the endolymph, into the bodies of the IHCs. Here the influx of potassium alters the hair cell membrane, and small parcels of chemicals are released from the base of the hair cell and cause the nearby nerves to become active and send pulsed signals towards the brain.

The cochlear nerves reach the cochlear nucleus in the brainstem as the first relay station on the way to perception. After this, half the fibres cross over to the other side of the brainstem and continue their journey to the higher auditory centres and conscious 'hearing' in the temporal lobe of the cerebral cortex. This journey is described in Chapter 4.

Acknowledgements

I am grateful to Kate Lay MSc, MIMI, RMIP, Medical Illustrator at the Ear Institute, Grays Inn Road, for her help in preparing some of the illustrations.

References

Alberti P (1964) Epithelial migration over tympanic membrane and external canal. *Journal of Laryngology and Otology* 78: 808–830.

Campos A, Betancor L, Arias A *et al.* (2000) Influence of human wet cerumen on the growth of common and pathogenic bacteria of the ear. *Journal of Laryngology and Otology* 114:925–929.

Sirigu P, Perra M, Ferreli C, Maxia C, Tumo F (1997) Local immune response in the skin of the external auditory meatus: an immuno-histochemical study. *Microscopy Research and Technique* 38:329–334.

Stone M, Fulghum R (1984) Bactericidal activity of wet cerumen. *Annals of Otology, Rhinology and Laryngology* 93:183–186.

Yoshiura K, Kinoshita A, Ishida T *et al.* (2006) A SNP in the *ABCC11* gene is the determinant of human earwax type. *Nature Genetics* 38:324–330.

The central auditory system

David McAlpine

4

Introduction

The process by which sound is transduced by the cochlea of the inner ear renders auditory information into trains of electrical events that, ultimately, form the neural code for hearing. This chapter describes the form and subsequent transformations of this neural code, from the primary auditory nerve fibres synapsing on the inner hair cells (IHCs) of the cochlea, to auditory cortical centres responsible for processing speech and other complex sounds (Figure 4.1).

The auditory nerve fibres

The passage of neural information both to and from the cochlea is made possible by means of the fibres of the VIIIth cranial nerve, often referred to as the auditory nerve or, more completely, the audiovestibular nerve, as it also contains fibres projecting from the vestibular organs of the inner ear. Fibres that constitute the cochlear division of the VIIIth cranial nerve – the primary auditory nerve fibres or ANFs – are classified as bipolar neurons (nerve cells). These are cells that have two projections arising from the cell body,

one receiving electrical impulses from the IHCs in the cochlea, the other taking impulses out of the cell to the next 'relay point' in the nervous system, the cochlear nucleus. In the case of the spiral ganglion neurons, their synaptic endings at one end are applied directly to the base of the IHCs, and those at the other end connect with the cochlear nucleus – the first part of the auditory brain proper. Because the cell bodies are contained within the spiral structure of the cochlea, ANFs are sometimes also referred to as spiral ganglion cells. ANFs exist in two distinct forms, type I and type II fibres. Type I ANFs, which are relatively large in diameter and well myelinated, comprise 95% of the *afferent* fibres in the cochlea (i.e. those that send information from the cochlea to the brain), and synapse with individual IHCs. There are about 3000 IHCs in the human cochlea and about 30,000 spiral ganglion cells. Each IHC receives nerve fibres from several spiral ganglion cells, but each spiral ganglion cell is connected to only one IHC. This one-to-one innervation of type I fibres is a critical factor in their ability to show the same sharp frequency tuning as the part of the basilar membrane they innervate. The thinner type II fibres constitute the remaining 5% of primary ANFs. These fibres innervate the base of multiple outer

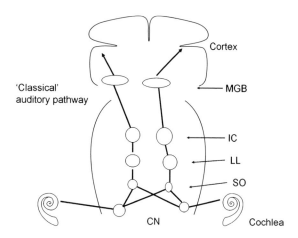

Figure 4.1 Diagram of the ascending auditory neural pathway in the brain. MGB: medial geniculate body; IC: inferior colliculus; LL: lateral lemniscus; SO: superior olivary complex; CN: cochlear nuclei. (Contributed by JM Graham with the help of Kate Lay MSc, MIMI, RMIP.)

hair cells (OHCs), their responses are only poorly characterised, and their function in hearing unknown. A third group of fibres conveyed within the auditory nerve represent the final stage of the cochlear *efferent* system, sending information down from the brain towards the cochlea. Arising from neurons in and around several of the main auditory brainstem nuclei, notably the medial and lateral superior olivary nuclei of the superior olivary complex (SOC), cochlear efferents synapse directly either on the base of the OHCs, or on the terminal endings of type I fibres that themselves synapse with IHCs.

The transmission of auditory information from the cochlea to the auditory pathways in the brain by means of the type I fibres represents a critical stage in brain processing of sound, and damage to these fibres generally leads to reduced hearing abilities. So too, damage to the cochlear hair cells, the most common cause of deafness, is reflected in the responses of type I fibres, which lose their sensitivity to, and selectivity for, different sound frequencies when the OHCs are damaged by noise, for example.

Tonotopicity, the representation of different frequencies at different anatomical sites, is present at all levels of the auditory system. In the cochlea,

high frequencies are detected at the basal end, nearest to the oval window (see Chapter 3), and if the cochlea were to be 'unrolled' it would be seen to be arranged like the keyboard of a piano, with high frequencies at one end and low frequencies at the other. This tonotopic arrangement is present at all levels of the auditory system, up to and including the auditory cortex in the brain (Figure 4.2).

The exquisite tuning of type I fibres reflects the tuning of the part of the basilar membrane that they innervate. Frequency-tuning curves (FTCs – see Figure 4.3a) plot the sound level that evokes activity above the background, or spontaneous, firing rate for each sound frequency. The characteristic frequency (CF) – the frequency at which responses occur to quietest sound – illustrates the sharpness of tuning for sound frequency of the healthy basilar membrane, with the best thresholds often around zero decibels of sound pressure level (SPL) in many species (Ruggero, 1973). Type I fibres typically show a wide range

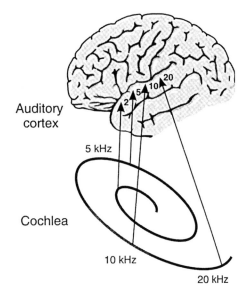

Figure 4.2 Tonotopic organisation of the cochlea, with individual frequencies projecting to the primary auditory cortex, to be represented there with a similar tonotopic organisation. (From Clark G (2003) *Cochlear Implants.* New York: Springer-Verlag, reproduced with kind permission of Professor Graeme Clark and the publishers, Springer Science and Business Media.)

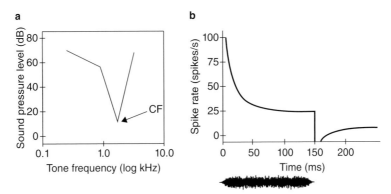

Figure 4.3 Responses of type I auditory nerve fibres. **a**, Representation of a normal frequency-tuning curve (FTC) for an auditory nerve fibre. The black curve outlines the range of sound levels and frequencies that evoke action potentials above the spontaneous, or background, level. **b**, Peristimulus time histogram (PSTH) of the response to a constant-level stimulus (here a burst of noise). The response (curve) adapts from an initial high discharge rate at stimulus onset to a steady-state level until the stimulus is terminated. The response then falls below the spontaneous rate, before recovering.

of spontaneous firing rates, up to 100 action potentials per second in some cases, activity that is generated by the spontaneous release of the neurotransmitter acetylcholine from the base of the IHC to stimulate the end of the nerve fibre leading to the spiral ganglion cell. Connections of this kind and those between neurons are called synapses. All ANFs show low thresholds for generating action potentials in the healthy cochlea, reflecting the sensitivity of the basilar membrane to quiet sounds, and generally tend to 'saturate' (show their maximal firing rate) by some 20–30 dB above threshold, maintaining this firing rate in spite of very high sound levels. Nevertheless, some distinction between fibres is normally made in this regard; those fibres with 'low', as compared to 'high', spontaneous rates tend to show somewhat higher thresholds, and a more sloping 'profile' to their firing rate *versus* sound level response, than do 'high spontaneous rate' fibres. This suggests a dichotomy into highly sensitive fibres that rapidly saturate their response, and less sensitive fibres that encode increasing sound intensity, with increasing firing rates up to high levels of sound. It should be noted, however, that these distinctions are not always clear-cut, nor is it clear that such distinctions can be made in all species. The summed activity of many type I fibres can be recorded as the compound action

potential of the electrocochleogram (see Chapter 7), or the early N1 potential of the auditory brainstem response (ABR). The probability of action potential firing in type I fibres is related to the magnitude of the receptor potential of the IHCs they innervate. This, in turn, reflects the magnitude (or velocity) of the basilar membrane vibration, and is related to the sound energy at that particular frequency. In response to a constant sound, such as a tone at CF, ANFs show an 'adapting' response profile, with an initially high discharge rate at stimulus onset adapting to a steady-state 'plateau' until the stimulus is terminated, whereupon the firing rate might briefly fall below that of the spontaneous rate before recovering. This pattern is best observed by averaging the response to a succession of identical stimuli to create a peri-stimulus time histogram (PSTH – see Figure 4.3b).

For sound frequencies below about 4 kHz in many mammals, type I fibres respond to the cycle-by-cycle changes in the membrane potential of the IHCs (itself reflecting the back-and-forth deflections of the hair-cell stereocilia) with action potentials that are 'phase locked' to the stimulus waveform (see Figure 4.4a). As sound frequency increases, however, the proportion of 'direct' to 'alternating' current carried in the receptor potential increases, so that by 4 kHz and above,

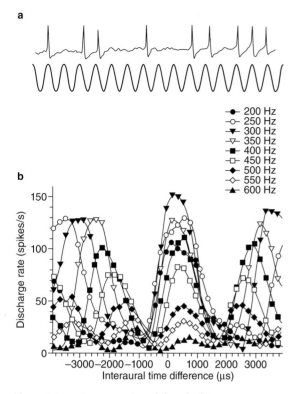

—●— 200 Hz
—○— 250 Hz
—▼— 300 Hz
—▽— 350 Hz
—■— 400 Hz
—□— 450 Hz
—◆— 500 Hz
—◇— 550 Hz
—▲— 600 Hz

Figure 4.4 **a**, Representation of phase locking to a pure tone. Action potentials (top trace) are not evoked to every cycle of the stimulus (bottom trace), but when they are evoked they occur only at a particular phase angle (point) within each cycle. **b**, Response of an ITD-sensitive neuron to a range of sounds leading either at the ear on the same side to the brain centre recorded (negative interaural time differences (ITDs)) or on the opposite side (positive ITDs). Note that for each pure tone frequency to which the neuron (here, in the IC) is sensitive, the response is cyclic, with peak responses separated by an interval that reflects the periodicity of the stimulus. The ITD at which the peaks are aligned (here the central peak) indicates the neuron's characteristic delay. (Adapted with permission from McAlpine D (2005) Creating a sense of auditory space. *Journal of Physiology* 566:21–28.)

the hair-cell response no longer follows the cycle-by-cycle changes in the stimulus waveform but only the 'envelope' of the sound. This is reflected in the responses of auditory nerve fibres, which show phase locking of their responses to the stimulus fine structure for frequencies below 4 kHz. This phase locking provides a potential cue for assessing pure-tone pitch, and is critical to the ability to localise the source of a sound in

the horizontal plane by means of calculating the difference in the arrival time of the sound at each ear (see next section).

The cochlear nucleus

Auditory nerve fibres entering the cochlear nucleus (CN) bifurcate, innervating both the ventral and dorsal aspects of the CN (VCN and DCN, respectively). The CN is the first postsynaptic stage after the hair cell synapse, and provides the possibility of both excitatory and inhibitory neurotransmission (hair cell and ANF synapses are purely excitatory), and the convergence of multiple inputs onto single neurons. The CN is characterised by a division of labour between and within its different subdivisions. Neurons of the VCN, particularly the spherical bushy cells (SBCs) of the anterior division (AVCN) and the globular bushy cells (GBCs), appear specialised for temporal processing, with large synaptic contacts and fast membrane kinetics. Indeed, the non-homogeneity of CN responses reflects the highly divergent morphologies, patterns of connectivity and biophysical properties within the CN. Given the homogeneity of its inputs, the CN represents a significant transformation in neural coding of sound. Nevertheless, the frequency-tuning characteristics of CN neurons largely reflect their ANF inputs.

The DCN is a laminated structure, comprising an outer, 'molecular', layer with a relatively low neural density, an adjacent fusiform layer, and a deeper central area containing a wide range of different cell types. A significant literature exists detailing the responses of neurons in the DCN, which appear particularly specialised for processing spectral cues that arise from the interaction of complex sounds with the head and the outer ear, and which constitute important cues for localising the source of a sound, particularly in the vertical plane (including distinguishing 'front' from 'back'). In particular, the responses of so-called 'type IV' neurons of the DCN appear to be determined by a dedicated neural circuit within the DCN itself. Type IV neurons show a small 'island' of near-threshold activation around their CF, with a much larger central inhibitory area at higher sound intensities, believed to be derived from the DCN's onset-chopper (Onset-C) neurons, which respond to a stimulus with a brief burst of large regularly spaced spike potentials, followed by a lower level of sustained activity, and act as broad-band inhibitors. The combination of excitatory inputs from ANFs, broad-band inhibition from the putative onset-C neurons, and inhibition derived from type II DCN neurons (themselves also thought to be the target of onset-C inhibition), renders type IV neurons particularly sensitive to (inhibited by) notches in the acoustic spectrum, presumably those generated by the interaction of sound with the head and pinna. How might such neurons encode the potential cues for sound-source elevation such notches provide? A potential answer lies in understanding the neurons to which type IV neurons project in the auditory midbrain nucleus of the inferior colliculus, which essentially respond in the opposite manner, being maximally activated by the notch in the sound spectrum (Davis *et al.*, 2003).

The predominant cell types of the VCN are the bushy cells, divided into globular and spherical bushy cell types (GBCs and SBCs, respectively). ANFs synapse with bushy cells by means of some of the largest synapses in the brain, the end bulbs of Held. Single ANF endings envelop the bushy cells, making multiple synaptic contacts, and ensuring a tight coupling between pre- and postsynaptic responses. Many bushy cells are 'primary like', in that they show response properties recognisable as being the same as those from the primary ANFs, with well-tuned, relatively simple V-shaped tuning curves, and PSTHs showing the classic onset response decaying to a steady state. Nevertheless, their tuning appears somewhat sharper than that of ANFs. Recordings made from the axons of SBCs in the anterior division of the VCN (AVCN) in particular, indicate improved synchrony and entrainment of phase locking relative to ANFs, especially for frequencies up to 1 kHz. This reflects their role in maintaining, and even enhancing, information about the fine temporal structure of sounds. The octopus cells of the posterior division of the VCN (PVCN), which receive bouton-like synaptic endings from ANFs, also show high temporal precision but respond mainly at stimulus onset, or in response to trains of modulated sounds. A further class of neurons that resides throughout the VCN, the multipolar cells, receive bouton-like synaptic inputs, and are characterised physiologically by a 'chopping' response pattern in response to tonal input, in which action potentials are generated at regular intervals. This chopping pattern reflects intrinsic cell temporal properties rather than the phase-locked responses to acoustic inputs seen in the ANFs.

Information leaves the CN carried by the three main output fibre tracts, the ventral, intermediate and dorsal acoustic striae. Axons from the DCN leave the CN via the dorsal acoustic stria (DAS), traverse the midline and project directly to the inferior colliculus (IC) on the opposite side of the brain, via the lateral lemniscus. The IC is the site of multiple convergent inputs, both ascending and descending. Fibres in the ventral acoustic stria (VAS – also known as the trapezoid body) leave the VCN to innervate the nuclei of the ipsilateral and contralateral superior olivary complex, where information from the two ears converges to create binaural sensitivity. Fibres leaving the VCN via the intermediate acoustic stria originate from octopus and multipolar cells. These tend to innervate the neurons of the periolivary nuclei and, after crossing the midline at the level of the medulla, the IC via the lateral lemniscal fibres. Fibres from octopus cells terminate in the ventral nucleus of the lateral lemnisus (VNLL), and thence to the IC.

Binaural hearing and the brainstem pathways

According to the duplex theory (Rayleigh, 1907), human sound localisation is subserved by two mechanisms: at low frequencies (<1500 Hz), sources of sounds are localised using interaural *time* differences (ITDs), whereas at high frequencies localisation is achieved by interaural *intensity* differences (IIDs). Sensitivity to ITDs and IIDs is referred to as binaural ('two-eared') hearing, and brainstem pathways underpinning binaural hearing are highly specialised, particularly those contributing to ITD sensitivity, which comprise some of the most temporally precise neural elements in the brain.

ITDs arise when the sound source is located closer to one ear than the other. For humans this is maximally 600–700 μs (*millionths* of a second), corresponding to a source located directly to the left or the right. ITDs are processed by neurons in the medial superior olive (MSO) of the SOC. Individual MSO neurons are innervated by SBCs from the cochlear nucleus on each side of the brain, and respond as binaural coincidence detectors, showing maximum firing rates at favourable ITDs – i.e. when phase-locked input from each ear arrives in temporal coincidence, and with lower firing rates at other ITDs (Figure 4.4b). Phase locking of action potentials to the stimulus fine structure is an absolute requirement for generating ITD sensitivity in MSO neurons, and various specialisations, particularly of the SBCs, ensure that phase locking is maintained until at least the level of the MSO. Nevertheless, the upper limit of phase locking is reduced in the ascending auditory pathway, so that by the level of binaural integration the upper limit lies around 2 kHz, rather than the 4–5 kHz seen in the ANFs. Certainly most mammals are insensitive to ITDs in the fine structure of a sound above this frequency.

By imposing an ITD on the stimulus waveform at each ear, a cyclic pattern of responses is evoked in MSO neurons, with response maxima occurring at those ITDs that represent intervals separated by the period of the pure-tone frequency presented (see Figure 4.4b and Yin and Chan, 1990). This cyclic response reflects the underlying binaural coincidence detection. MSO neurons also receive bilateral inhibitory inputs via some of the largest and most reliable synapses in the brain, including the calyx of Held in the medial nucleus of the trapezoid body (MNTB), and recent studies (Brand *et al.*, 2002) indicate these inhibitory inputs to be critical in determining the preferred ITD tuning of individual MSO neurons.

Interaural intensity differences, the second binaural cue, arise when the passage of sound is impeded by the head, creating an acoustic 'shadow' at the ear further from the source.

Unlike ITDs, which are largely independent of the sound frequency (the speed of sound is constant for all frequencies), IIDs increase with increasing sound frequency; the head creates a larger acoustic shadow at shorter and shorter wavelengths of sound (see Chapter 5). Thus, IIDs are a more effective cue for localisation at higher than at lower sound frequencies. Lateral superior olivary (LSO) neurons are innervated by excitatory inputs originating from the SBCs on the ipsilateral (same) side and by inhibitory inputs via the ipsilateral MNTB, which itself receives excitatory input from GBCs in the opposite CN. LSO neurons respond maximally to stimulation of the ipsilateral ear, and this response is increasingly inhibited by increasing stimulation of the contralateral ear. Thus, LSO neurons encode IID in the form of a 'rate code', with the spike rate being determined by the relative sound level between the ears; sounds located closer to the ipsilateral ear generate near-maximal rates, with the rate falling as the source moves around the head closer to the inhibitory ear. With a LSO located in each brain hemisphere, the relative activity of the two LSOs, acting in a 'push–pull' fashion, represents a simple code for the location of the sound source generating that activity.

The major excitatory output from the MSO is primarily to the ipsilateral midbrain nucleus of the inferior colliculus (IC), while that from the LSO is to the contralateral IC.

The cochlear efferent system

A significant proportion of the total fibre density in the auditory system projects from higher brain centres to lower ones. The most explored of these is the cochlear efferent system. Fibres of the cochlear efferent system originate from cells in and around the major nuclei of the auditory brainstem, the LSO and MSO. Hence, the efferent system is divided into lateral and medial divisions, the lateral olivocochlear (LOC) and medial olivocochlear (MOC) pathways. The relatively thin, unmyelinated LOC fibres project largely to the ipsilateral cochlea, synapsing on the synaptic terminals of type I ANFs innervating the IHCs.

The thicker, more myelinated MOC fibres project largely to the contralateral cochlea, terminating directly on the OHCs. These latter fibres form the crossed olivocochlear bundle (COCB). Electrical stimulation of the COCB, access to which is achieved from the floor of the fourth ventricle, leads to a shift in the sensitivity of the cochlea to sound stimulation, through an inhibitory effect on the OHCs. Effectively, the gain of the cochlear amplifier generated by the active process in the OHCs is reduced, ultimately shifting sensitivity of individual ANF fibres to higher sound levels. This can be observed as a reduction in the magnitude of the compound action potential (the N1 component of the ABR).

The inferior colliculus

From an anatomical perspective, the IC occupies a pivotal position in the auditory brain. As the major auditory nucleus of the midbrain, the IC receives input from numerous ascending pathways in the auditory brainstem. Although many basic responses of IC neurons have been characterised (see Irvine, 1992 for review), specific roles for the IC in auditory processing remain to be determined. The IC also receives a significant descending input from the cortex and auditory thalamus via the corticofugal pathways, the functions of which remain largely unexplored. Pharmacologically, the IC hosts a potent cocktail of neurotransmitters and neuromodulators, including serotonin and opiates. Taken together, this suggests a level of complexity in the IC that potentially provides for a significant processing of auditory information beyond that of the sensitivity to relatively low-level acoustic cues observed in the lower brainstem. It is surprising, therefore, that evidence for any specific contribution of the IC to hearing is lacking, although it is often accessed for *in vivo* experimental recordings.

The IC comprises several relatively distinct subregions, including the central nucleus (ICC), the external nucleus (ICX) and the dorsal shell (DIC). The ICC, part of the main ascending auditory pathway, is tonotopically organised, with neurons generally showing increasing CF along the dorsoventral axis. Neurons in the other subdivisions are generally less well tuned for sound frequency, often responding better to noise than to tones, and may also show habituating responses to repeated stimulation. It is also clear that by the level of the IC, a considerably greater proportion of neurons show non-monotonic rate-level functions compared with lower brain centres. In addition, a significant reduction in spontaneous activity occurs at successive stages in the ascending pathways and, by the level of the IC, single neurons show very low spontaneous firing rates indeed. Part of this is undoubtedly due to the filtering of spontaneous activity by binaural brainstem nuclei. Since the majority of anatomical projections to the IC are derived from the superior olive and the nuclei of the lateral lemniscus, brain nuclei in which neurons are often binaurally sensitive, it follows that the majority of IC neurons also show such sensitivity, and it is commonly assumed that the IC is critical for sound localisation. How IC responses differ from those in the lower brainstem, however, appears to be a matter of degree, rather than of type.

In addition to binaural sensitivity, the ability of IC neurons to follow modulations in the amplitude of an acoustic waveform (amplitude modulation or AM) has been studied extensively. Neural sensitivity to AM is not unique to the IC, nor even are IC neurons especially sensitive to AM compared with neurons in other auditory centres. The general consensus, although by no means conceded universally, is that the main difference between the processing of AM signals in the IC and their processing in other brain regions lies in the upper frequency at which individual neurons can phase lock their spike output to the modulated waveform – being lower than is commonly observed in the brainstem nuclei, and higher than in thalamus or cortex.

Significant contributions to our understanding of the IC as a functional unit come from investigations of auditory processing in highly adapted auditory species such as echo-locating bats and barn owls (Wagner *et al.*, 2007). Indeed, the field is indebted to such studies, since they have, on the whole, provided for a framework around which it is possible to construct a functional understanding of IC processing. Nevertheless, a significant drawback in employing such exotic species in experimental studies of auditory processing is that, for these species, sound localisation is the critical factor in hearing. Although in humans sound-source localisation is undoubtedly important, other functions such as the processing of complex pitch information, in speech, are likely to be more important in the organisation of the human brain.

Perhaps an over-arching principle of collicular processing lies in the abundance of inhibitory inputs, glycinergic but especially GABA-ergic, that appear to influence a wide range of stimulus response properties. The source of inhibitory inputs to the IC is widespread, and includes intrinsic connections, input from the dorsal nucleus of the lateral lemniscus (DNLL) in particular, and descending input from the cortex and thalamus. The role of some of these inhibitory circuits is reasonably well described in echo-locating bats, less so in more general mammals, although a consensus view is that GABA-ergic inhibition at least, with its longer, less temporally precise time course, may control the gain of the IC. The role of the more temporally precise glycinergic input, some of which is derived from the LSO, remains to be determined.

The auditory thalamus and cortex

Unlike the visual system in which the organisational principles and response properties of the thalamus and cortex are well understood, or at least well described, those of the auditory system are only poorly understood. In part this is due to the more extensive precortical processing that exists in the auditory compared with the visual pathway.

The auditory thalamus, which is an obligatory station in the ascending pathway, relaying input from the IC to the cortex, comprises three main divisions, the ventral, medial, and dorsal medial geniculate body (MGB). The ventral (v)MGB is organised tonotopically, and constitutes the major lemniscal division of the MGB. Neurons in the vMGB show a range of frequency-tuning characteristics – many are narrowly tuned for a single sound frequency although they can also be multilobed or broadly tuned – with relatively short response latencies. The primary role of the vMGB is thought to be in relaying frequency, intensity and spatial (binaural) information to the auditory cortex. Neurons of the medial division of the MGB (mMGB) show more diverse response patterns than those of the ventral division, tend to be more labile in their responsiveness, and show considerably longer response latencies to sound stimulation than vMGB neurons. Neurons in the dorsal MGB are generally only broadly tuned for sound frequency and only poorly responsive to individual frequencies.

Fibres leaving the MGB do so via the auditory radiations to terminate on thalamo-recipient neurons in layers 3 and 4 of the primary auditory cortex. The primary auditory cortex in humans lies on the anterior transverse temporal gyrus, corresponding to Brodman areas 41 and 42. As in other sensory cortices, auditory cortex is a six-layered laminar structure, with specific input, output and intracortical layers. Neurons appear to be organised in columns, with neurons in each column showing similar CFs, although the concept of CF is less strict than in lower brain centres. Generally, it is well established in mammals that the two major auditory fields are primary auditory cortex (A1) and the adjacent anterior auditory field (AAF), and from experimental recordings in a range of species, these fields appear to be tonotopically organised, with mirror-imaged frequency maps, with A1 and AAF abutting each other at the high-frequency end of the tonotopic gradient. As with higher cortical areas in other sensory modalities, there are a number of areas related to hearing that lie beyond the primary auditory cortex (extra-primary areas). There are also projections to the area of Wernicke, which lies posterior to the primary auditory cortex and is responsible for the understanding of speech, and Broca's area, anterior to the primary cortex, responsible for normal speech production.

Despite the relatively less-well-developed understanding of cortical processing in hearing compared with that of vision, considerable progress has recently been made in elucidating functional divisions of the cortical fields through the use of functional magnetic resonance imaging (fMRI) and other brain-imaging/recording techniques such as magneto-encephalography (MEG). These studies suggest evidence for divisions according to sound properties such as complex pitch (musical notes and voice pitch), for example, as well as spatial location of sound sources, and pathways leading away from the primary areas organised according to 'where' and 'what' an auditory stimulus might be (Griffiths *et al.*, 2004; Micheyl *et al.*, 2007). The MEG technique in particular is well suited to studying temporal aspects of auditory processing, and is beginning to reveal how the temporal structure of sounds might be encoded and organised across space (i.e. neural tissue) and across time.

Summary

The neural process of hearing starts at the synapse of the auditory nerve fibres with the IHCs. Sound frequency, the primary feature encoded by the sensory epithelium in the cochlea, is maintained, through tonotopicity, as the major organisational principle in the central auditory nervous system, to the level of primary cortex and beyond. The auditory pathways comprise many subcortical structures; some have well-defined functions such as the binaural brainstem nuclei responsible for coding sound-source location; others, such as the IC, have less-well-defined roles, which nevertheless appear to play a substantial role in hearing by virtue of their extensive anatomical projections and diverse response properties. A significant increase in our knowledge of cortical function with respect to hearing is unfolding, with the advent, and now widespread availability, of brain-imaging tools.

References

Brand A, Behrend O, Marquardt T, McAlpine D, Grothe B (2002) Precise inhibition is essential for microsecond interaural time difference coding. *Nature* 417:543–547.

Clark G (2003) *Cochlear Implants*. New York: Springer-Verlag.

Davis KA, Ramachandran R, May BJ (2003) Auditory processing of spectral cues for sound localization in the inferior colliculus. *Journal of the Association for Research in Otolaryngology* 4:148–163.

Griffiths TD, Warren JD, Scott SK, Nelken I, King AJ (2004) Cortical processing of complex sound: a way forward? *Trends in Neurosciences* 27:181–185.

Irvine DRF (1992) Physiology of auditory brainstem pathways. In: Fay RR, Popper AA, eds. *Springer Handbook of Auditory Research, Vol 2, The Mammalian Auditory Pathway: neurophysiology*, pp 153–231. New York: Springer.

McAlpine D (2005) Creating a sense of auditory space. *Journal of Physiology* 566:21–28.

Micheyl C, Carlyon RP, Gutschalk A *et al.* (2007) The role of auditory cortex in the formation of auditory streams. *Hearing Research* 229:116–131.

(Lord) Rayleigh (1907). On our perception of sound direction. *Philosophical Magazine* 13: 214–232.

Ruggero MA (1973) Response to noise of auditory nerve fibers in the squirrel monkey. *Journal of Neurophysiology* 36:569–587.

Wagner H, Asadollahi A, Bremen P *et al.* (2007) Distribution of interaural time difference in the barn owl's inferior colliculus in the low- and high-frequency ranges. *Journal of Neuroscience* 27:4191–4200.

Yin TC, Chan JC (1990) Interaural time sensitivity in medial superior olive of cat. *Journal of Neurophysiology* 64:465–488.

An introduction to acoustics: clinical implications

5

Richard Knight

Introduction

The aim of this chapter is to give an introduction to acoustics, in particular focusing on how it relates to audiology. A good scientific basis to our understanding of audiology helps our appreciation of the most important aspects of the auditory environment and the hearing process, and also helps us in the fields of hearing assessment, instrumentation and hearing aids. However, 'physics' is often a subject that strikes fear into the hearts of those for whom it is not home territory, therefore the intention here is to provide a descriptive overview of the main concepts applicable to audiology, without going too deeply into the mathematics.

There are various basic concepts in acoustics that are relevant for audiology, and a brief introduction will be given here, followed by a brief discussion of some audiological applications in which acoustical concepts can be applied.

Acoustic parameters and units of measure

Periodic sounds

Sound can be categorised as *periodic* or *aperiodic*. Periodic sounds repeat in a regular time interval, and examples include a sine wave or a musical note.

There are some parameters by which we can characterise periodic sounds.

Period

Anything that repeats at a regular time interval can be characterised by the time interval between each repeat. Periodic audible sounds repeat in a small fraction of a second: periods between about 0.05 and 0.00005 s lie within the audible range for humans. However, in practice, it is easier to deal with the reciprocal of period, which is frequency.

Frequency *versus* pitch

The frequency of a sound is how often it repeats per second, and the unit of measure is Hertz (Hz) (HR Hertz: German physicist, 1857–94) (1 Hz = 1 repeat per second). Period and frequency can therefore be calculated from each other as follows:

$$\text{Period (seconds)} = \frac{1}{\text{Frequency (Hz)}}$$

$$\text{Frequency (Hz)} = \frac{1}{\text{Period (s)}}$$

Frequency is the more usual quantity with which to define a periodic sound.

A word about pitch

The pitch of a sound is the psychological correlate of frequency. In other words, the listener's perception of 'high' and 'low' pitch correlates with 'high' and 'low' frequency. However, the terms frequency and pitch are not entirely interchangeable, as the perceived pitch of a tone can alter somewhat with intensity, while the frequency remains unchanged. Also, a complex sound containing energy at a series of different frequencies may still be perceived as a single pitch, as is the case with a single note from a musical instrument containing a series of higher harmonics. This is demonstrated in Figure 5.1a, in which a waveform which would be perceived as a single note is seen to contain a series of higher harmonic frequencies.

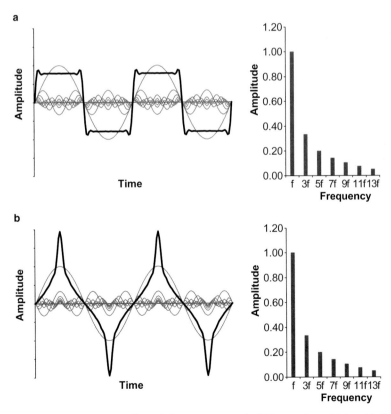

Figure 5.1 Summation of harmonics and the effect of phase. **a**, Series of odd harmonics, which, added together, produce an approximate square wave. The left-hand chart shows the waveform in time, the right-hand chart shows the frequency spectrum. **b**, If alternate harmonics are inverted, the wave produced approximates to a triangular wave, although the same frequencies are present.

Phase

When used in the context of a sound wave, the term phase usually refers to the stage in its cycle at a given moment in time. Phase is measured in degrees or radians, with one cycle being 360° (degrees) or 2π c (radians), although when using radians the units (c) are often omitted as it is technically a dimensionless quality.

By convention, a phase of zero is often considered to be when the wave is at its midpoint going positive. For example, in Figure 5.2 the thick line is at 0° at the left of the chart, and goes through two full cycles by the right side of the chart. Without a clear starting point, we often cannot resolve between whole cycles of phase: in Figure 5.2, the thinner curve lags behind the thicker curve by one-quarter of a cycle, but could equally lag by additional whole cycles or even lead by three-quarters of a cycle, and so on.

Phase can be relevant to perception, for example when comparing Figure 5.1a and Figure 5.1b, the only difference is a 180° phase shift given to alternate harmonics, but the effect is to change the resultant waveform shape from a square wave to a triangular wave.

Wavelength

The wavelength of a periodic sound is dependent on its frequency, but also the speed with which it is travelling, and that depends on what it is travelling through. The speed of sound in air is usually considered to be around 343 m/s, and this is the case at 20°C at normal atmospheric pressure, but the speed of pressure waves in most liquids and solids is far higher than this, and hence the wavelength is longer for the same frequency.

The speed of sound in air is also not constant, being slower at lower temperature and lower air pressure, and this can be relevant when considering sound propagation over large distances.

Wavelength can be calculated as follows:

$$\text{Wavelength (metres)} = \frac{\text{Velocity (m/s)}}{\text{Frequency (Hz)}}$$

Aperiodic sounds

If periodic sounds are sounds that repeat in a regular time interval, then aperiodic sounds are all the other sounds that do not fall into this category. Aperiodic sounds do not repeat regularly, and examples include continuous sounds such as pink or white noise, and brief transient bursts of sound such as clicks. In fact, most everyday sounds that we encounter are aperiodic. (Of course in many tests used in audiology, clicks are often presented repeatedly at regular time intervals. Nevertheless, these are normally presented with enough of a time interval between them for them to technically be considered as individual events.)

While periodic sounds contain sound energy at comparatively few discrete frequencies, aperiodic sounds tend to contain sound energy at a continuous range of frequencies, and this is the case with both continuous random noises and clicks.

Sound pressure level

The ear is able to respond to an impressively wide range of sound pressures. The quietest sound that a normal human ear can hear in the most sensitive part of the audible frequency range (1–5 kHz) is about 20 µPa (Pa = Pascals). However, typical speech at 1 m may be 200 times this, and the loudest sound that the human ear

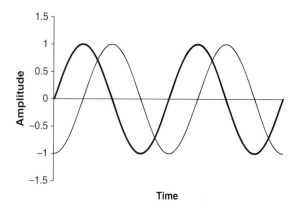

Figure 5.2 The thick curve shows a sine wave; the thinner curve is the same sine wave but delayed by one-quarter of a cycle.

can resolve is 20 Pa, i.e. 1 million times greater than the quietest sound detectable (note although that damage to the ear would soon result from noise levels this high – see Chapter 14).

As pitch is the psychological correlate of frequency, so loudness is the psychological correlate of sound pressure. However, once again the terms are not interchangeable, as the ear is not equally sensitive to all frequencies, and also perceived loudness increases more rapidly with increasing sound pressure at the extremes of the frequency range, particularly below 200 Hz. In people with a hearing loss resulting from damage in the cochlea, perceived loudness will often increase more rapidly than expected with increasing sound pressure.

The decibel (dB)

Dealing with values for sound pressure in Pascals is not especially convenient in audiology, partly because quite a few noughts can be involved which may be misread, but also because the subjective response to loudness is more related to ratio changes in sound pressure than to the pure numerical change. For example, the ear would be unlikely to notice a sound pressure change from 10 Pa to 11 Pa, whereas a change from 0.0001 Pa to 1.0001 Pa would be perceived as a huge increase.

Therefore a base-10 logarithm is taken of the sound pressure in Pascals, using the formula shown below:

$$\text{Sound pressure level (dB SPL)}$$
$$= 20 \times \text{Log}_{10} \frac{(\text{Sound pressure (Pa)})}{(2 \times 10^{-5} \text{ (Pa)})}$$

(Note the value of 2×10^{-5} Pa is chosen to result in a value of 0 dB SPL at normal hearing threshold at 1 kHz. Therefore, negative values of sound pressure level are possible, although normally inaudible. The multiplier 20 is simply to make the numbers a more convenient scale, it is 20 rather than 10 because the formula was really generated for sound intensity, which is related to sound pressure squared. Bringing the square out

from the bracket results in an additional multiplier of 2.)

Further distancing our units from their pure physical references, in audiology we usually apply a frequency weighting to SPL in order to have hearing thresholds at 0 dB for normal hearing subjects across the frequency range of interest. When this weighting has been applied, our sound pressure level in decibels is labelled as dB HL. Other frequency weightings are also in use and are designed to reflect the frequency response of the human ear at different sound pressure levels: dB(A) is quite similar to dB HL and is most appropriate for describing the subjective response to quiet sounds; dB(B) and dB(C) are less often used and are appropriate for describing the subjective response to louder sound levels.

Propagation of sound

Types of propagating waves

There are two main types of propagating waves: *transverse* and *longitudinal*. In transverse waves, the motion of individual particles in the medium is at right angles to the direction in which the wave is travelling, oscillating around an equilibrium resting point. An imperfect example is of waves on water, where the wave travels along the water surface although the water surface travels up and down (the example is imperfect because water waves also contain some forward–back movement).

In longitudinal waves, the motion of individual particles is in the direction that the wave is travelling, oscillating forward and back about an equilibrium resting point. The wave propagates by each particle, as it moves, altering the pressure applied to the next particle, causing it also to move. Sound waves in air are longitudinal waves. In fact, air molecules are continually on the move with random thermal movements (known as Brownian motion), so sound waves are in fact more-organised movements superimposed on this.

It is common to see longitudinal waves represented graphically as transverse – this is because of the difficulty in illustrating longitudinal displacement on the same axis as the direction of wave propagation.

There are other waveform types that are possible, especially in solid materials, such as torsional waves and combination types of wave.

Reflections and impedance

An important aspect of sound propagation is what happens when a sound wave encounters a boundary, as this is when a reflection may occur.

First, we need to consider what a boundary is in acoustical terms, and this requires some understanding of impedance. The acoustic impedance of a material is a measure of how much energy, in the form of sound pressure, it takes to make particles in the material move. An abrupt change in impedance between one material and the next results in imperfect onward transmission of the travelling wave, with some energy being reflected back. A more gradual transition between different impedances results in more efficient transfer of the travelling wave with less energy reflected.

Examples of this can be seen in rooms with hard surfaces, where the hard walls reflect sound back into the room, resulting in reverberation and potentially a noisy environment in which it can be difficult to hear clearly against the reverberant field. Softer furnishings offer a smaller impedance step and therefore allow a greater proportion of incident sound energy to enter the material and be absorbed, with the result that less sound energy is reflected.

In acoustics, an example of an attempt to achieve a gradual impedance change is seen in a horn fitted to a loudspeaker driver to provide a gradual transition from the high impedance of the driver to the comparatively low impedance of free air. The ideal shape for this is exponential, although in practice this shape is usually compromised, with the horn becoming linear as it widens to control the directivity.

There are also impedance transformations in the ear, which will be discussed shortly.

Standing waves

Standing waves are seen when successive waves are reflected back by an impedance step. The reflected wave 'interferes' with the incident wave, adding up where they are in phase, and cancelling out where they are out of phase. The result of this is areas of large waves (antinodes) which seem to go up and down without going anywhere, with becalmed areas (nodes) in between. Although the waves appear to be not travelling, in fact they are made of two waves travelling in opposite directions. This is illustrated in Figure 5.3.

Repeated reflections can occur backwards and forwards between two reflecting surfaces, which can add in phase if the path length is equivalent to a whole number of wavelengths.

It is worth mentioning that a reflection can also occur at a boundary with a step-down

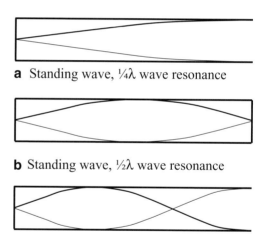

a Standing wave, ¼λ wave resonance

b Standing wave, ½λ wave resonance

c Standing wave, ¾λ wave resonance

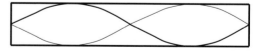

d Standing wave, 1λ wave resonance

Figure 5.3 Illustrations of different standing waves that can be supported in tubes; **a** and **c** require different boundary conditions at each end; **b** and **d** require the same conditions at each end (can be either both open or both closed, the nodes and antinodes swap places depending on the boundary conditions). The two waves shown indicate different moments in time. λ = wavelength.

change in impedance. A relevant example of this is that sound waves travelling in air in a tube can be reflected by the open end, because the impedance of air in an enclosed space is greater than that of free air. This means that a standing wave can, and does, occur in the ear canal.

Diffraction

We are quite familiar with the idea that light travels in more or less straight lines. If an opaque barrier is between us and an object, we don't see the object. However, sound can bend around a barrier in order to be heard even when line-of-sight is blocked. This is because sound has a much greater wavelength than light, and the amount that a wave bends around objects is a function of the wavelength compared to the size of the obstruction. If the wavelength is small compared to the barrier, a fairly effective 'shadow zone' is created behind the barrier. On the other hand, if the wavelength is large compared to the barrier, the waves bend around much more, and a less effective shadow zone is created. This is illustrated in Figure 5.4.

A related effect is seen in sound propagation from a single-driver loudspeaker, with low-pitched sounds being radiated much more broadly than high-pitched sounds, which tend to be directed in a narrow beam straight ahead.

Refraction

The direction of sound propagation can also bend even without obstructions being present. This is because, as mentioned previously, the speed of sound propagation in air increases with temperature and air pressure. If one end of a wave front travels faster than the other end, the direction of travel becomes bent towards the side that was travelling slower. In light, this effect occurs in a lens. A generic illustration is shown in Figure 5.5.

In sound, this effect is especially noticeable over large distances, where temperature gradients can direct sound upwards or downwards.

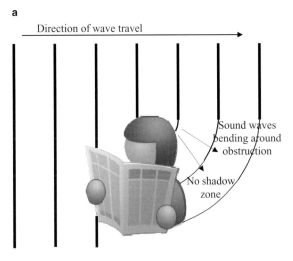

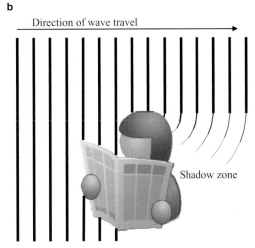

Figure 5.4 Diffraction of waves passing around an obstruction. In **a**, the wavelength is long compared to the obstruction, and the waves therefore bend around behind the obstruction resulting in no effective shadow zone, whereas in **b**, the wavelength is small compared to the obstruction and the waves tend to continue in a straight line with less invasion into the shadow zone.

Air pressure reduces with altitude and also causes sound to refract upwards. Changing wind speed or direction with altitude can also result in significant refraction of sound. Taken together, these effects can have a considerable effect on sound propagation over large distances.

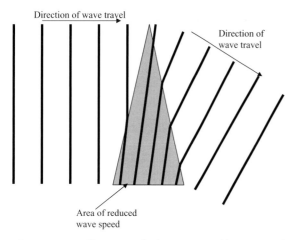

Direction of wave travel

Direction of wave travel

Area of reduced wave speed

Figure 5.5 An illustration of refraction caused by an area of reduced wave speed. The part of the wave with a shorter path at reduced speed ends up ahead of the rest of the wave, with the result that the orientation of the wave front is altered and therefore the direction of propagation changes.

The hearing process

The function of the human ear involves a variety of physical processes which will be described briefly in mechanical terms here. A fuller description of the workings of the ear with detailed anatomy can be found in Chapter 3.

The outer ear is essentially involved in the collection of sound and directing it to the tympanic membrane. There is a resonance in the concha area, which enhances sound in the 5–6 kHz region, and another resonant peak at around 2.5 kHz as a result of a quarter-wave resonance of the ear canal, resulting in a gain of 15–20 dB at the eardrum. See Shaw (1974) for more details. The pinna and concha are also important for front/back and up/down directional discrimination, which is achieved by sound from different directions exciting different resonances in the ear and therefore having different tonal characteristics. Of course, a lot of directional information is also obtained from timing and level differences in the sound received by the two ears.

Resonances of the concha are lost with a hearing-aid earmould, and therefore some impairment of directional ability is inevitable. Occlusion by an earmould also moves the ear canal resonance to a far higher frequency, partly because of a shortening of the air space in the ear canal but also because it becomes a resonance between two closed ends rather than between a closed and an open end, which means it becomes more of a half-wavelength rather than a quarter-wavelength resonance. This effect is corrected for in the output of the hearing aid. As ear canals vary in size and shape, it is necessary to verify hearing aid settings with measurements of sound levels 'in-the-ear' beyond the tip of the earmould near to the tympanic membrane.

The middle ear can be thought of as an impedance-transforming device designed to improve the transmission of sound energy from the relatively low-impedance medium of air to the higher-impedance medium of the fluid-filled inner ear. It seems that the primary way in which this is achieved is in the difference in surface area between the tympanic membrane and the footplate of the stapes, so that the vibrations from a large surface (tympanic membrane) are focused onto a smaller surface (stapes footplate). However, there are also thought to be additional impedance transformations obtained by a lever action of the middle ear bones and also through a buckling or hinging motion of the tympanic membrane (Khanna and Tonndorf, 1972).

The motion of the stapes footplate results in movement of the oval window, behind which is the inner ear, filled with an incompressible fluid. The inner ear is a hard-walled enclosure, and the only other flexible window is the round window. Therefore the round window is forced to move in the opposite direction to the movements in the oval window. The basal end of the basilar membrane lies between these two windows, and therefore is also deflected by movement of the stapes.

A transverse wave 'ripple' then runs along the basilar membrane. The detailed physics of this are complex. In descriptive terms, from base to apex the basilar membrane becomes broader and more compliant, with the result that low frequencies can propagate further towards the apex than can higher frequencies. The amplitude of the travelling wave caused by a single frequency grows to a peak, before diminishing rapidly once the point is reached at which the basilar membrane is too compliant to support the travelling wave at that frequency. The peak of this travelling wave is greatly enhanced by the activity of the outer hair cells, whose action can be considered to be to counteract the damping effects of the friction associated with the travelling wave motion and to amplify the travelling wave.

All this process is aimed at producing a deflection of the stereocilia of the inner hair cells, allowing ions to enter through gates at the stereocilia tip links, which in turn causes a depolarisation of the cell and encourages the nerve to fire from the base of the cell.

Beyond this lies a neural auditory pathway which is discussed in Chapter 4.

Speech perception and production

Speech production

The wide range of sounds present in speech are generated by a process in which sound generated by a source is modified by a filter (called the 'source-filter model').

Source

For most speech sounds, the initial sound source is provided by vibration of the vocal folds in the larynx. These sounds can be referred to as 'voiced'. The flow of air from the lungs pushes the vocal folds apart, but then muscular tension and the rapid passage of air between the folds pulls them closed again. The continuing flow of air then forces them open again. This repeated opening and closing produces a sound with a fairly low-frequency note (about 125 Hz for an adult man, 250 Hz for an adult woman) derived from the frequency at which the folds open and close. There is also higher-frequency sound energy present because the motion of the folds is

not perfectly sinusoidal and also because of the air rushing through the constriction at the vocal folds.

There are also some speech sounds for which the vocal folds do not generate the sound source. These sounds are sometimes referred to as 'unvoiced'. In this case, the sound source is provided by a constriction or closure elsewhere, mostly between various parts of the tongue and palate or with the teeth and lips at the front of the mouth. This produces a sound source with a wide frequency spectrum and no clear 'pitch', often like a hissing in the case of a constriction, or a clicking sound in the case of a brief obstruction to the air flow.

Filter

Once generated, the sound from the source is modified by a 'filter'. This filter consists of the entire vocal tract lying between the source and the lips. Therefore, voiced sounds, where the sound source is at the vocal folds, are modified by the throat, mouth and nasal cavity above this. Unvoiced sounds, typically generated in the mouth, are only modified by structures further out ('downwind') than this, and therefore the throat is not involved.

Voiced speech contains energy at a wide range of frequencies, but the resonances of the vocal tract result in an enhancement of the sound at particular frequencies called 'formant frequencies'. Changes in the shape of the 'filter', such as changing the size of the cavities in the throat, mouth and nasal cavity, or introducing constrictions along the vocal tract, can give rise to great changes in the tonal quality of the speech sound by changing these formant frequencies, and this allows the wide range of voiced sounds present in speech to be produced.

The range of unvoiced sounds are generated by constrictions at the back, middle or front of the mouth. Plosive sounds are formed by closure of the vocal tract followed by a release of the air flow, for example the plosives /p/ and /b/ are formed by closure of the lips, whereas /c/ and /g/ are formed by closure at the back of the mouth.

Speech perception

In order to hear and fully understand speech, we need to be able to pick up on some quite subtle changes. Changes needing to be detected include movements in the formant frequencies, the presence or absence of voicing, and subtle timing differences such as the time to the onset of voicing after a plosive sound such as /p/ (long time to the onset of voicing) or /b/ (short time to the onset of voicing).

It is also possible to decode different speakers' voice characteristics arising from different-sized vocal folds and vocal tracts and also from different accents. Fortunately, the brain is superb at lifting the important features out of running speech and also resolving ambiguities from the context and from lipreading cues.

Effect of hearing impairment

The excellence of the brain at making sense of speech means that mild hearing losses often seem to have little or no impact on communication, as the brain can seamlessly fill in missing sounds from speech with very few errors. The telephone is a good example of this, as the limited frequency range of the telephone doesn't usually prevent complete understanding of what is being said. However, there comes a point when the extent of hearing loss means that too much speech information is missing and hearing difficulty increases. This difficulty is partly a result of failure to hear speech cues, and also results from the reduced resolution of frequency and timing information which often occurs with impaired hearing sensitivity.

As hearing loss commonly occurs predominantly at the higher frequencies, and these are the sounds that are produced in the front of the mouth and lips, often lip reading can be very helpful in resolving speech ambiguities caused by high-frequency hearing loss.

Effect of hearing loss on development of speech

Development of speech sounds is heavily dependent on the ability to hear the sounds in the speech of others and then to monitor the production of one's own speech. Therefore, the speech of an individual with a severe hearing loss predating speech development can be unclear or missing some speech sounds if it has not been possible to provide access to these sounds through hearing aids.

For this reason, hearing aid fittings for children have slightly different aims compared to those for adults. Children's hearing aid prescriptions attempt to give audibility to as wide a range of sounds as possible, whereas in adults the emphasis is usually on amplifying high-frequency sounds, to maximise speech intelligibility.

Acoustical considerations in hearing aids

Hearing aids are discussed in detail in Chapter 19; however, some relevant acoustical issues will be discussed next.

Frequency range

The full range of sounds present in speech covers a wide frequency range from as low as 100 Hz up to 8 kHz. However, the lowest octave or two of this range seems to be less important for speech clarity and can also be dominated by unwanted background noise, and therefore hearing aid prescription formulae for adults tend to emphasise the higher frequencies in order to maximise speech intelligibility.

Recruitment and compression

The activity of the outer hair cells in amplifying the travelling wave is primarily effective for quiet sounds, as the outer hair cell response saturates at higher levels and becomes proportionately less significant. Therefore, individuals whose hearing loss is mainly related to the loss of outer hair cell function notice a loss of hearing sensitivity for quiet sounds but hear louder sounds with a near-normal sensation of loudness. As sounds become louder, the experience is of abnormally rapid growth of loudness. This is called 'recruitment', and in order to prevent amplified loud sounds becoming uncomfortably loud, the appropriate hearing aid for such a hearing loss will amplify quiet sounds but leave louder sounds comparatively unchanged, a characteristic called compression. There are various parameters surrounding compression, including how rapidly the compression is activated following the onset of a loud sound, and how quickly the compression is released after the loud sound finishes.

Ear canal resonances

As mentioned previously, the physical presence of a hearing aid earmould has an impact on outer ear resonances, with an inevitable loss of gain, which needs to be accounted for in the hearing aid output and tailored individually to the hearing aid user because of variations in ear canal sizes and shapes.

Feedback

In general, feedback occurs when the gain of the hearing aid exceeds the attenuation of sound passing from the hearing aid output back to the microphone. Under these conditions, sound can repeatedly travel through the hearing aid, becoming louder each time, and becomes detectable as a single frequency tone (or family of tones).

The simple solutions are either to reduce the gain of the hearing aid or increase the attenuation afforded by the earmould. However, modern hearing aids employ various signal-processing techniques to allow more gain-before-feedback than would have been the case historically. As these techniques can have an adverse effect on music, as sustained musical notes can be mistaken by the hearing aid itself for feedback, some hearing aid users appreciate a dedicated 'music setting' in which the feedback suppression is removed and the amplification of high frequencies is moderated.

Conclusion

In this chapter I have attempted to give an accessible introduction into acoustical considerations that are relevant in audiology and to discuss some of the main practical applications. It is my hope that this will be helpful in developing a working understanding of the physics basis for our activities in audiology, which may inform and aid clinical decisions.

Acknowledgements

I would like to thank David Baguley for his helpful advice and suggestions regarding this chapter.

References

Khanna SM, Tonndorf J (1972) Tympanic membrane vibration in cats studied by time-averaged holography. *Journal of the Acoustical Society of America* 51:1904–1920.

Shaw EAG (1974) The external ear. In: Keidel WD, Neff WD, eds. *Handbook of Sensory Physiology*, Vol 5/1, pp 455–490. Berlin: Springer.

Subjective audiometry

Judith Bird and Rachel Humphriss

6

Introduction

Subjective audiometry describes a range of hearing assessment procedures where the subject gives a conscious response to an auditory stimulus. This chapter will mainly consider pure tone audiometry as this is the mainstay of current audiological assessments. This provides information about the level of hearing and nature of hearing loss and is used in decisions about diagnosis, treatment and rehabilitation. Test techniques and prerequisites will be explained and the reader will be led through interpretation of results. In addition, more complex procedures will be discussed.

History

The first step in diagnosing and describing a patient's hearing loss is to obtain a good history. The clinician should establish the length of history, whether the loss was sudden or gradual in onset, which ear(s) are affected, whether there was any obvious antecedent event (e.g. viral illness, head trauma, etc), whether there are other associated otological symptoms such as vertigo, tinnitus, otalgia or discharge, and whether the patient has a history of recent or past noise exposure. In addition, it is imperative that a good history of the psychosocial aspects of the patient's hearing loss is obtained, so that the clinician can begin to construct a rehabilitative strategy for that patient.

During the history, the clinician will be able to gain a subjective impression of the patient's ability to hear. This subjective impression will then guide expectations of the result of subsequent audiometry; if inconsistent, a number of techniques can be used to assess the 'non-organic' patient, some of which are described later in this chapter (see also Chapter 15).

Tuning-fork tests

Tuning-fork tests are used widely by many clinicians as the initial stage in describing a patient's hearing loss. Typically, low-frequency tuning forks of 256 or 512 Hz are used (Figure 6.1). Activation of the tuning fork is achieved by hitting the prongs onto a dull surface (such as the bone just below one's flexed elbow) while holding the stem. To assess air conduction, the

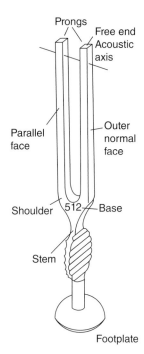

Prongs
Free end
Acoustic axis
Parallel face
Outer normal face
Shoulder
512
Base
Stem
Footplate

Figure 6.1 Tuning fork.

fork is then held in front of the ear. To assess bone conduction, the footplate is placed onto the mastoid bone (the bone behind the ear) or the forehead. There are two tests in common usage, which are briefly described below.

Weber's test

This test was developed by Ernst Heinrich Weber of Wittenberg (1795–1878), and works on the principle that bone-conducted sound will be heard either in the *better* hearing ear in the case of unilateral sensorineural hearing loss, or in the ear with the *greatest* conductive hearing loss. The footplate of the vibrating tuning fork is simply placed on the forehead and the patient is asked which ear he hears the sound in. If hearing is normal or there is a symmetrical sensorineural hearing loss, then the sound will be heard either in the centre of the head or in each ear equally. In the case of unilateral sensorineural hearing loss, then the sound will be heard in the better hearing ear. With unilateral conductive hearing

loss, then the sound will be heard in the ear with the conductive hearing loss.

Rinne's test

Adolf Rinne of Gottingen first described this test in 1855. Its purpose is to distinguish conductive from sensorineural hearing loss. The vibrating prongs of the tuning fork are held in front of the patient's ear (without touching it), and the patient is asked whether he can hear the tone. The footplate of the tuning fork is then placed on the mastoid bone behind that ear and the patient asked which of the two tones was the louder. If the air-conducted sound is louder, the response is described as Rinne positive; if the bone-conducted sound is louder then it is Rinne negative. A Rinne positive response indicates normal hearing or a sensorineural hearing loss, a Rinne negative response a conductive hearing loss. One potential source of error to be aware of is that if the patient has a severe sensorineural hearing loss in the test ear, then a falsely negative Rinne response may be recorded, as the bone-conducted sound may be heard by the opposite cochlea due to cross-hearing (see 'Inter-aural attenuation' below). A Rinne response can be confirmed as false negative by repeating the test while introducing a loud masking noise (see below), for instance from a Bárány box, into the opposite ear to the one being tested.

Pure tone audiometry

The most widely used procedure for describing hearing thresholds is pure tone audiometry (PTA), a behavioural technique which is used in routine clinical practice. This technique is highly standardised and based on the 'Hughson–Westlake' method (Hughson and Westlake, 1944) which is used globally. The international standard for audiometry is ISO 8253. The British Society of Audiology (BSA) Recommended Procedure (BSA, 2004) described in this chapter should be taken as a typical example, and the reader is referred to this for the detailed test

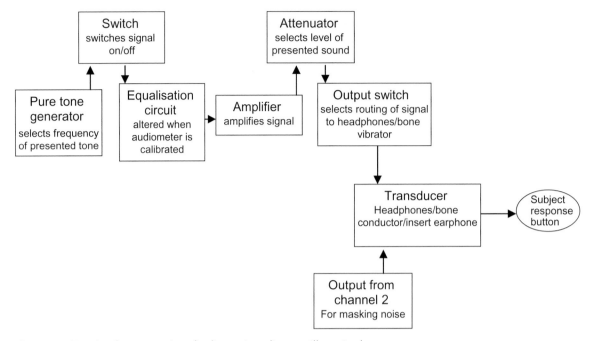

Figure 6.2 Functional representation of a diagnostic audiometer illustrating key components.

procedure. Audiometry should only be carried out by appropriately trained clinicians, with careful adherence to procedures, as inaccurate results could lead to inappropriate management decisions with potentially harmful consequences.

Equipment

For all the tests described in this chapter, signals are presented through an audiometer. This device controls the test signals and is built to precise national and international standards (IEC 60645-1). The key components are illustrated in Figure 6.2.

Traditionally, audiometers have been manufactured as stand-alone units (Figure 6.3). More recently, PC-based audiometers have become available (Figure 6.4a). These use the same basic hardware components, but data are stored in the database rather than recorded manually. This has the advantage that results are easily transferable into other software packages, for example

for hearing aid fitting. Sound is transferred from the audiometer to the subject via a transducer. The most common transducer is the earphone, which can either rest on the ear (supra-aural shown in Figure 6.4b) or cover the ear (circumaural shown in Figure 6.4a) or be inserted into

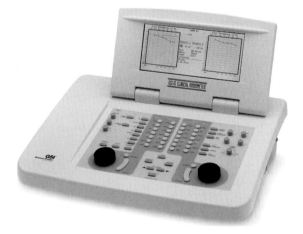

Figure 6.3 Clinical diagnostic audiometer (with permission from Cardinal Health).

a

b

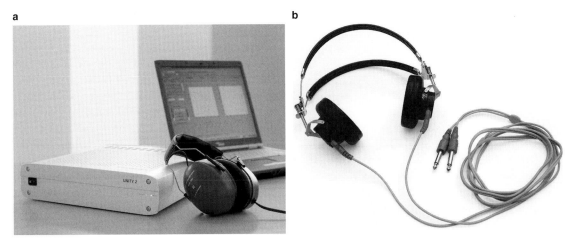

Figure 6.4 Earphones. **a**, PC-based clinical audiometer (with circum-aural earphones) (with permission from Siemens Hearing); **b**, supra-aural earphones.

the ear canal (insert earphones). This is testing hearing by *air conduction*. In addition, a bone vibrator can be used that sits on the mastoid, and sound passes to the inner ear by *bone conduction*. All these transducers have to be calibrated with a particular audiometer and cannot be transferred to another set of equipment.

Calibration

To ensure continued accuracy of results, the following protocol for calibration should be used (BSA Recommended Procedure (BSA, 2004)).

Stage A checks

This is a daily check of the audiometer and involves a listener with normal or known hearing levels performing a listening check at all frequencies through headphones and the bone conductor. This involves checking the audiometer output at very low levels and across all frequencies, listening for distortion at raised levels, a visual check for signs of wear of all components, and a functional check of switches and displays.

Stage B checks

This is the objective calibration carried out at an interval of up to 12 months. It involves measure-

ment of the output from the headphones and bone conductor using acoustic or mechanical couplers, and comparison with relevant standards.

Stage C checks

This is a more detailed objective check usually only used after a serious fault or after equipment has been in use for a long time.

Objective calibration has to be carried out to internationally agreed standards as set out in ISO 389 parts 1–5. Threshold measurements from a large group of young otologically normal subjects have been used to calculate average normal hearing levels and the equivalent sound pressure level (SPL) expressed in decibels (dB; see Chapter 5) in a particular ear simulator for a certain type of headphone. These levels are known as the reference equivalent threshold sound pressure levels (RETSPLs). It is these values that are used in audiometer calibration. These thresholds define the 0 dB line on a pure tone audiogram (see below), and therefore thresholds are expressed in dB HL (dB hearing level). Similarly, measurements have been made to define normal thresholds for bone conduction (reference equivalent threshold force levels, RETFLs).

Environment

The test room should be such that the tester is clearly able to see the patient; conversely, the patient should be seated so that he is unable to see the tester adjust the audiometer controls. These controls should also be used in such a way that extraneous noise does not result. It is also extremely important that the environment is quiet, to enable accurate testing. To achieve the stringent noise requirements required to achieve accurate threshold measurements in otologically normal young adults, a sound-treated booth is required. The levels required are specified in ISO 8253-1 and described in BSA Recommended Procedure (BSA, 2004).

Some environments where costs of sound-proofing are prohibitive will not achieve the required levels, and therefore screening testing down to a clinically relevant level of 20 dB HL is sometimes carried out (Smith and Evans, 2000). It is vital for audiometry in such conditions that as much care as possible is taken in reducing ambient noise. This will involve use of double glazing, soft furnishings to dampen sound, and a location away from noise. As a general rule, levels should not exceed 35 dB(A) and this can be measured easily with a sound level meter.

Test procedure

Following otoscopic examination, a minimal history about factors that have the potential to directly affect test administration is taken: any recent noise exposure, current tinnitus, and whether the patient has a better hearing ear. The patient is then instructed about the task: he is to respond to sounds that he hears through the headphones by pressing a button; he should keep the button pressed for as long as he hears the sound; he should respond however faintly he hears the sound and regardless of which ear he hears it in. If the patient is unable to press the response button then another inaudible response system should be used, such as raising a finger. The earphones can then be carefully placed over the patient's ears, being careful to remove any

hearing aids, spectacles or earrings that may affect this. Most centres use supra-aural headphones, although insert earphones are also common.

The tester then finds air-conduction (AC) thresholds for frequencies 1 KHz, 2 KHz, 3 KHz, 4 KHz, 6 KHz, 8 KHz, 500 Hz, 250 Hz in that order (3 KHz and 6 KHz may be omitted). In brief, once the tester has established that the patient can clearly hear the tone, the intensity is reduced in 10 dB steps until the tone is no longer heard. The intensity is then raised in 5 dB steps until the listener responds. The intensity is then reduced by 10 dB and the ascending 5 dB steps repeated. Threshold is recorded when the listener responds at the same level on two out of every two, three or four responses (i.e. 50% or more) on the ascent. It is important to vary the length of time between tones as well as their duration; regular presentation will allow the subject to guess when the next tone is coming and therefore give a false response. When the difference in the thresholds of the two ears is greater than the inter-aural attenuation, then cross-hearing may occur and masking must be used.

The same technique is used for determining bone-conduction (BC) thresholds, the bone conductor being placed on the mastoid bone behind the ear with the poorer hearing. The test order is similar to that for AC testing except that it is limited to the 500 Hz to 4 KHz range. One of the limitations of bone vibrators is that they tend to emit more airborne sound than vibration at frequencies greater than 2 KHz. For that reason it is recommended that the test ear is occluded with either a supra-aural earphone or earplug when testing 3 KHz and 4 KHz. Another limitation is that at low frequencies, the patient may feel rather than hear the sound. These 'vibrotactile' thresholds may be as low as 55 dB at 500 Hz, and it is important that these are differentiated from true hearing thresholds when recorded.

Inter-aural attenuation

Although the use of earphones appears to test the hearing of each ear separately, the phenomenon of cross-hearing means that this is not always the case. This particularly applies when the hearing in each ear is very different. When testing the hearing of the poorer ear, the sound may actually be detected by the better ear, albeit at a lower intensity. This attenuation of the sound as it travels across the skull to the better hearing ear is known as 'inter-aural attenuation' or 'trans-cranial transmission loss'. The minimum inter-aural attenuation for air conduction is 40 dB when using supra-aural headphones, and 55 dB when using insert earphones. Therefore, a signal of 70 dB using supra-aural headphones (for example) will be heard at approximately 30 dB in the non-test ear (depending on the individual and on the frequency of the tone). For bone conduction, there is no inter-aural attenuation, i.e. the signal will be heard at approximately the same intensity in each ear regardless of which ear the bone vibrator is placed behind. Therefore masking will frequently be required to determine true bone-conduction thresholds for each ear.

Masking

Masking involves temporarily raising the hearing threshold of the non-test ear by a known amount so that the true threshold of the test ear can be measured. This is achieved using 'masking noise' which is a narrow band noise with a centre frequency coinciding with that of the test tone and bandwidth of one-third to one-half of an octave. The masking noise is presented into the non-test (better) ear at an intensity which prevents that ear from hearing the test tone, and the apparent pure tone threshold of the test ear is then remeasured. The intensity of the masking noise is then increased by 10 dB and the threshold-finding procedure repeated. This procedure is repeated until at least four measurements have been recorded and until three successive levels of masking, 10 dB apart, give the same pure tone threshold (or until the output of the audiometer is reached or the patient finds the level of the masking noise uncomfortable). This level is termed the 'plateau' and is the true pure tone threshold at that frequency. The previous apparent pure tone threshold can then be recorded as a 'shadow' point (symbol given in Table 6.1). In

order to mask bone conduction, ideally the masking noise will be delivered by an insert earphone, although in practice many centres use supra-aural headphones, which can be cumbersome with the bone conductor also being in place.

The three rules of masking

These are listed in the BSA Recommended Procedure (BSA, 2004), and if applied correctly ensure that the true pure tone thresholds for each ear are found without fears that cross-hearing may have occurred.

Rule 1: Air-conduction audiometry
Masking is needed at any frequency where the difference between the left and right not-masked air-conduction thresholds is 40 dB or more (headphones) or 55 dB or more (insert earphones).

Rule 2: Bone-conduction audiometry
Masking is needed at any frequency where the not-masked bone-conduction threshold is more acute than the air-conduction threshold by 10 dB or more.

Rule 3: Air-conduction audiometry
Masking is needed where rule 1 has not been applied but where the bone-conduction threshold of the better ear is more 'acute' by 40 dB (headphones) or 55 dB (insert earphones) or more than the not-masked air-conduction threshold attributed to the worse ear. The worse ear would then be the test ear and the better, non-test ear should be masked.

The audiogram

The results of pure tone audiometry are plotted on a chart called an audiogram (Figure 6.5). This has the appearance of an 'upside-down' graph. The horizontal axis gives frequency (Hz) in octave bands (a useful analogy would be that of going up the piano keyboard in octaves, doubling the frequency with each octave rise). The vertical axis gives the intensity of sound (in dB

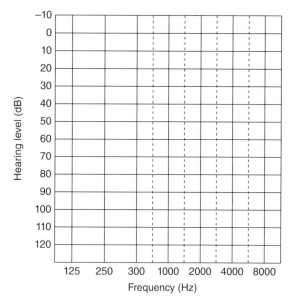

Figure 6.5 Pure tone audiogram chart.

HL). Therefore, the further down the chart, the louder the intensity. Thus, normal hearing is at the top (20 dB HL or better), with the hearing becoming progressively worse the further down the chart that thresholds are recorded.

Hearing thresholds are plotted using standardised symbols which are used to denote the ear being tested, whether the threshold was found using air or bone conduction, and whether masking was used (Table 6.1). Some example audiograms are given in Figure 6.6.

Table 6.1 Symbols used in pure tone audiometry.

	Right	Left
Air conduction, masked if necessary	○	✕
Air conduction, not masked (shadow point)	●	✖
Bone conduction, not masked		△
Bone conduction, masked	⎡	⎤

Audiometric descriptors

Clinicians will usually describe audiograms in general terms rather than specifying the threshold at each individual frequency. Descriptors are used to denote the severity of any hearing loss as well as its nature (i.e. sensorineural, conductive or mixed) and configuration. Table 6.2 gives the four audiometric descriptors that relate to severity of hearing loss.

The *nature* of a patient's hearing loss, relates to the site of the lesion causing that hearing loss. A conductive hearing loss originating from middle ear pathology is identified when bone-conduction thresholds are found to be better than air-conduction thresholds (termed the air–bone gap) (left ear in Figure 6.6a). In the case of a sensorineural hearing loss (due to cochlear or neural pathology), there will be little, if any, difference between air- and bone-conduction thresholds (Figure 6.6b). With a mixed hearing loss, bone-conduction thresholds will be poorer than normal, which is the sensorineural component of the hearing loss, and, in addition, there will be a demonstrable air–bone gap (Figure 6.6c).

The *configuration* of a hearing loss denotes the shape of the audiogram. Terms such as 'high frequency', 'sloping', 'flat', 'reverse slope', 'peaked', 'cookie-bite', '4 KHz notch' and 'trough' are in common usage and these, when combined with information about the site of lesion, can provide vital information in the determination of diagnosis. Descriptors such as 'bilateral', 'unilateral', 'symmetrical' and 'asymmetrical' also allow the results from the two ears to be combined. For example, Figure 6.6a can be termed a 'unilateral moderate flat conductive hearing loss', whereas Figure 6.6b shows a 'symmetrical mild to severe high-frequency sensorineural hearing loss'. At present, there is no standardisation for the use of these terms, and in fact experienced clinicians often disagree on how to describe an audiogram. In an attempt to address this, Margolis and Saly (2007) have recently developed a classification system which is validated and fully automated. This patented system, known as AMCLASS™ consists of 161 rules and claims to have better consensus with a

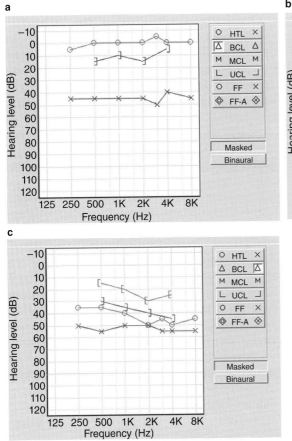

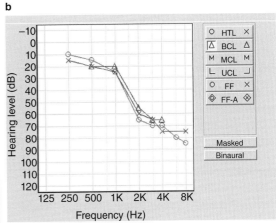

Figure 6.6 Describing an audiogram: the nature of the hearing loss. **a**, Conductive hearing loss; **b**, sensorineural hearing loss (symmetrical); **c**, mixed hearing loss (bilateral).

panel of experts than the average agreement between two experts alone.

As a final point, it is paramount that whatever descriptors the clinician employs, they are *not*

Table 6.2 Descriptors used when describing severity of hearing loss.

Audiometric descriptor	Hearing threshold level (dB)[a]
Mild hearing loss	20–40
Moderate hearing loss	41–70
Severe hearing loss	71–95
Profound hearing loss	In excess of 95

[a]Based on the average of pure tone hearing thresholds at 250, 500, 1000, 2000 and 4000 Hz. (BSA (2004) *Recommended Procedure for Audiometry*.)

used to either describe or assume the degree of disability or handicap that a patient might be experiencing as a result of their hearing loss. Previous studies have shown that hearing handicap and disability correlate only weakly with audiometric configuration (Eriksson-Mangold and Carlsson, 1991; Newman *et al.*, 1997).

Special cases – variation of technique

The elderly

Care should be taken with elderly subjects that tones are not presented too quickly and that there are long enough intervals between stimuli, otherwise inaccuracies may arise. Manual dexterity and the ability of the subject to make the required physical response should be briefly assessed prior to the test. Fatigue may affect the reliability of results, so a short break can be used if required.

Children and subjects with special needs

An experienced tester can reliably carry out pure tone audiometry in children down to and below five years of age. However, some modification of technique can be used to maintain the level of the child's concentration and motivation and to maximise information gained in a short space of time. Play audiometry (sometimes called performance audiometry) involves conditioning a child to respond with a play activity (e.g. putting a peg in a board) on hearing a test tone. The ability to elicit responses is therefore not dependent on acquired language skills. Any reduction in the number of frequencies tested or tone presentation at levels above the expected threshold will compromise the accuracy of the test; therefore any changes to conventional technique should be noted on results. McCormick (2004) gives more detail on paediatric hearing tests, and concludes that by the age of three years, it should be possible to record thresholds very close to adult values if the child is conditioned appropriately. (More detail on hearing testing in children is found in Chapter 12.)

In extreme cases, subjects with severe physical or mental impairment may be carefully observed for any consistent, repeatable physical responses (change in facial expression, for example) to sound presentations.

Non-organic hearing loss (see also Chapter 15)

There will be occasions where results of audiometry do not match with observed clinical hearing ability. In such instances, technique can be modified by ascending to threshold from silence and by using longer stimulus duration and interstimulus intervals (Cooper and Lightfoot, 2000). Bowdler and Rogers (1989) discuss various methods of obtaining more accurate thresholds including the Fournier technique where presentation levels are repeatedly altered by large increments up to 25 dB. The Stenger test is a useful tool to evaluate an apparent unilateral hearing loss where hearing is suspected of being better than at levels initially recorded. This is based on the principle that if two tones at the same frequency are simultaneously presented to both ears, only the louder one will be heard. Tones are played simultaneously at 10 dB above the threshold in the better ear and 10 dB below the threshold in the worse ear. If a response is obtained, the louder tone in the worse ear is not heard, confirming the hearing loss is genuine. Where a response is not elicited, this suggests that the threshold in the 'worse' ear is better than the responses given. Martin (2002) gives a helpful review of this complex area.

Automatic audiometry

A self-recording form of audiometry was developed by Békésy in 1947 and for decades was used widely both for the recording of hearing thresholds and in the identification of retrocochlear pathology (Green and Huerta, 1994). Latterly, it was particularly used for industrial audiometry. Computer-driven audiometry systems have now superseded this technique.

The Audioscan system uses an alternative algorithm to conventional audiometry, in that it sweeps across the frequency range at a constant hearing level rather than changing intensity within each frequency. The result is a hearing test which is highly sensitive to inter-octave frequencies (it can theoretically record 64 frequencies per octave) (Zhao *et al.*, 2002). The test time in patients with hearing losses, however, is lengthy, making this technique more applicable to research than to clinics (Zhao *et al.*, 2002).

Another system known as AMTAS™ (Automated Method for Testing Auditory Sensitivity) is currently under development. A clinical audiometer is controlled by a computer, and the sequence of stimulus levels follows those used in conventional audiometry. This technique does, however, differ from conventional audiometry in a number of ways: the bone conductor is placed on the forehead under a headband (of calibrated force); circum-aural rather than supra-aural earphones are used; the stimulus is presented in a time interval that is specified for the listener rather than there being no clearly specified time interval; masking noise is always applied to the contralateral ear; and the listener responds by means of a touch screen. The sequence of tones is punctuated by no-sound trials or 'catch trials', which allows the determination of False Alarm Rate, one of a number of quality control measures that the system combines to give a measure of overall quality at the end of the test (Qual-ind™ quality assessment method, Margolis *et al.*, 2007). The AMTAS™ system allows up to four people to be tested at once and by personnel who do not have to have the expertise of a qualified audiologist. This system therefore offers potential efficiency savings to the audiology clinic.

Limitations of results of audiometry

In many cases, results of audiometry will give a good indication of ability to hear complex information, such as speech. However, occasionally, because of other pathology in the hearing mechanism, ability to hear and understand speech is worse than predicted from the pure tone audiogram. One example of this is where cochlear dead regions are present (Moore *et al.*, 2000; Moore, 2004). This term is used when a part of the cochlea tuned to one frequency region has no surviving inner hair cells. Pure tones at those frequencies may still be detected as a result of the broad frequency tuning of the ear at loud intensities. However, studies have shown that sound presented at a pitch where dead regions exist may contribute little to speech discrimination and may indeed have a negative impact (Vickers *et al.*, 2001).

Cases have been also been described of patients with normal pure tone thresholds who report considerable difficulty in auditory tasks. This condition has historically been called obscure auditory dysfunction, King–Kopetsky syndrome or central auditory processing disorder, but the preferred term is auditory processing disorder. Much debate exists around the cause, diagnosis and management of this condition (see Chapter 22).

Sound field testing

In addition to the transducers already described, it is also possible to present signals through loudspeakers. Pure tones are not suitable in normal clinical environments, as standing wave patterns may result and therefore frequency-modulated tones are used (warble tones). Due to the absence of calibration RETSPLs for sound field warble tones, the issues surrounding calibration are complex and may involve biological calibration with otologically normal subjects.

The main clinical application is in the testing of children by obtaining conditioned responses to auditory signals (see Chapter 12). Sound field aided threshold testing is generally no longer used in adult hearing rehabilitation. This is because of the complex multichannel signal processing used in modern digital hearing aids. Testing with tones may give thresholds that do not reflect how the hearing aid will perform with a complex real-world signal such as speech.

Supra-threshold tests

Speech audiometry

Given some of the limitations described above, sometimes speech signals are used rather than pure tones to give a greater indication of real-world hearing ability rather than just hearing sensitivity.

Equipment and speech material

Occasionally material for speech discrimination testing is presented using live voice. However, given that speech is a variable signal, for accuracy and repeatability of results, it is usually preferable to use recorded material. Material can be of many forms, from phonemes and simple words to complex sentences (e.g. Arthur Boothroyd word lists or Bamford–Kowal–Bench sentences) and is available in many different languages. Audiovisual presentations of test words and test sentences such as City University of New

York (CUNY) sentences are also available on DVD with and without lip reading. Signals are sometimes presented with competing noise. Response can be by forced choice (for example, choosing one response from four options given) or repetition of what was heard. Calibration of speech material is outlined in ISO 8253-3. Standardised speech material is required to have a calibration signal included in the recording. This enables the level to be set through the audiometer. The correct use of masking is important, particularly where there is asymmetry in hearing. This needs to be broad-band speech-shaped noise and the level needs to take any air–bone gap into account.

Terminology

Variations in terminology occur across different countries, but the current international standard specifies speech recognition in preference to speech discrimination or speech intelligibility. The following terms are in common use:

- *speech recognition threshold* (SRT): the level at which 50% of test material is correctly identified
- *maximum speech recognition score*: the maximum score (usually expressed as a percentage) correctly identified from a list of recorded words, regardless of level of presentation. This is sometimes called optimum discrimination score
- *optimum speech level*: the speech level at which the maximum score is obtained.

Figure 6.7 gives an example of a speech audiogram.

Clinical applications

Speech audiometry is widely used in the assessment of patients' suitability for cochlear implants. This is usually performed using sound field, recorded material and hearing aids, with and without lip-reading. Results are used to assess if benefit from a cochlear implant is likely to be greater than the use of optimised hearing aids.

Speech audiometry is also sometimes used in hearing rehabilitation before hearing aids are

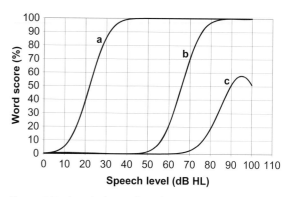

Figure 6.7   A typical speech audiogram. **a**, Normal speech curve; **b**, typical results obtained in a subject with conductive hearing loss; **c**, example of results in a subject with sensorineural hearing loss.

fitted. Evidence does not support its use as an accurate predictor of hearing aid benefit (Killion and Gudmundsen, 2005). However, it is sometimes used to identify patients with particularly poor discrimination ability who may benefit from further counselling about the expected benefit from hearing aids and detailed information about hearing tactics.

Results of speech audiometry are also used in combination with pure tone audiometry when making decisions about ear surgery. For example, in patients with vestibular schwannoma, it is not unusual for someone to have good hearing thresholds but poor discrimination ability. Results of speech audiometry are used in making decisions about potential benefits of a surgical approach to preserve residual hearing.

Uncomfortable loudness levels (ULLs)

The test for ULLs (sometimes known as loudness discomfort levels, LDL) aims to find the quietest level that is judged uncomfortably loud. There is significant intra-subject variability and there may be poor repeatability for such a test, and it is very important that standardised wording is used (BSA Recommended Procedures (BSA, 2004)). A pure tone is presented and the level raised in 5 dB steps. The subject has to indicate either by pressing a button or by raising a hand as soon as the sound reaches a level that is uncomfortable. Care needs to be taken when carrying out this test because of the loud sound intensities used, especially in patients with tinnitus as this may be exacerbated. The levels obtained can give some indication of recruitment or hyperacusis. While there has been some debate on the usefulness of this test, Munro and Patel (1998) concluded that there is good correspondence with real-world loudness discomfort. The main application is in setting the maximum output of hearing aids, which can be done more precisely than by using a hearing aid manufacturer's default settings. For each case, the clinical usefulness needs to be balanced against any risks. An example of a pure tone audiogram showing ULLs is given in Figure 6.8.

Conclusion

This chapter has attempted to give an overview of subjective audiometry procedures and interpretation. For those embarking on clinical prac-

tice, it is strongly recommended that national standards and procedures referenced here are referred to for more detail. When carried out accurately, audiometry is a powerful tool for the evaluation of hearing.

References

Bowdler DA, Rogers J (1989) The management of pseudohypacusis in children. *Clinical Otolaryngology* 14:211–215.

British Society of Audiology (2004) *Recommended Procedure. Pure tone air and bone conduction threshold audiometry with and without masking and determination of uncomfortable loudness levels.* Reading: British Society of Audiology.

Cooper J, Lightfoot G (2000) A modified pure tone audiometry technique for medico-legal assessment. *British Journal of Audiology* 34: 37–46.

Eriksson-Mangold M, Carlsson SG (1991) Psychological and somatic distress in relation to preceived hearing disability, hearing handicap, and hearing measurements. *Journal of Psychosomatic Research* 35:729–740.

Green DS, Huerta L (1994) Tests of retrocochlear function. In: Katz J, ed. *Handbook of Clinical Audiology*, 4th edn, pp 178–179. Baltimore: Williams and Wilkins.

Hughson W, Westlake H (1944) Manual for program outline for rehabilitation of aural casualties both military and civilian. *Transactions – American Academy of Ophthalmology Otolaryngology* 48(suppl):1–15.

Killion MC, Gudmundsen GI (2005) Fitting hearing aids using clinical prefitting speech measures: an evidence-based review. *Journal of the American Academy of Audiology* 16:439–447.

Margolis RH, Saly GL (2007) Toward a standard description of hearing loss. *International Journal of Audiology* 46:746–758.

Margolis RH, Saly GL, Le C, Laurence J (2007) Qualind™: a method for assessing the accuracy of automated tests. *Journal of the American Academy of Audiology* 18:78–89.

Martin F (2002) Pseudohypacusis. In: Katz J, ed. *Handbook of Clinical Audiology*, 5th edn,

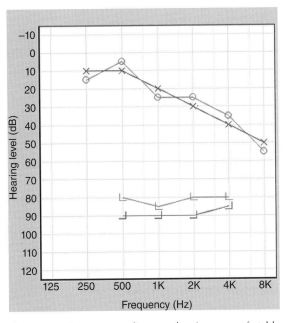

Figure 6.8 Pure tone audiogram showing uncomfortable loudness levels.

pp 584–604. Baltimore and Philadelphia: Lippincott Williams and Wilkins.

McCormick B (2004) Behavioural hearing tests for infants in the first five years of life. In: McCormick B, ed. *Paediatric Audiology 0–5 Years*, 3rd edn, pp 67–109. London: Whurr.

Moore BC (2004) Dead regions in the cochlea: conceptual foundations, diagnosis, and clinical applications. *Ear and Hearing* 25:98–116.

Moore BC, Huss M, Vickers DA, Glasberg BR, Alcántara JI (2000) A test for the diagnosis of dead regions in the cochlea. *British Journal of Audiology* 34:205–224.

Munro KJ, Patel RK (1998) Are clinical measurements of uncomfortable loudness levels a valid indicator of real-world auditory discomfort? *British Journal of Audiology* 32:287–293.

Newman CW, Jacobson GP, Hug GA *et al.* (1997) Perceived hearing handicap of patients with unilateral or mild hearing loss. *Annals of Otology, Rhinology, and Laryngology* 106: 210–214.

Smith and Evans (2000) BSA Recommended Procedure. Hearing assessment in general practice, schools and health clinics: guidelines for professionals who are not qualified audiologists. *British Journal of Audiology* 34:57–61.

Vickers DA, Moore BC, Baer T (2001) Effects of low-pass filtering on the intelligibility of speech in quiet for people with and without dead regions at high frequencies. *Journal of the Acoustical Society of America* 110:1164–1175.

Zhao F, Stephens D, Meyer-Bisch C (2002) The Audioscan: a high frequency resolution audiometric technique and its clinical applications. *Clinical Otolaryngology* 27:4–10.

Standards relating to audiometry

IEC 60318-1:1998 *Electroacoustics – Simulators of Human Head and Ear. Part 1: Ear simulator for the calibration of supra-aural earphones*. Geneva: Geneva International Electrotechnical Commission.

IEC 60318-2:1998 *Electroacoustics – Simulators of Human Head and Ear – Part 2: An interim acoustic coupler for the calibration of audiometric earphones in the extended high-frequency range*. Geneva: Geneva International Electrotechnical Commission.

IEC 60318-3:1998 *Electroacoustics – Simulators of Human Head and Ear. Part 3: Acoustic coupler for the calibration of supra-aural earphones used in audiometry*. Geneva: Geneva International Electrotechnical Commission.

IEC 60645-1 (2001) *Audiological Equipment. Part 1: Pure tone audiometers*. Geneva: Geneva International Electrotechnical Commission.

IEC 60645-2 (1993) *Audiometers. Part 2: Equipment for speech audiometry*. Geneva: Geneva International Electrotechnical Commission.

ISO 389 Parts 1–5 (1: 1998; 2: 1994; 3: 1994; 4: 1994; 5: 2006) *Reference Zero for the Calibration of Audiometric Equipment*. Geneva: International Standards Organisation.

ISO 8253-1 (1989) *Acoustics – Audiometric Test Methods. Part 1: Basic pure tone air and bone conduction audiometry*. Geneva: International Standards Organisation.

ISO 8253-2 (1992) *Acoustics – Audiometric Test Methods. Part 2: Sound field audiometry with pure tone and narrow-band test signals*. Geneva: International Standards Organisation.

ISO 8253-3 (1996) *Acoustics – Audiometric Test Methods. Part 3: Speech audiometry*. Geneva: International Standards Organisation.

Useful websites

- British Cochlear Implant Group: www.bcig.org.uk
- The British Society of Audiology: www.thebsa.org.uk
- International Organization for Standardization (ISO): www.iso.org
- International Electrotechnical Commission (IEC): www.iec.ch

Objective audiometry

Neil Donnelly and William Gibson

7

Introduction

The term objective audiometry describes a variety of tests that do not rely on the active cooperation of a subject. They are not a true measure of hearing, which is a subjective sensation. The aim is to demonstrate auditory function by recording physiological data rather than behavioural responses. Most objective audiometric tests only provide information about part of the hearing mechanism. The information they provide allows for certain deductions to be reached regarding a subject's ability to hear. Therefore, objective audiometric tests can be used to estimate the threshold of hearing and to assist with the diagnosis of neuro-otological disease (Table 7.1).

Airborne sound waves arriving at the tympanic membrane are transmitted via the tympanic membrane and ossicles to the perilymph fluid within the inner ear. The middle ear overcomes some of the impedance mismatch between air and perilymph by acting as a mechanical transformer. Within the inner ear, the sound waves are separated into their constituent frequencies and amplified by the tonotopical properties of the basilar membrane and active movement of the outer hair cells. The inner hair cells convert this mechanical vibration into electric currents, which pass via the cochlear nerve to the brainstem and higher auditory centres.

Objective audiometry tests can be classified according to the part of the hearing mechanism they evaluate. This review will discuss the various tests, beginning at the middle ear and progressing towards the higher cortical levels.

Impedance audiometry

Impedance audiometry refers to tests that measure changes in the compliance of the middle ear mechanism. Compliance is the ease with which energy flows through an acoustic system. Changes in compliance of the middle ear can be observed in disease states or can be induced by a sound stimulus which causes a contraction of the stapedius muscle.

Tympanometry

Tympanometry is a test that measures the compliance of the tympanic membrane and ossicular chain. Used as a clinical test, it can provide

Table 7.1 Clinical applications of objective audiometric tests.

	Middle ear assessment	Estimate of hearing threshold	Neonatal hearing screening	Neuro-otological diagnosis
Impedance audiometry				
Tympanometry	✓	✗	✗	✗
Acoustic reflex testing	✗	✗	✗	✓
Otoacoustic emissions	✗	✗	✓	✗
Auditory evoked potentials (AEP)				
Electrocochleography	✗	✓	✗	✓
Auditory brainstem responses	✗	✓	✓	✓
Middle-latency AEP	✗	✓	✗	✓
Long-latency AEP	✗	✓	✗	✓

information regarding the state of the tympanic membrane and middle ear cleft, ossicular chain integrity and mobility, and Eustachian tube function. It does not provide information about the inner ear, and therefore any inferences regarding hearing must be made with information from other tests.

For the middle ear to function as an efficient mechanical transformer, the compliance must be optimal. Under normal circumstances the tympanic membrane is intact, the ossicular chain is mobile and the pressure within the middle ear is equal to that in the external ear canal. The compliance of the middle ear mechanism will be altered if any of these factors are altered. The effect of a reduced compliance of the middle ear system is to decrease the efficiency of the transformer mechanism, which will decrease the amount of sound entering the ear (admittance), and increase the amount of sound prevented from entering (impedance).

A tympanometer is the instrument used to measure middle ear compliance. It contains a sound generator, a microphone and a pump, each connected via tubing to a small ear probe. The probe is placed in the ear canal to form an airtight seal. A 226 Hz sound stimulus is passed down the ear canal to the tympanic membrane. In infants younger that 4 months, a probe tone of 1 kHz is used as it provides more reliable results, because of the physical characteristics of the soft external ear canal in children of this age. Depending on the compliance of the tympanic membrane, some of the sound is absorbed into the ear while some of the sound is reflected. The microphone detects the amount of sound reflected, which is measured in terms of the volume that would reduce the sound intensity proportionately. Simultaneously, the tympanometer alters the pressure within the ear canal. As the pressure in the ear canal is altered, the eardrum becomes stiffer and more of the sound is reflected. The test shows the highest compliance (the 'peak'), measured as volume, at a pressure equal to that of the middle ear pressure. The tympanometry measurement is plotted as a tympanogram. Tympanograms are most commonly described according to the Jerger system of classification (Jerger, 1970) (Figure 7.1).

Type A demonstrates a compliance peak between +100 and −150 daPa and suggests normal middle ear function. The admittance is normally between 0.2 and 2.5 cm³. A reduced admittance volume (Type As – a lower peak than normal) can be observed when ossicular chain fixation is present, while an increased admittance (Type Ad – a higher peak than normal) may be observed in cases of ossicular discontinuity or atelectasis of the tympanic membrane.

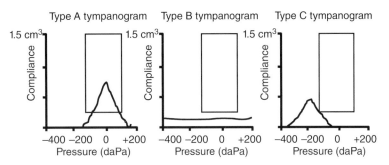

Figure 7.1 Jerger classification of tympanograms.

Type B is a flat trace representing no compliance peak. The interpretation of this finding depends upon the measured ear canal volume, which is normally less than 1 cm^3 in a child and less than 1.5 cm^3 in an adult. In the presence of a normal ear canal volume, the type B tympanogram is likely to represent a middle ear effusion. If the ear canal volume is increased, then the finding is likely to represent a tympanic membrane perforation or presence of a patent grommet, since the volume of the whole middle ear space and mastoid air cells is connected, via the perforation, with the external ear canal.

Type C demonstrates a compliance peak at less than −150 daPa. This finding most commonly represents Eustachian tube dysfunction or a partial middle ear effusion.

Acoustic reflex measurements

When a loud sound enters the ear, it can cause a reflex contraction of the stapedius muscle. This is called the acoustic reflex (AR), and the quietest sound that triggers the reflex is considered the acoustic reflex threshold. The acoustic reflex threshold (ART) is about 60–70 dB HL above the subjective pure tone audiogram (PTA) threshold in a normal ear. The acoustic reflex is observed simultaneously in both ears due to the stapedial reflex pathway having both ipsilateral and contralateral projections. The afferent arc involves the ipsilateral cochlea, auditory nerve and brainstem, while the efferent arc involves both facial nerves and both stapedial muscles.

The contraction of the stapedial muscle stiffens the tympanic membrane, causing a change of impedance recorded by the tympanometer; this change continues while the loud sound persists, as normally the stapedius muscle continues to contract. ARTs are usually measured at 500, 1000, 2000 and 4000 Hz.

The range for the ART is 70–100 dB nHL (hearing level) in normal hearing. A conductive hearing loss results in the ART being elevated by a similar level to that of the conductive deficit, or not being recordable if there is an effusion (type B tympanogram) or stapes fixation (when, in spite of contraction of the stapedius muscle, the stapes itself fails to move, so no movement is recorded at the tympanic membrane). A conductive hearing loss with type A tympanogram and absent AR can help establish a diagnosis of stapes fixation secondary to otosclerosis. When there is a sensory hearing loss which causes recruitment, the gap between the audiometric threshold and the ART is reduced. The finding of recruitment can help differentiate sensory (cochlear) hearing losses from neural hearing losses due to retrocochlear pathology, such as a vestibular schwannoma. If there is a retrocochlear problem, the acoustic reflex may show an abnormal adaptation to a prolonged stimulus. This adaptation does not usually occur in a purely cochlear hearing loss.

AR testing can prove useful in cases where a non-organic hearing loss is suspected. In this situation, an ART may be encountered at a better threshold level than expected for the reported hearing loss.

Retrocochlear pathology is more thoroughly investigated by recording both the ipsilateral and contralateral AR for each ear. The pattern of results obtained can help pinpoint the location of the lesion within the reflex arc. AR testing is not only applicable to investigating hearing loss, but can also help investigate the site of a facial nerve injury when combined with a lacrimal (Schirmer's tear production) test.

One limitation of AR testing is that the reflex may be absent in as many as 5% of individuals with normal hearing.

Otoacoustic emissions

Otoacoustic emissions (OAEs) are generated by outer hair cells. When a sound is introduced to the cochlea, the motor properties of the outer hair cells increase the basilar membrane movement to amplify and sharply tune the sound signal to the appropriate part of the cochlear partition. This constant contraction and expansion generates an echo, first discovered by Kemp (Kemp, 1978), which can be recorded from a microphone placed in the ear canal. OAEs are classified into two groups, spontaneous and evoked. Spontaneous OAEs are found only in approximately 50% of individuals with normal hearing, so nothing can be inferred from their absence.

Evoked OAEs are divided into transient evoked OAEs (TEOAEs), distortion product OAEs (DPOAEs) and stimulus frequency OAEs (SFOAEs). Clinically, only TEOAEs and DPOAEs are used. Both tests can be performed in a quiet setting with easily transportable equipment and without extensive training. These factors have helped make OAE a popular hearing screening tool. An insert is placed in the ear and attached to an OAE machine containing the sound generator and microphone. A sound is generated and the ensuing emission measured.

TEOAEs are typically evoked by broad-band clicks at approximately 80 dB. It is possible to separate the OAE from the stimulus because of the slight delay (1 ms) in its onset. The recorded data are stored in two separate memory banks. Data that correlate between the two memory banks are considered a response. They provide information in a broad frequency range from 500 Hz to 4 kHz (Figure 7.2).

DPOAEs are a harmonic evoked by two different pure tone stimuli at two different intensities. The relationship between the different frequencies and intensity levels dictates the frequency response of the OAE.

Evoked OAEs are present in a vast majority of individuals with hearing thresholds better than 40 dB nHL. Because of this, OAEs have been widely used as a screening tool to detect normal hearing. A number of newborn hearing screening

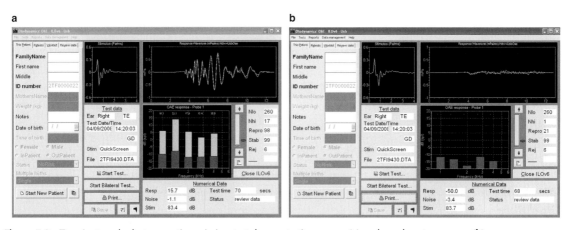

Figure 7.2 Transient evoked otoacoustic emission test demonstrating a pass (**a**) and an absent response (**b**).

programmes have been implemented to test all newborns with TEOAEs within the first days or weeks of life. Of course, although a child without OAEs may have a hearing loss, the test does not give any information about the degree of loss, which can range from moderate to profound. If there are associated risk factors such as prematurity or a family history of hearing loss, an auditory brainstem response (ABR) is performed as well as or instead of TEOAE.

The use of OAE as a screening tool is not without its problems. If the ear canal or middle ear space is blocked, the child will fail the test and this can lead to a referral for further audiological assessment when in fact the child has normal hearing (*false positive*). The false-positive rates can be reduced by a second test performed 2–3 weeks later. *False negatives* can also occur, especially in premature infants. These can pass the test, as the outer hair cells may survive despite the loss of inner hair cells resulting in hearing loss. False negatives may occur in up to 10% of children who are not deemed high risk enough to have an ABR (Rea and Gibson, 2003). For this reason some countries, including Australia, have not implemented OAE as the basis for their newborn screening programmes.

Auditory evoked potentials

Auditory evoked potentials (AEPs) describe the electrical activity within the cochlea and along the auditory pathway in response to auditory stimulation. The classification of AEPs is based on the response time (latency) relative to the onset of a stimulus. AEPs are described as short-, middle- or long-latency responses.

AEPs are recorded with special equipment. The aim is to differentiate auditory activity (signal) from other types of electrical activity that are not of interest (noise). An auditory stimulus is presented to the ear via a transducer (earphone or loudspeaker). This generates an electrical response in the auditory pathway. A recording system is used to detect these tiny potentials. The subject is attached to the recording apparatus using electrodes. The electrodes are paired, with

one being non-inverting and the other inverting. A third electrode acts as the ground electrode. The electrodes pass the electrical information to a differential amplifier, which amplifies and filters the potential difference between pairs of recording electrodes. High- and low-pass filters favour the electrical activity which contains the auditory signal and helps to reject noise. The principal method used to improve the signal to noise ratio is averaging. This relies on repeated presentation of the stimulus and measurement of the electrical activity that follows. This electrical activity contains the evoked potential, which occurs at a constant time after the stimulus (latency). The noise occurs at random intervals, which differ between each individual recording. Averaging aims to reduce the random noise to almost zero.

Electrocochleography

The electrocochleogram (ECochG) is a short-latency response and measures the electrical activity within the cochlea and first-order cochlear nerve fibres in response to sound. The test is performed with an electrode placed either in the ear canal (extratympanic) or with an electrode placed through the eardrum (transtympanic), so that the tip of the electrode lies on the promontory close to the round window niche. The amplitude of the ECochG recordings declines logarithmically as the distance from the round window increases. Extratympanic recordings have been used for diagnostic purposes but lack the robustness of transtympanic recordings.

The ECochG records three normal potentials, the cochlear microphonic (CM), the summating potential (SP) and the action potential (AP) (Figure 7.3). The CM is derived from the hair cells and has the same waveform as the stimulus, as seen in the first two traces in Figure 7.5. The SP is a direct current potential derived from the shift in the baseline of the CM, which continues for the duration of the stimulus. The AP is a compound neural potential that is derived from the afferent auditory nerve fibres leaving the cochlea and represents an algebraic summation of the AP of many individual nerve fibres.

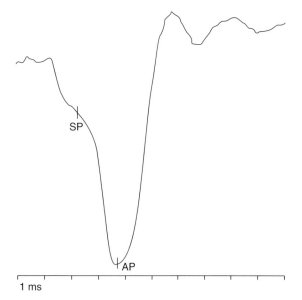

Figure 7.3 Electrocochleography waveform. AP, action potential; SP, summating potential.

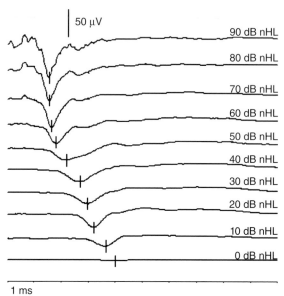

Figure 7.4 Click electrocochleography used to establish hearing thresholds.

A variety of stimuli can be used to elicit the ECochG, depending on the particular indication for the test. These include clicks and more frequency-specific stimuli, such as tone pips or tone bursts.

The AP can be used to estimate the threshold of hearing. Using a click stimulus, the AP mostly reflects the activity in the basal turn of the cochlea as the nerve fibres within the basal coil of the cochlea fire faster and with better synchrony than the more apical fibres. The threshold of the click ECochG gives an overall estimate of hearing for audiometric frequencies above 2 kHz (Figure 7.4). Frequency-specific tone pips from 500 Hz to 8 kHz can be used to obtain a better estimate of the hearing for individual frequencies (Figure 7.5). The ECochG is especially useful for estimating the hearing loss in very young or uncooperative children (Wong *et al.*, 1997). Transtympanic testing is often performed during general anaesthesia using a needle electrode, but there is an advantage in using an electrode with a larger tip, such as the 'golf club' electrode which provides larger recordings. The 'golf club' electrode is placed through a posterior myringotomy, so that the tip of the electrode sits in the round window niche.

The CM has a limited usefulness as the threshold of the response does not relate to the hearing

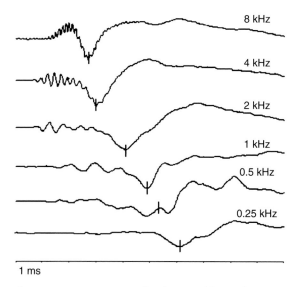

Figure 7.5 Frequency-specific electrocochleography traces recorded at 70 dB HL.

level. Large abnormal CMs are recorded from children suffering with 'auditory neuropathy'. These abnormal CMs generate an abnormal positive direct current (DC) potential (O'Leary *et al.*, 2000). This correlates with the unexpected presence of OAEs in the ears of these children with a hearing loss. The large CMs and OAEs may be due to survival of outer hair cells despite the loss of inner hair cells.

The SP is useful for determining the presence of endolymphatic hydrops (increased endolymph volume) and for confirming the diagnosis of Ménière's disease. This is because the SP is increased when there is an asymmetric CM, probably related to basilar membrane displacement caused by the hydrops. In the past, a ratio of the amplitude of the click SP *versus* the click AP has been used to diagnose hydrops. Various ratios have been suggested: most commonly when there is a SP/AP ratio greater than 40%. However, the click SP/AP ratio has poor sensitivity and specificity. A better correlation of ECochG findings with endolymphatic hydrops can be obtained by measuring the absolute amplitude of the SP in response to tone bursts, most significantly at 1 kHz (Conlon and Gibson, 2000).

Further applications for ECochG include intraoperative use during stapedectomy surgery to demonstrate hearing gain and show any adverse changes. With the advent of middle ear devices such as the floating mass transducer (FMT; see Chapter 21), which can be placed in the round window niche or on a total ossicular chain prosthesis (TORP; see Chapter 9), ECochG may have a role is demonstrating that the correct coupling has been achieved.

Auditory brainstem responses

The auditory brainstem response (ABR – synonym brainstem electric response: BSER) is a series of five to seven waves occurring within 10 ms of the onset of a stimulus (Figure 7.6). Wave I occurs 1.5–2 ms after the onset of the stimulus, with subsequent waves following at 1–2 ms intervals. It is generally agreed that wave I is generated by

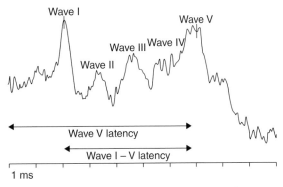

Figure 7.6 The auditory brainstem response waveform.

the distal portion of the auditory nerve in the cochlea. It is similar to the AP of the ECochG. Wave II is considered to arise in the vicinity of the cochlear nucleus. Wave III is attributed to the superior olivary complex within the lower pons. Wave IV is not always identified and is often partially merged with wave V. This IV–V complex is attributed to the lateral lemniscus and inferior colliculus within the midbrain.

An ABR can be obtained using click stimuli, but the response is mostly derived from frequencies about 2–3 kHz. Better frequency-specific information is obtained using tone pips. The recording electrodes are placed on the ipsilateral earlobe or mastoid (inverting electrode) and on the vertex of the head (non-inverting electrode). The ABR waveform is present from the third trimester in pregnancy and is measurable in premature infants as early as 27 weeks' gestational age, but has prolonged latencies due to the immaturity of the auditory system. In a neonate, the waveform consists of three component peaks, with longer latencies than those seen in adults. The waveform gradually assumes the adult waveform by the age of two years, as the auditory pathway matures.

The ABR has many clinical uses. The IV–V waveform is particularly useful for estimating the hearing threshold. The potentials are smaller and more difficult to judge than those of the ECochG, but there is the advantage that testing can be performed either while the subject is awake or during sleep or sedation. The ABR is commonly used for diagnostic testing in infants who have been referred after failing OAE or automated ABR (AABR) hearing screening.

AABR is used for neonatal hearing screening in some countries. The ABR for full-term babies is fairly consistent, so a template of the response enables automatic detection of the waveform. Screening AABR apparatus is commercially available. The apparatus is easily applied and uses a 35 dB nHL click. The presence of a hearing response is shown by a green light (pass), while absence of a response shows a red light (refer). The advantage of AABR screening compared to OAE screening is that it is less susceptible to middle ear problems and will not give a false positive for auditory neuropathy. The referral rate with AABR is less than 2% after a second test, thereby reducing the number of children referred for diagnostic testing. The apparatus is more expensive than that for OAE and the test time is longer; however, the reduction in referrals (false positives) makes the test cost-effective. In infants who fail either OAE or AABR, a full ABR is then performed to establish the likely hearing threshold.

The ABR has other diagnostic uses. The latency of each of the components from wave I to wave V is precise. A pathological condition affecting the cochlear nerve will delay the transmission and the latency of wave V. This has provided a screening test for a vestibular schwannoma, but has now largely been replaced by contrast-enhanced magnetic resonance imaging (MRI). The ABR waveform is also affected by brainstem lesions, in which a delay between waves III and V may be evident. Multiple sclerosis may cause disordered and poorly repeatable ABR waveforms. 'Auditory neuropathy' appears to provide a widened wave I with no ensuing waveform, but the abnormal waveform is not neural, and relates to the abnormal positive DC potential seen on the ECochG.

An ABR can also be elicited in response to bone conduction stimuli, usually clicks. This can be useful in estimating cochlear function in infants undergoing hearing aid prescription, and in those with congenital microtia.

Steady-state evoked potentials

Steady-state evoked potentials (SSEPs – synonym: auditory steady-state response, ASSR) is a test that records any early electrical potentials that are phase locked to the stimulus. Analysis of the time window suggests that wave V of the ABR is the main source. The stimulus is amplitude modulated at a rate of 71 Hz for young children. The response is measured statistically until it is judged that a positive event has occurred. The original concept was that SSEPs could be used as a simple automated means of determining hearing thresholds. There are, however, some concerns. SSEPs in children are best recorded during sleep, under sedation or even general anaesthesia. The SSEP thresholds do not appear to be accurate if the hearing loss is mild (e.g. less than 40 dB HL). Not knowing the source of the electrical potentials is also a concern. Non-hearing potentials such as abnormal vestibular evoked myogenic potentials (VEMPs) or the abnormal positive potentials seen in auditory neuropathy may mistakenly result in a false-positive result.

Middle-latency potentials

Middle-latency auditory evoked potentials (MLAEPs) occur with latencies ranging from roughly 18 to 80 ms. They consist of a biphasic waveform with a negative wave occurring at about 20 ms (Na), a positive wave at about 30 ms (Pa), a second negative wave at about 40 ms (Nb), and a second positive wave occurring at about 50 ms (Pb). Generators are thought to include the thalamocortical projections to primary and secondary auditory cortices. In order to obtain reliable middle-latency recordings, it is necessary that a constant subject state is maintained, either light sleep or wakefulness. This has limited the clinical popularity of MLAEPs. Potential clinical uses include threshold estimation, evaluation of cochlear implant candidates and monitoring of the depth of anaesthesia.

Long-latency auditory potentials

AEP responses occurring beyond 50 ms are referred to as long-latency auditory evoked potentials (LLAEPs) or cortical auditory evoked potentials (CAEPs). They span the transition from obligatory to cognitive responses.

The obligatory responses have three major components. P1, occurring between 55 and 80 ms; N1, occurring between 90 and 110 ms and P2, occurring between 145 and 180 ms (Figure 7.7). They are generated at the level of the primary auditory cortex and the auditory association areas of the temporal lobes. They can be generated using a frequency-specific tone burst. The accurate correspondence with perceptual hearing thresholds and the frequency-specific information make this a useful test in medico-legal assessment of hearing for compensation cases and for diagnosis in suspected non-organic hearing loss. Another clinically useful obligatory evoked potential is the mismatch negativity (MMN). It is elicited when a deviant stimulus is presented in a sequence of standard stimuli. It reflects the ability of the central nervous system to compare the deviant stimulus to the previous standard set stored in short-term memory.

Cognitive evoked potentials vary with the cognitive tasks assigned while responses are recorded. The N2 response is the first cognitive evoked potential. The P3 (or P300) response is another such potential. It occurs in internal higher-level brain processing associated with stimulus recognition and novelty. It is largely a research tool and can be used in the study of memory disorder, information processing and decision making.

The LLAEP and the cognitive evoked potentials are very sensitive to both attention and subject states. LLAEPs require a conscious and cooperative subject, and may be unrecordable if the subject becomes drowsy or is sedated. These potentials are time consuming to obtain, thus limiting their clinical usefulness.

Electrically evoked auditory potentials

There are now a growing number of cochlear implant recipients (see Chapter 20). Electrically evoked auditory potentials enable assessment of cochlear nerve function prior to surgery and provide a useful means of assessing the function and effectiveness of the implant once inserted. These tests can be classified according to the part of the hearing mechanism they evaluate, in a similar manner to the AEPs.

Electrically evoked compound action potentials

Equipment to record electrically evoked compound action potentials (ECAPs) is now available from the commercial cochlear implant manufacturers. These responses are termed as neural response telemetry (NRT) by Cochlear Ltd, as neural response imaging (NRI) by Advanced Bionics and as auditory nerve response telemetry (ART) by Med-El. One of the electrodes in the intracochlear array is stimulated, and the first-order neural response recorded from an adjacent electrode. Initially it was hoped that

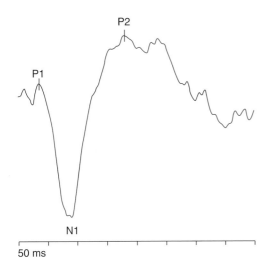

Figure 7.7 Long-latency auditory evoked potential obligatory responses.

this would provide an indication of the threshold of each electrode to aid programming, especially in young children. Unfortunately, the artifact resulting from electrical stimulation occurs at the same time as the response. To remove the electrical artifact, a number of procedures are undertaken but it is still difficult to identify the response in some subjects, and the ECAP thresholds do not bear a reliable relationship to the behavioural responses.

Electrically evoked stapedial reflex thresholds

The stapedial reflex can be elicited by stimulating any one of the intracochlear electrodes. The reflex is either observed by the surgeon using the operating microscope, or it can be recorded using a tympanometer after placing the probe in the contralateral ear canal. Electrically evoked stapedial reflex thresholds (ESRTs) provide useful information at the time of surgery, showing that the electrodes are placed within the cochlea. The ESRTs also provide some information about the expected comfortably loud levels, which can be helpful when mapping the implant postoperatively.

Electrically evoked auditory brainstem responses

The ABR waveform can be elicited by an electrical stimulus. The electrically evoked auditory brainstem response (EABR) can be obtained without electrical artifact contamination (Game *et al.*, 1990). A series of peaks is obtained similar to the acoustically elicited ABR response. This is helpful in determining if there is any retrocochlear problem affecting the auditory pathway in the brainstem. The threshold of wave V of the EABR is more sensitive than the ECAP but still does not always accurately predict the behavioural thresholds. Nevertheless, if excellent EABRs are obtained, these usually predict a good cochlear implant outcome.

Electrically evoked long-latency auditory potentials

Electrically evoked long-latency auditory potentials (ELLAEPs), like the cortical potentials, occur at 100–300 ms. These potentials show maturation of the auditory cortex in hearing children up to the age of 4 years. This maturation begins at a later age in children who have received a cochlear implant. The ELLAEPs are tedious to obtain, but the test procedure can usually be completed in 30–60 minutes in a cooperative subject.

The stimulus can be a sound stimulus, but this often causes problems because electrical artifact often obscures the LLAEP. It is much easier to use a train of pulses generated electrically through the cochlear implant. The technique can be used to investigate the cortical function in individuals who fail to make good progress with their cochlear implant despite good EABR waveforms. In implant recipients with multiple disabilities, the ELLAEP can provide threshold levels in the absence of behavioural responses.

Summary

Objective audiometric tests can provide highly accurate information regarding hearing mechanisms. That the tests are 'objective' rather than 'subjective' does not mean that they are not subject to error. The tests depend upon specialist equipment that requires careful maintenance and calibration. Skilled individuals are needed to perform the tests and to interpret the findings. Any deductions made from data must be considered in the context of each individual patient's history.

References

Conlon BJ, Gibson WP (2000) Electrocochleography in the diagnosis of Ménière's disease. *Acta Otolaryngologica* 120:480–483.

Game CJ, Thomson DR, Gibson WP (1990) Measurement of auditory brainstem responses evoked by electrical stimulation with a cochlear implant. *British Journal of Audiology* 24: 145–149.

Jerger J (1970) Clinical experience with impedance audiometry. *Archives of Otolaryngology* 92:311–324.

Kemp DT (1978) Stimulated acoustic emissions from within the human auditory system. *Journal of the Acoustical Society of America* 64:1386–1391.

O'Leary SJ, Mitchell TE, Gibson WP, Sanli H (2000) Abnormal positive potentials in round window electrocochleography. *American Journal of Otology* 21:813–818.

Rea PA, Gibson WP (2003) Evidence for surviving outer hair cell function in congenitally deaf ears. *Laryngoscope* 113:2030–2034.

Wong SH, Gibson WP, Sanli H (1997) Use of transtympanic round window electrocochleography for threshold estimations in children. *American Journal of Otology* 18:632–636.

The radiological assessment of hearing loss

Simon Lloyd and Patrick Axon

8

Introduction

Deafness can arise as a result of pathology affecting any part of the auditory pathway from the ear canal to the central auditory cortex. Thus, the underlying aetiology of deafness is varied. Historically, identification of the location of any lesion has relied on audiological and psychoacoustic testing as well as clinical examination. In the early part of the last century, plain x-rays were introduced and, together with tomographical and angiographic techniques, became a useful adjunct in the investigation of these patients. The work of Godfrey Hounsfield in the early 1970s led to the introduction of computerised tomography (CT) and began a revolution in the ability to accurately image the head and neck region, assigning most of the plain radiographic techniques to the history books. Over the past 30 years, extraordinary advances in CT and magnetic resonance imaging (MRI) technology have produced considerable strides forward in the quality of the images produced using these techniques. With this has come an enhanced ability to investigate the aetiology of deafness.

Principles of radiological techniques

Both CT and MRI produce cross-sectional images of the target tissues in a variety of different planes. Each has its advantages and disadvantages (Table 8.1), but broadly speaking CT provides excellent visualisation of bony anatomy, whereas MRI is ideal for imaging soft tissues. Each works in a different way. A detailed description of this is beyond the scope of this chapter but a brief summary is outlined below.

Computerised tomography

CT relies on the differential absorption of x-rays by different tissues. A narrow beam of radiation is produced by an x-ray tube. The x-ray passes through the target tissue and the attenuated beam is recorded by a series of detectors. By rotating the beam through 360°, a detailed greyscale image of the target can be created. An example of a normal high-resolution CT scan of the temporal bone is shown in Figure 8.1.

An initial scout view is taken to identify the skull base, and the scanner is tilted by 10–15° to

Table 8.1 Advantages and disadvantages of computerised tomography and magnetic resonance imaging.

	CT	MRI
Advantages	Excellent imaging of bony structures Fast acquisition time Not claustrophobic Cheap	No ionising radiation Excellent imaging of soft tissues Excellent multiplanar image resolution
Disadvantages	Poor imaging of soft tissues Uses ionising radiation Lower-resolution reformatted multiplanar images	Poor imaging of bony structures Claustrophobic[a] Noisy Long acquisition times More expensive than CT

[a]Open scanners are increasingly available.

allow for the angulation of the skull base relative to the horizontal plane. The images are usually acquired in the axial (horizontal) plane at slice widths as small as 0.5 mm, and scanning extends from the mastoid tip to the floor of the middle cranial fossa. Coronal and sagittal reconstructions (these terms relate to the vertical plane viewed from the front and the side respectively) can then be created by manipulating the axial data, and, using modern high-resolution scanners, these reformatted images have a resolution approaching that of the original axial images (Figure 8.2). Three-dimensional reconstructions

can also be produced. The images can then be adjusted in order to provide the best resolution of bony structures.

There have been a number of technological improvements in CT scanning over the past few years. Modern scanners have several parallel rows of detectors that allow the acquisition of multiple slices for each rotation. In addition, rather than having to stop between scans to move the position of the patient, continuous data acquisition is now possible using modern spiral CT scanners. This has resulted in much faster acquisition times and a reduction in movement

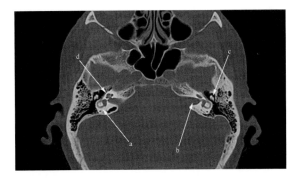

Figure 8.1 A high-resolution axial CT scan displaying the structures of the middle and inner ears. On both sides the lateral semicircular canal (**a**) is clearly visible, as are the internal auditory meati (**b**) and the head of the malleus and body of the incus (**c**). On the right, the apical turns of the cochlea are also visible (**d**).

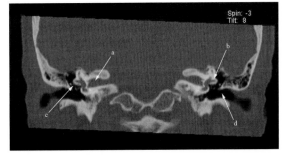

Figure 8.2 A coronal CT reconstruction of a normal temporal bone. The internal auditory canal is seen on both sides (**a**). The lateral semicircular canals are also visible (**b**); the middle ear (**c**), and the external auditory canal (**d**) are also seen.

artefact. Until recently, CT scanners have been bulky devices requiring purpose-built accommodation. However, progressive reduction in the size of the scanners has allowed the introduction of office CT scanners that are particularly suited to imaging of the head and neck.

Magnetic resonance imaging

MRI differs from CT in that it does not use ionising radiation. Using a high-field-strength superconducting magnet, a strong magnetic field is generated. Within this, the nuclei of molecules align themselves with the magnetic field. In the case of clinical MRI, hydrogen nuclei are used because they are abundant within tissues. The nuclei are then exposed to radiofrequency energy which deflects the hydrogen nuclei out of alignment with the magnetic field (excitation). On returning to their original alignment (relaxation), energy is released and this can be measured in order to produce an image. Because hydrogen nuclei are used, any tissue that contains water will be visible on the scan. This makes MRI an excellent modality for imaging soft tissues but it is unable to image bone as it only contains small amounts of water.

There are, broadly speaking, two main types of image produced by MRI, called T_1-weighted and T_2-weighted images. T_1 and T_2 are decay constants which determine how quickly the nuclei return to their resting state. The speed of relaxation is dependent on the tissue type. Thus, certain tissues are better imaged with T_1-weighted imaging and vice versa. T_2-weighted imaging is excellent for scanning tissues with a high water content.

In addition, a paramagnetic material called gadolinium-DTPA can be injected prior to the investigation. This is particularly useful for enhancing intracranial tumours while using T_1-weighted sequences.

The excitation pulses used in MRI can be applied in a number of different ways, called pulse sequences. Examples include spin echo sequence, short tau inversion recovery (STIR) sequence, echo planar imaging (EPI) and non-echo planar imaging (non-EPI).

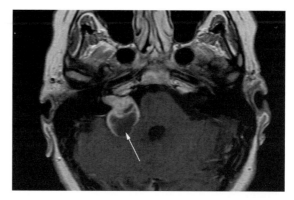

Figure 8.3 A T_1-weighted axial MRI scan with gadolinium-DTPA enhancement, showing a large right-sided vestibular schwannoma with cystic change within it (arrow).

MRI produces multiplanar imaging and allows slice thicknesses as small as 0.3 mm. Over recent years, improvements in coil technology and greater field strengths have reduced acquisition times and improved resolution. Similarly, more powerful software has allowed more effective three-dimensional (3D) reformatting of images.

The commonest use for MRI in patients with deafness is for the identification of vestibular schwannomas. Protocols vary from institution to institution, but in the authors' institution a T_1-weighted sequence with gadolinium-DTPA enhancement is used (Figure 8.3).

Functional MRI, which measures neuronal activity within the brain, has been used in a research setting for the investigation of prelingually deafened children.

Children

Both MRI and CT are usually well tolerated by adults, but children require special consideration. Under 3 months a child can often be scanned during natural sleep. However, children between 3 months and 5 years usually require general anaesthesia or sedation. Children older than 5 years can usually be scanned in the same way as an adult.

Assessing the imaging

Axial CT and MRI scans are, by convention, shown with the front of the head at the top of the page and the back of the head at the bottom of the page. The right ear is on the left side of the page and the left ear is on the right side of the page, as if viewing the scan from below.

A structured anatomical approach to assessment of any imaging is essential in order to ensure that pathology is not missed. Assessment should be divided into external ear, middle ear, inner ear and intracranial contents. In the assessment of the deaf patient, the focus should be on the temporal bone and the adjacent intracranial structures. As previously mentioned, CT is ideal for assessment of the bony anatomy of the temporal bone and MRI provides excellent anatomical data regarding the soft tissues, particularly those of the internal auditory canal (IAC) and the cerebellopontine angle (CPA).

Specific conditions

Congenital hearing loss

Congenital abnormalities of the ear often result in hearing loss and may involve the external, middle or inner ears, or a combination of these (20% of cases). External and middle ear abnormalities are much more common than inner ear abnormalities and frequently occur together. It is unusual for middle and inner ear abnormalities to occur together, as they have different embryological origins.

Congenital abnormalities of the inner ear

Congenital abnormalities of the inner ear form a spectrum of abnormalities that range from complete aplasia of the labyrinth (Michel deformity), through the common cavity deformity in which there is a primitive cochlear sac (Figure 8.4), to the Mondini deformity with incomplete partitioning of the distal turns of the cochlea. These are thought to represent arrest of cochlear development at progressively later stages during foetal

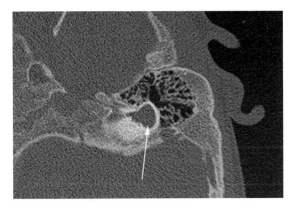

Figure 8.4 An axial CT scan showing a left common cavity deformity of the inner ear (arrow) in a child with profound bilateral sensorineural hearing loss.

development. These abnormalities are often bilateral. Some hearing may be present in patients with a Mondini deformity, but more severe dysplasias usually result in profound sensorineural deafness from birth. Other abnormalities of the inner ear include a bulbous internal auditory canal, abnormally angulated internal auditory canal, absence of the partition between the internal auditory canal and labyrinth, and a wide vestibular aqueduct (Figure 8.5). All these abnormalities can be identified on high-resolution CT imaging, but T_2-weighted MRI is useful in assessing the contents of the IAC and may be used in place of CT to assess cochlear and endolymphatic abnormalities. Many children with these abnormalities are candidates for cochlear implantation.

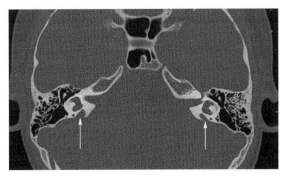

Figure 8.5 An axial CT scan showing bilateral wide vestibular aqueducts (arrows). The right side is wider than the left.

Congenital abnormalities of the middle ear

Abnormalities of the middle ear usually manifest as ossicular malformations and may be associated with abnormalities of the course of the facial nerve. The stapes is the ossicle most frequently affected. It may be absent, fixed or have a crural deformity. The incus and malleus may be fixed or deformed (Figure 8.6), and there may be ossicular discontinuity. These abnormalities are associated with a conductive hearing loss. CT scanning is the ideal modality for identifying abnormalities of the middle ear.

Congenital abnormalities of the external ear

Deformities of the external ear may involve the pinna, the ear canal or both and may be of variable severity. Ear canal atresias may be complete or incomplete and may involve all or part of the ear canal. They may be bony or made up from soft tissues or, more commonly, a combination of both. These abnormalities are often associated with abnormalities of the middle ear and are best imaged with CT scanning. There are several classification systems, but the most frequently used is that described by Altmann which grades the severity of aural atresia from I to III. Grade I is the mildest grade of aural atresia and consists of a small external ear with a fairly normal middle ear space. Grade II consists of an absent ear canal and a small middle ear space, with abnormalities of the ossicles. Grade III is the most severe grade and consists of an absent ear canal and a small or absent middle ear space. The ossicles may be absent.

Radiological abnormalities of specific syndromes

Congenital hearing loss of any type may be associated with one of a large number of syndromes. The more common ones are outlined below.

- In *Treacher Collins' syndrome*, radiological abnormalities are symmetrical and include an unpneumatised mastoid and small attic and antrum in all patients. Around 50% have microtia and atresia of the external ear canal. Ossicular abnormalities are also common, as is an altered course of the facial nerve. Some patients have dysplasia of the lateral semicircular canal.
- *Crouzon's syndrome* is characterised by external ear canal atresia, ossicular anomalies, an

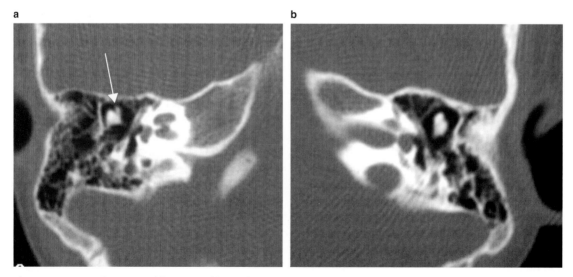

a　　　　　　　　　　　　　　　　　b

Figure 8.6　An axial CT scan of the temporal bone showing congenital hypoplasia of the malleus (**a**, arrow); **b** shows a normal malleus for comparison.

underpneumatised middle ear and dysplasia of the semicircular canals.

- In *Goldenhar's syndrome*, also called hemifacial microsomia, there is microtia, meatal atresia and middle ear abnormalities in almost all cases. Other radiological features include a low tegmen and an underpneumatised middle ear.
- *CHARGE association* (an acronym standing for coloboma, heart defects, atresia of the choanae, retardation of development, genital abnormalities, ear abnormalities) is associated with a number of radiological abnormalities. The most common is absence of the semicircular canals. Other abnormalities include external ear canal atresia, ossicular anomalies and the Mondini deformity.
- In *branchio-oto-renal syndrome*, 60% have external, middle or inner ear abnormalities. Radiological findings include a short upward-pointing petrous pyramid, ossicular abnormalities (the stapes is often affected and is most commonly monopodial and fixed in the oval window), hypoplasia of the distal turns of the cochlea and a short bulbous internal auditory canal.
- *Pendred's syndrome* may be associated with the Mondini deformity, enlargement of the vestibule and deficient modiolus and a widened vestibular aqueduct.
- The *wide vestibular aqueduct syndrome* results from a wider than normal vestibular aqueduct (Figure 8.5). The calibre of the vestibular aqueduct should be around the same diameter as that of the posterior semicircular canal. A widened aqueduct may be defined as an increase in the anteroposterior diameter of the mid-portion of the descending limb of greater than 1.5 mm. It may be associated with X-linked deafness, Pendred's syndrome and branchio-oto-renal syndrome.
- X-linked deafness is usually a bilateral, symmetrical, mixed deafness which only affects males. There is congenital fixation of the stapes and a progressive sensorineural hearing loss. Radiological features include a widened lateral end of the internal auditory canal, producing a bulbous appearance, and a deficient bony plate between the lateral end of the

internal auditory canal and cochlea. There may be high perilymph pressure, and attempts at stapes surgery have a high risk of producing a stapes gusher, causing total loss of hearing if hearing was present before surgery. Similarly, in cochlear implant surgery there may be rapid flow of perilymph and cerebrospinal fluid from the cochleostomy.

Chronic otitis media

Historically, it has been felt that imaging in patients with chronic otitis media has been unnecessary. However, recently, CT imaging has gained popularity as a useful adjunct in the assessment of disease extent, and gives useful information regarding the status of the ossicular chain and the degree of erosion of the temporal bone (Figure 8.7).

In addition, attempts have been made to utilise imaging techniques to assess ears that have undergone mastoid surgery in order to exclude the presence of recurrent or residual cholesteatoma and avoid the need for additional unnecessary surgery. It was initially hoped that CT would be accurate enough to fulfil this role, but it has

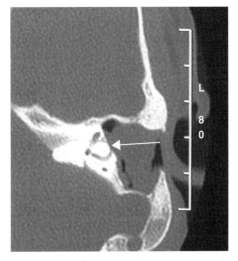

Figure 8.7 An axial CT scan showing significant bony erosion of the lateral semicircular canal resulting from cholesteatoma (arrow).

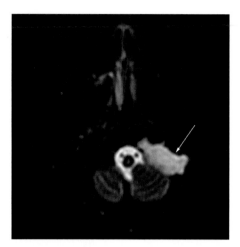

Figure 8.8   A non-echo planar imaging MRI of an extensive left temporal bone cholesteatoma which has destroyed the entire otic capsule and extends to the petrous apex (arrow).

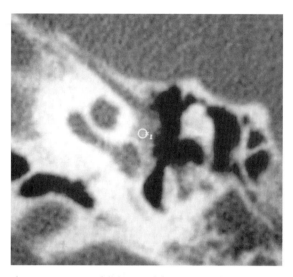

Figure 8.9   An axial CT scan of the temporal bone showing otospongiosis of the region of the *fissula ante fenestram*. The marker illustrates the area of otospongiosis.

become clear that this technique is not reliable in this setting. Similar hopes have surrounded the use of MRI, especially non-echo planar imaging MRI (Figure 8.8). The evidence base for the use of this technique is in its infancy at present, but outcomes following clinical trials are awaited with interest.

Otosclerosis

Radiology does not usually play a role in the day-to-day management of otosclerosis, but it is possible to visualise the abnormal bone laid down in this condition, termed otospongiosis, on CT imaging as this bone is relatively demineralised (Figure 8.9). The abnormal bone is most often focused around the anterior part of the oval window, a region termed the *fissula ante fenestram*. However, otospongiosis can be much more extensive and may involve the entire otic capsule (Figure 8.10). Using CT densitometry, it is possible to assess the degree of demineralisation and confirm the diagnosis of otosclerosis, although this has found limited application in clinical practice.

The majority of prostheses used in stapes surgery consist of a fluroplastic piston and a metal wire. The most commonly used metals are stainless steel and platinum. If a patient who has had stapes surgery is undergoing an MRI, it is important to know what type of prosthesis has been used, as it is potentially possible for the magnetic field of the scanner to dislodge the prosthesis and cause either a conductive or a sensorineural hearing loss. In practice, however, almost all modern prostheses are MRI safe.

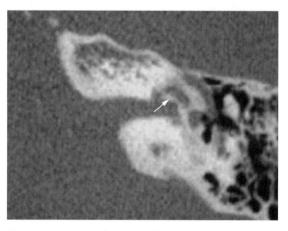

Figure 8.10   An axial CT scan showing extensive left peri-cochlear otospongiosis (arrow).

Tumours

The most common neoplasm in otological practice is the vestibular schwannoma. MRI scanning has revolutionised the investigation of patients with this condition and has become the gold standard method of imaging for any patient with unilateral or asymmetrical sensorineural hearing loss. Most units dealing with these tumours on a regular basis use T_1-weighted imaging with gadolinium-DTPA enhancement. The tumours enhance well with the gadolinium-DTPA, providing maximum contrast to the low signal intensity of the temporal bone, and medium signal intensity of the cerebrospinal fluid on T_1-weighted imaging (Figure 8.3).

MRI is also used for the investigation of patients with neurofibromatosis type 2. These patients have bilateral vestibular schwannomas together with other intracranial and spinal cord tumours which include meningiomas and schwannomas of other cranial nerves (Figure 8.11).

Other tumours of the temporal bone are extremely rare but mention should be made of

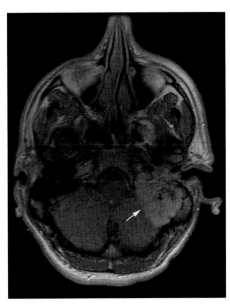

Figure 8.12 An axial T_1-weighted MRI with gadolinium-DTPA enhancement showing a large left glomus jugulare tumour (arrow).

glomus tumours. The imaging of these highly vascular tumours is complex and usually involves both CT and MRI as well as angiography (Figure 8.12). Radiological techniques can also be used to embolise these tumours, either as a primary treatment or, more often, as a prelude to surgical removal.

Temporal bone trauma

Temporal bone trauma can result in a conductive, sensorineural or mixed hearing loss. High-resolution CT is the mainstay for assessment of temporal bone trauma and allows identification of fracture lines and the presence of ossicular disruption. It also allows assessment of the facial nerve in cases where there is an associated facial weakness.

The most common abnormality seen is dislocation of the incus, which is usually displaced inferiorly. However, with severe head injuries, fractures of the temporal bone can occur.

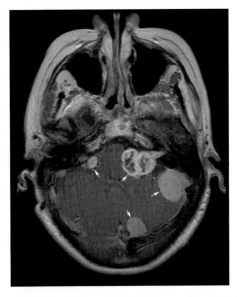

Figure 8.11 An axial T_1-weighted MRI scan with gadolinium-DTPA enhancement showing bilateral vestibular schwannomata and multiple meningiomas (arrows) in a patient with neurofibromatosis type 2.

Fractures have historically been catagorised as longitudinal or, less frequently, transverse, depending on their orientation relative to the long axis of the temporal bone. However, in practice most fractures have features of both these types (Figure 8.13). A detailed anatomical description of the injury is more useful than a broad catagorisation into longitudinal or transverse types.

Diseases of the temporal bone

There are a number of rare bone dysplasias that can affect the temporal bone and cause both conductive and sensorineural hearing loss.

In *osteogenesis imperfecta* there is demineralisation of the temporal bone which is indistinguishable on CT imaging from severe cochlear otospongiosis. The ossicles may be thin, predisposing them to fracture, which causes a conductive hearing loss.

Fibrous dysplasia causes expansion of the temporal bone and this process may involve any part of the temporal bone. On CT the bone has a characteristic expanded, 'ground glass' appearance (Figure 8.14).

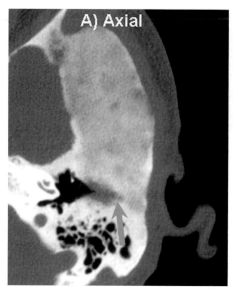

Figure 8.14 An axial CT scan showing fibrous dysplasia of the left temporal bone (arrow).

Meningitis

Meningitis can cause ossification of the labyrinth, termed labyrinthitis ossificans. This begins as fibrous obliteration as early as 2 weeks following the insult and progresses to ossification. The initial fibrous reaction usually manifests as patchy reduced signal within the cochlear duct on T_2-weighted MRI (Figure 8.15b), but in some cases there may be a generalised mild reduction in signal which reflects not fibrosis but the presence of thick fluid within the cochlear duct. At this stage there may be no visible changes on CT. Later on, once true ossification has occurred, narrowing or complete obliteration of the cochlea duct can be identified on high-resolution CT imaging. In those patients who are deaf following meningitis, it is important to image the cochlear ducts early and consider early cochlear implantation, as ossification can occur at any point up to 5 years after the initial infection. Implantation in patients who have ossification can be difficult, although the radiological findings often overestimate the degree of ossification, especially in those patients who have a more generalised reduction in signal within the cochlear ducts on MRI.

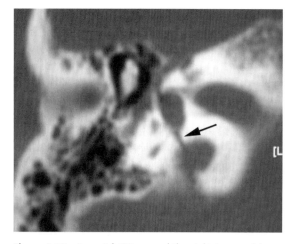

Figure 8.13 An axial CT scan of the right temporal bone showing a transverse fracture through the vestibule (arrow) and involving the horizontal portion of the facial nerve.

a

b

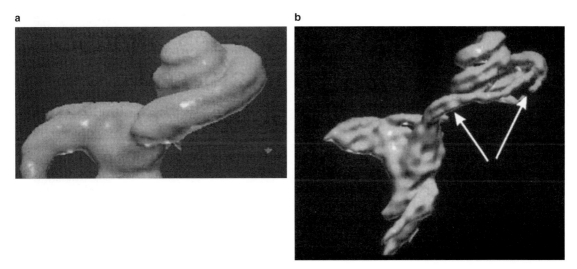

Figure 8.15 Three-dimensional MRI reconstruction of a normal cochlea (**a**) and a cochlea displaying labyrinthitis ossificans (**b**, arrows).

Imaging and cochlear implantation

Imaging of patients being considered for cochlear implantation is vital. However, the best method of imaging is still under discussion, some units advocating CT as the imaging modality of choice, some advocating MRI, and some advocating both. CT provides excellent visualisation of the bony structure of the cochlea and internal auditory canal, although it is not able to visualise the cochlear nerve itself. MRI, on the other hand, has the advantage that it displays the contents of the IAC as well as giving structural information regarding cochlear duct anatomy. Most units performing cochlear implantation would perform a heavily weighted T_2 MRI in children, allowing identification of a cochlear nerve. In postlingually deafened adults, not deafened by meningitis, an MRI is not necessary but a CT scan should be performed.

Ironically, the last bastion of the plain x-ray is within the field of cochlear implantation. In order to check the position of the implanted cochlear implant electrode postoperatively, a plain x-ray of the temporal bone taken in the reverse Stenver's position is used. This should show coiling of the electrode within the cochlear duct (Figure 8.16).

New developments

Over the past 5 years, otologists have become increasingly aware of a condition called superior semicircular canal dehiscence syndrome. This condition is characterised by dizziness which may be induced by loud sound (Tullio's phenomenon), an awareness of one's own bodily sounds

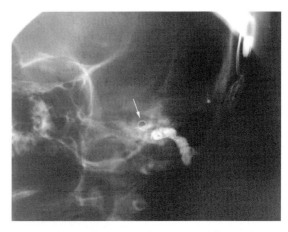

Figure 8.16 A plain x-ray of the temporal bone taken in Stenver's position, showing the expected coiling of the electrode (arrow) within the cochlear duct following cochlear implantation.

(autophony), and may be associated with an apparent conductive hearing loss. It results from a dehiscence of the bone overlying the apex of the superior semicircular canal. This defect can usually be identified with high-resolution oblique coronal CT imaging through the long axis of the superior semicircular canal (Figure 8.17).

Another interesting condition is pulsatile tinnitus. Historically, this phenomenon has been under-investigated, but there are a number of specific causes that may be identified and treated. Imaging plays a role in the identification of vascular causes for pulsatile tinnitus. These include peripheral vascular disease, vascular otological tumours such as glomus tumours, dural fistulae and abnormalities of the venous drainage of the cranial cavity, such as superior sagittal sinus stenosis. MR venography, CT venography and angiography all have a place in the investigation of these patients. Similarly, interventional radiological procedures are available for embolisation of vascular anomalies, and stenting may be performed to treat stenoses.

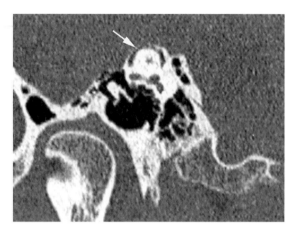

Figure 8.17 An oblique coronal CT scan of the superior semicircular canal, illustrating superior semicircular canal dehiscence (arrow).

The aetiology and management of conductive hearing loss in children and adults

William Hellier

9

Introduction

The external and middle ear are responsible for collecting sound and transforming it from air pressure waves in the outside environment to fluid pressure waves in the perilymph of the cochlea. During this process, a degree of amplification of the sound energy occurs. Any disease process or structural change in the external ear, tympanic membrane, middle ear or ossicles (Figure 9.1) will reduce the transfer of sound energy to the neural component of the cochlea and give a conductive hearing loss (CHL). Unlike most sensorineural hearing losses, conductive hearing losses are potentially reversible medically or surgically. In a purely conductive hearing loss, there is also the retention of the neural ability to discriminate sound well, so this type of hearing loss can respond very well to amplification of sound, with the use of a hearing aid or other amplification device. The degree of CHL can vary according to the pathology, but may range from a mild 20–30 dB hearing loss, to a 60 dB hearing loss, which is the maximal CHL that can occur.

The cause of a CHL can be external or middle ear disease, and therefore these will be discussed separately.

External ear disease

Any process that occludes the external ear canal will lead to a CHL. This will usually be easily identifiable by clinical examination, as excellent visualisation of the external ear and canal is possible with the modern otoscope and microscope.

Congenital external ear deformity

Children can be born with growth failure of one or both external ears. This can involve the pinna (*microtia*; Figure 9.2), the external canal (*meatal atresia*), or both.

The sensorineural hearing is often normal, as the cochlea develops from separate origins and at a different time from the external ear, but there can be associated middle ear anomalies. If

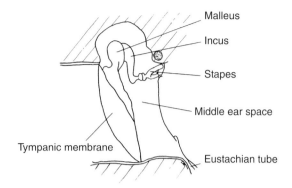

Figure 9.1 Anatomy of the middle ear.

both ears are affected, the child will have up to a 60 dB hearing loss, which will have a profound effect on hearing and speech development. In the very young child, bone-conduction auditory brainstem response (ABR) testing is needed urgently to assess the sensorineural thresholds, and a bone-conducting hearing aid is fitted if appropriate. The aid can be a traditional bone-conducting aid or a bone-anchored hearing aid (BAHA), initially held on a soft band (see Chapter 21). Treatment options for children with severe microtia and meatal atresia are either surgery to create a new meatus, or permanent BAHAs. Reconstructive surgery has a variable hearing outcome, and in many cases the new meatus will re-stenose or heal poorly. The mainstay of reha-

bilitation in the UK is the insertion of titanium screws into the mastoid at around the age of 4–5 years (when the skull is thick enough), to allow the attachment of a BAHA aid. The cosmetic aspect of the microtia can be treated with pinna reconstructive surgery, or the mounting of a prosthetic ear with the BAHA on the titanium abutments.

A child with only one ear affected, and a normal hearing ear on the other side, will usually develop normal speech and hearing without the need for urgent aiding. A BAHA, prosthetic ear or surgical reconstruction can be considered, if desired by the child and parents, as the child grows.

Acquired external canal stenosis

In adults or, rarely, children, the external canal can become narrowed, stenotic, or completely occluded (Figure 9.3). The main causes of this are infection, trauma, including surgery, or bony outgrowths of the canal called exostoses.

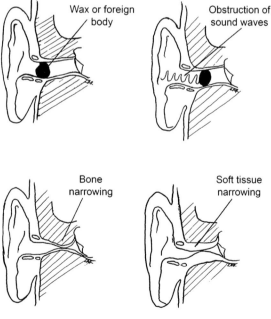

Figure 9.3 Obstruction of the external auditory canal by wax, bony or soft tissue. Sound waves cannot reach the tympanic membrane.

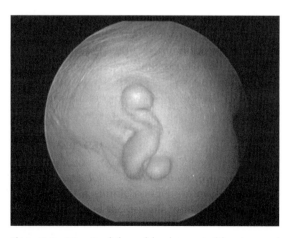

Figure 9.2 Microtia: failure of development of the pinna and external auditory canal.

Recurrent otitis externa causes granular changes in the canal and scarring. Cold water exposure, often in swimmers or surfers, causes periosteal irritation and bony overgrowths which can block the ear directly, or secondarily due to failure of skin and wax migration past the deep exostoses.

The hearing loss due to *stenosis* can be mild, but a total occlusion will cause a maximal loss. If the stenosis is incomplete, or a short segment, bony or cartilaginous, meatoplasty surgery can widen the canal with improvement in the hearing. Longer stenoses or total occlusion often will need meatoplastic widening with skin grafts to bring in new epithelium. Circular structures, however, tend to heal with scarring and re-stenosis, and the more severe stenoses can re-narrow quite rapidly. The alternative management of these conditions is a bone-conducting hearing aid, or a formal BAHA, which can give excellent results.

External meatal *exostoses* can be treated surgically by drilling down the bony outgrowths with a bony meatoplasty. If there is careful preservation of the deep canal skin, the outcome is usually very satisfactory, with a widened meatus, normal hearing and improved migration of the deep skin. Care has to be taken not to touch the tympanic membrane or malleus with the drill, as this can cause a sensorineural loss or perforation of the tympanic membrane.

Wax, infection or foreign body

Wax and desquamating epithelium are continually produced by the external canal. Usually this slowly migrates like a 'conveyor belt' laterally out of the ear canal. Wax can become impacted if pushed back into the canal as often occurs with cotton buds. Regular use of cotton buds to 'clean' the ear is normally not necessary. As well as preventing the natural outward migration of wax, there is a risk of damage to the tympanic membrane and skin of the external ear canal. Wax will not cause a major hearing loss until it completely occludes the canal. Removal can be achieved with drops such as sodium bicarbonate, which dissolves the wax, by syringing, or by suction using the microscope. Syringing can occasionally further impact wax and cause infection, and at this point microsuction can be needed, followed by antibiotic drops.

Rarely, a patient's epithelial 'conveyor belt' can break down, and the wax and keratin build up in the deep ear. This is referred to as keratosis obturans and can cause not only a CHL, but also slow erosion of the deep bony canal. Regular suction toilet of the ear is needed to prevent problems.

Otitis externa causes obstruction due to build-up of infected debris and skin, and often a mild CHL. Managment is with antibiotic/steroid ear drops and microsuction.

Middle ear disease

If the external meatus is clear, the tympanic membrane is usually easily seen. Using the otoscope or microscope, the tympanic membrane can be inspected, and if it is, as it should be, mildly translucent, some of the structures of the middle ear can be assessed. Any middle ear pathology may cause a CHL.

Embryologically, the middle ear is an outpouching of the nasophayrnx and first branchial pouch. The tympanic membrane separates the middle ear from the external canal, and the Eustachian tube links it to the nose and allows ventilation of the middle ear cleft. Management of middle ear disease, and the CHL caused, needs to recognise the importance of the Eustachian tube (Chapter 3).

Otitis media with effusion/glue ear

Otitis media with effusion (OME)/glue ear is usually a self-limiting condition in children and is due to the failure of adequate ventilation of the middle ear cleft by the Eustachian tube. The middle ear mucosa absorbs oxygen and possibly other gases, which must be replaced to allow equalisation of middle ear pressure with the external atmospheric pressure across the tympanic membrane. Failure of adequate ventilation may occur when there are problems with the function of the Eustachian tube, or possibly due to increased gas absorption by the middle ear mucosa (Figure 9.4).

Aetiology and incidence of otitis media with effusion in children

The exact causes of OME are not known, but there are a number of known associations. OME is more common under the age of 5 or 6 years and affects boys slightly more than girls. Allergy or atopy is associated with an increased risk of middle ear effusion, and there is evidence of bacterial 'biofilm' infection in the middle ear fluid. Recently, there have also been suggestions that reflux of acid from the stomach into the nasopharynx may have a role in some cases of OME. Children with cleft or abnormal palates have a very high incidence of OME, as do those with Down's syndrome and certain skull base abnormalities. Children who attend a nursery or a daycare facility, and those in homes where there is parental smoking are also more likely to have OME.

There are two peaks of incidence of OME in children: at approximately 2 and 5 years of age. The most common presentation is that of hearing loss. This may be noted by the parents or by the school, or picked up during screening hearing testing. Maternal observation is often, but not always, reliable, and the aphorism that 'a child should be judged to have a hearing loss until proved otherwise if it is suspected by their mother' is well founded. Some children may present with the sequelae of hearing loss – speech delay or behavioural changes, and some with recurrent acute otitis media on the background of persistent OME.

The diagnosis of OME can often be made clinically by inspection of the tympanic membranes with a good-quality otoscope with magnification. The classic features are of a dull, possibly indrawn drum, often with a fluid level and a slightly golden hue. Tympanometry confirms the diagnosis and measures the middle ear pressure reliably and quickly. Good-quality paediatric audiology testing is vital to assess the exact hearing thresholds and estimate the disability caused by the effusions.

The natural history of OME is usually one of resolution with improvement of Eustachian tube function and middle ear ventilation as the child grows. This fact needs to be borne in mind when discussing the management of OME.

Management of otitis media with effusion in children

The three main management possibilities for OME are those of watchful waiting, hearing aid provision, or insertion of tympanostomy tubes such as grommets. A number of other treatments have been tried, including antibiotics, antihistamines and systemic and topical decongestants. Trials confirm they have no major effect on OME and no real place in its management. Topical nasal steroids may have a place in treatment of a child with OME and marked rhinitis, but their place in OME alone is uncertain and the subject of ongoing trials.

It is important to assess the degree of CHL caused by the OME in a child, and also the amount of disability. Some children can be relatively unaffected by a mild hearing loss, and if so, a watchful waiting policy, waiting for the child to spontaneously recover with growth, is

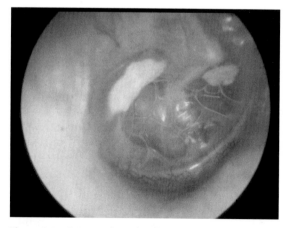

Figure 9.4 Otitis media with effusion or glue ear. There are air bubbles in the fluid behind the tympanic membrane. Two patches of tympanosclerosis can also be seen (see also Figure 9.6). (This figure was kindly provided by Professor Tony Wright.)

usually the most appropriate treatment. If a child with OME is having problems with the CHL, speech development or education, intervention is important. Severe retraction and thinning of the tympanic membrane can also occur imperceptibly unless the ears are checked otoscopically from time to time.

Myringotomy, or an incision in the tympanic membrane with aspiration of the middle ear fluid, is the simplest way to surgically treat OME. This can lead to a short-term improvement in ventilation of the middle ear and improvement in hearing to normal levels. The myringotomy soon heals, however, and the middle ear effusion returns. If a plastic tube is placed in the myringotomy this will hold open the incision and allow longer-term ventilation of the middle ear space by 'bypassing' the Eustachian tube. Placement of a tympanostomy tube such as a grommet will lead to a longer-term improvement in the hearing while this is in place and the lumen patent (Figure 9.5).

The tube is slowly extruded, like any foreign body, from the tympanic membrane over a period of 9 to 18 months. If the Eustachian tube function has matured over this period (the child has 'grown through' their OME), the hearing should remain good. Middle ear fluid, however, can return as the grommet falls out, and further intervention may be needed.

Studies have shown that on average the improvement in hearing due to a ventilation tube

lasts from 6 to 9 months, with an average hearing improvement of 8–12 dB. The Medical Research Council (MRC) in England has been investigating OME with the TARGET (Trial of Alternative Regimes for Glue Ear Treatment) trial. This has shown benefits from grommet insertion for children with OME and hearing loss, and confirms improvements in hearing loss to well within normal limits (10–15 dB HL) (Haggard M, personal communication). In the UK, the National Institute for Health and Clinical Excellence (NICE), a government body that reviews the clinical and cost-effectiveness of medical interventions, has recommended the use of grommets in any child with persistent OME and hearing thresholds of 25–30 dB or worse.

Tympanostomy tube insertion in children needs to occur under a general anaesthetic, and this must be considered in the decision on whether to operate. Maintaining a persistent perforation in the tympanic membrane does lead to infection if water enters the middle ear although the grommet. Grommets reduce the risk of middle ear infection from upper respiratory tract infections but, should an infection occur, pus, sometimes with blood, may discharge through the grommet into the external ear. Discharge from a grommet may occur in up to 20% of children, and in 2–4% can be persistent. This will usually settle with topical antibiotic/steroid ear drops or, occasionally, oral antibiotics. Uncommonly, the tubes will need to be removed if the discharge does not settle, or progress is complicated by granulation tissue around the grommet.

When the tubes are extruded from the tympanic membrane, the underlying perforation normally heals spontaneously. However, there can be a residual perforation in 1–4% of cases. This can act as a natural grommet, if the child still has poor Eustachian tube function, but if persistent may need to be surgically closed once the child has grown. T-tubes or Permavents are designed to stay in the tympanic membrane far longer than simple grommets. They are, however, associated with a greater incidence of residual perforation, in 10–25% of cases in some studies. Bleeding in the layers of the tympanic membrane at surgery, and the presence of the grommet may lead to scar tissue or tympanosclerosis being laid down in the

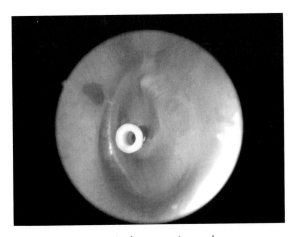

Figure 9.5 Grommet in the tympanic membrane.

eardrum (Figure 9.6). Although visible, this does not commonly cause a problem with the hearing unless there is any inflammation or scarring around the ossicles.

Adenoidectomy may be used as an adjuvant procedure with grommet insertion. A number of studies have shown benefit from the addition of adenoidectomy, and the TARGET trial showed a reduction in the rate of recurrent OME and also a general health benefit. This benefit seems to be greatest in the 4–8-year-old age group, in whom the adenoids often seem to be at the peak of their size. Removal of the adenoids is thought to give benefit from both improvement in ventilation of the nose and Eustachian tube, as well as a reduction in bacterial colonisation of the adenoidal pad, which may be implicated in OME. The existence of bacteria in an inert 'planktonic' state, described as a *biofilm*, is being recognised as a possible causative factor in OME. Adenoidectomy may clear tissue that harbours biofilms, and therefore help OME resolution.

The alternative management of OME to surgical intervention is the provision of hearing aids. Children will often tolerate aids well in moderate or severe conductive and sensorineural hearing losses, and they can provide good amplification in the mild loss associated with OME. The conductive loss caused by the effusion, however, may fluctuate in its severity, which leads to problems with aid programming. For the mild loss,

and with the option of a straightforward surgical alternative, there can be issues of acceptance of the aid with both parents and children, and most families whose child has symptomatic OME will opt for grommet insertion. Hearing aids are very helpful where surgery is contraindicated due to other health problems, or when there are specific reasons to avoid ventilation tube insertion, such as recurrent infections when tubes are in place.

Otitis media with effusion in adults

Adults can also suffer from middle ear effusion. This classically can follow an upper respiratory tract infection leading to Eustachian tube dysfunction. The CHL and feeling of fullness produced can be very irritating, even although the loss is quite mild. It is always illuminating how quickly an adult will complain about OME, while a child's condition may not be recognised for some months. As with children, OME in adults is often self-limiting and commonly resolves after 2–6 weeks. Persistent OME, if not troublesome, may be managed conservatively, but many adults prefer to have a ventilation tube inserted. Longer-term ventilation tubes are sometimes necessary as adults, unlike children, may not grow through their OME. It is important to check the post-nasal space of any adult that presents with OME, as rarely it can be caused by compression of the Eustachian tube by a malignant tumour. The Chinese have a higher incidence of post-nasal space squamous carcinoma than Europeans, and this often presents as unilateral OME.

Chronic otitis media

Acute middle ear infection normally clears up within 3 weeks. If the infection fails to subside after 2–3 months, the infection is said to be 'chronic', healing is less likely to occur, and long-term damage may be present.

Chronic otitis media (chronic suppurative otitis media; CSOM) is traditionally separated into two types. In COM without cholesteatoma there is a perforation of the tympanic membrane and possibly damage to the ossicles, with CHL.

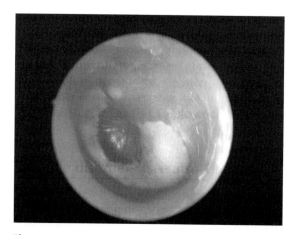

Figure 9.6 Tympanosclerosis in the tympanic membrane.

There may also be a persistent discharge from the middle ear. If this continues for a long time it can cause further damage to the contents of the middle ear; in a very few cases it may also produce cochlear damage, with sensorineural hearing loss. In the other type, a pathological process called cholesteatoma develops, and this form is therefore called COM with cholesteatoma.

Cholesteatoma forms when part of the tympanic membrane, possibly weakened by infection, becomes sucked into the middle ear space, forming a 'pocket'. This typically occurs either in the pars flaccida (see Chapter 3) or in the posterior part of the pars tensa, where the stapes and round window lies. This pocket is, of course, lined with the same epithelium that covers the surface of the tympanic membrane. When the outer layer of epithelium dies and falls off, instead of migrating outwards along the ear canal, it becomes trapped in the pocket. Once the pocket is full of dead epithelial cells, more cells continue to be produced, the contents of the pocket become infected, and the pocket swells under the pressure of the extra cells, inflammation and pus. The pocket is inside the middle ear space, so that when it expands it will erode the contents of the middle ear. Cholesteatoma can therefore be very dangerous, destroying ossicles, eroding inwards to damage the facial nerve and destroy the bone protecting the cochlea and semicircular canals, thus producing sensorineural deafness, and even travelling upwards or backwards to enter the cranial fossa, with a risk of meningitis and cerebral abscess.

There is also a congenital form of cholesteatoma, produced probably by epithelial cells deposited in the anterior middle ear space in the foetus, anterior to the malleus handle. This can expand in the same way as the acquired type of cholesteatoma described above, and cause damage and infection, usually in childhood and in the absence of previous middle ear infections.

Cholesteatoma surgery

Cholesteatoma must be treated surgically. The mass of cholesteatoma is dissected out from the middle ear. The traditional method is by *radical mastoidectomy*, drilling away all the mastoid air cells and the posterior wall of the external ear canal to expose and remove the disease. In *modified radical mastoidectomy*, the tympanic membrane is then grafted and some attempt may be made to repair damage to the ossicles (see information on ossiculoplasty later in this chapter). The 'open' mastoid cavity can be inspected in the clinic and any recurrence of the disease identified and removed. However, the mastoid cavity may be prone to recurrent infection and also does not clean itself automatically, as occurs in the normal external ear canal. This means that the patient will have to make regular visits to the ear, nose and throat (ENT) clinic to have wax and dead skin removed. A more recent technique is *intact canal wall mastoidectomy* (synonyms: *combined approach tympanoplasty*, or *canal wall-up mastoidectomy*). Here, the mastoid bone is drilled to expose the cholesteatoma, leaving the posterior wall of the canal intact. The tympanic membrane is elevated, using the technique described for myringoplasty, ossiculoplasty and stapedectomy, below, and a window, called a posterior tympanotomy, is drilled from the mastoid cavity, forward, into the middle ear, medial to the level of the tympanic membrane. This exposure allows any disease to be dissected out, while leaving the external ear canal intact. The tympanic membrane is grafted. After an interval of 9 months or more, the mastoid is re-explored; any residual cholesteatoma that may have grown, will easily be visible, and can be removed, and if necessary ossicular damage repaired to improve the hearing. In contrast to radical mastoidectomy, the external ear canal is preserved, without the need for regular clinic visits for cleaning.

Tympanic membrane perforation

The majority of tympanic membrane perforations follow an episode of acute otitis media, with non-healing of the epithelial layers (Figure 9.7). Trauma and perforations after ventilation tubes account for the other causes. The CHL that results can vary in level, from no appreciable loss in very small perforations, to up to 50 dB in subtotal ones. The possibility of a degree of the CHL being caused by an ossicular problem must

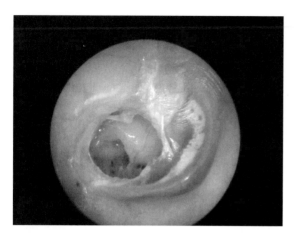

Figure 9.7 Perforation of the tympanic membrane. The stapes head and thinned long process of the incus is just visible through the perforation: the stapedius tendon is visible to the left of the stapes head.

always be borne in mind when assessing any perforation, as often the original inflammatory event(s) will have involved the ossicles as well.

The CHL with tympanic membrane perforations is usually greatest in the lower frequencies, and greater with increasing perforation size. The site of perforation seems not to be significantly related to the degree of hearing loss in a recent study, but depends more on the volume of the middle ear and mastoid, with smaller middle ear clefts showing greater conductive losses (Mehta *et al.*, 2006).

Management of the CHL associated with tympanic membrane perforation can be with hearing aids, or surgical with a tympanoplastic procedure. *Tympanoplasty* is a general term used to describe a surgical procedure designed to remove pathology and repair defects in the middle ear and tympanic membrane. An operation to repair a defect of the tympanic membrane is described as *myringoplasty*; repair of ossicular damage is described as *ossiculoplasty*.

In a persistently inactive or dry perforation, where the patient prefers not to have surgery, or is unsuitable for surgery because of age or for medical reasons, a hearing aid can give good amplification of sound, and hearing improvement. Wearing an occlusive hearing aid mould, however, can change the environment of the

external and middle ear in some patients and lead to discharge and infection – the ear becomes 'active'. If this does occur, the hearing aid mould must be changed to a more non-occlusive style or may have to be discontinued. At this point, reconsideration of surgical tympanoplasty should occur. The other option in the scenario of the non-intact tympanic membrane, persistently wet ear and CHL is the BAHA (see Chapter 21). This can be fitted to a behind-the-ear abutment, and allows the ear canal and middle ear to remain open and ventilated while providing bone-conduction aiding. This can prove very effective and give a good hearing improvement in such difficult situations.

Tympanoplastic surgery aims to graft the tympanic membrane and allow healing to occur. A perforation arises when the epithelial edges of the hole in the drum stop migrating towards one another and leave a defect. The graft material, although it is usually incorporated into the drum, probably acts as 'scaffolding', allowing the freshened epithelial edges to grow over a solid structure to heal the hole. The first part of the procedure, therefore, is excision of the edge of the perforation to expose fresh epithelium that will restart the natural healing process.

A number of materials can be used to act as a graft material for myringoplasty. The grafts that are currently most commonly used are the fascia covering the temporalis muscle above and behind the ear, periosteum from the mastoid bone, and perichondrium from the cartilage of the tragus or pinna. All are autologous (using the patient's own tissue), tough connective tissue layers that are easily accessible when operating on the ear. In the past, other synthetic materials and also tissue from cadavers have been used, but these graft materials are not now used in the UK, especially cadaveric tissue, due to the risk of infection with Creutzfeldt–Jakob disease. In small perforations, occasionally fat from the ear lobe is used to plug the perforation after the edges are freshened.

The tympanic membrane can be approached directly down the canal or using an incision behind (postaural) or in front of the ear (endaural). A flap of external meatal skin is lifted, and the annulus of the tympanic membrane identified. This is then elevated to enter the middle ear cleft. The chorda tympani nerve is often exposed at this point, but care is taken to preserve it, to avoid the disturbance of taste that is caused if it is divided. The malleus, incus and stapes are inspected and probed gently to assess their normality of movement.

The graft material can be placed over the perforation, an onlay graft, under the perforation, an underlay graft, or between the layers of the tympanic membrane, an interlay graft. The problem that can occur with onlay grafting is that any pressure generated in the nose, blowing it for example, will be transferred to the middle ear, and may push off the onlay material. There is also a risk of trapping epithelium beneath the graft, leading to cholesteatoma. The underlay graft has the benefit that positive middle ear pressure will push it more firmly against the undersurface of the tympanic membrane. Care must be taken with an underlay graft that it is well supported against the drum, otherwise it can fall back into the middle ear. The tympanic membrane is elevated, so that the graft can be placed between the bony annulus of the ear and the drum to give the required stability (Figure 9.8). Gelatine sponge that slowly dissolves can be used in the middle ear space to support the graft in some cases.

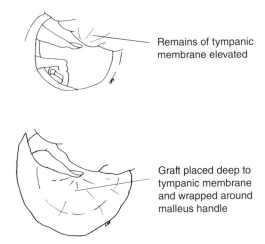

Remains of tympanic membrane elevated

Graft placed deep to tympanic membrane and wrapped around malleus handle

Figure 9.8 Tympanoplasty or grafting of the eardrum. The tympanic membrane is elevated and a graft placed medial to the drum and malleus handle.

The success rate after tympanoplastic surgery is good, with 70–95% perforation closure. Hearing improvement is also good; in 60–70% of ears the air–bone audiometric gap is closed to 10 dB, and to 20 dB in around 80%.

There is some debate regarding the lower limit of age at which one should attempt tympanoplasty. Many surgeons suggest that a child should be 10 years or over before surgery. Some studies have shown that there is an increase in graft success rate over this age. This is probably related to the improvement of the Eustachian tube function with increasing age, and a reduction in the rate of acute otitis media (AOM), both of which will influence the long-term success rate of the surgery. An older child also is far more able to accept and help with his or her treatment. Surgery can be beneficial in younger children, however, if the perforation is very active, giving a lot of symptoms, or the CHL is marked. In some patients there can be residual Eustachian tube dysfunction, which was probably instrumental in the initial otitis media, and up to 7–8% of ears can have persistent OME after perforation repair.

Ossicular fixation or discontinuity

Fixation or erosion of any of the three ossicles can occur within the middle ear cleft and will give a CHL of varying degree. This can occur congenitally or due to a number of middle ear pathologies.

Congenital anomalies of the ossicles usually occur in combination with changes in the external ear and tympanic membrane, but occasionally can occur in isolation. There can also be an underlying sensorineural hearing loss, so careful audiology needs to be performed. Fixation of any of the bones may occur. Congenital stapes fixation can be associated with an abnormal communication of the inner ear with the intracranial cerebrospinal fluid (CSF) space. Surgery in such cases carries the risk of cochlear damage, with sensorineural deafness following a perilymph 'gusher' where the inner ear fluid comes out at pressure, and care must be taken if operative intervention is considered.

Structural abnormalities of the ossicles can also be seen, with fused ossicles or missing bony elements. Surgery for the hearing loss can play a part if the abnormality is localised, but often, especially if there are associated external ear canal or tympanic membrane changes, the use of a hearing aid, either conventional or bone anchored, is favoured.

Acute otitis media, *trauma* and *cholesteatoma* can all lead to ossicular changes and a CHL. AOM, either a single severe episode or recurrent, can cause scarring and fixation of the ossicles. Tympanosclerosis is the term used to describe the hyaline changes that occur in the tympanic membrane, but also the calcification around the ossicles that can occur after AOM. Any inflammatory process, either infective with AOM, or with cholesteatoma, can stimulate osteogenesis and bony overgrowth especially seen around the malleus, or can lead to erosion of the bony ossicular structures.

The most common area of erosion is the long process of the incus, which can be partially or completely destroyed. If the bony damage is complete, a 60 dB maximal CHL may occur. Stapes erosion, usually of the crura (often the head can remain intact due to its blood supply from its tendon), is the next most common ossicular change, most often due to cholesteatoma. Erosion of the malleus head and incus body may occur with cholesteatoma, but loss of the handle of the malleus is uncommon. Trauma, be it either direct or concussive, may fracture or dislocate any of the ossicles (Figure 9.9).

Management of the conductive hearing loss associated with ossicular damage

This will depend on the exact pathology and the integrity of the tympanic membrane. The underlying cause of the ossicular change will need to have been addressed and the ear should be stable and dry. This means that for middle ear changes caused by AOM or CSOM, the tympanic membrane should be intact, after either spontaneous healing or grafting, and after cholesteatoma the disease should have been totally removed, and the eardrum should be healed, intact and stable.

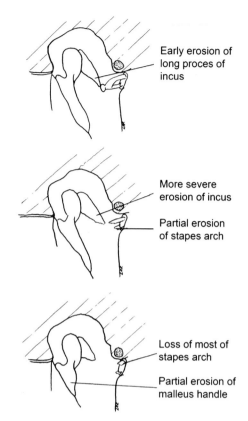

Early erosion of long proces of incus

More severe erosion of incus

Partial erosion of stapes arch

Loss of most of stapes arch

Partial erosion of malleus handle

Figure 9.9 Erosion of the ossicles due to chronic suppurative otitis media or cholesteatoma. Incus erosion is the most common, but progressive erosion of the other ossicles may occur.

Commonly after inflammatory changes, there are adhesions, consisting of scar tissue in the middle ear, and with chronic ear disease there can be ongoing dysfunction of the Eustachian tube. If there is persistent middle ear fluid due to chronically poor Eustachian tube ventilation, even if the ossicular mechanism is restored there will still be a residual CHL. Recurrent retraction of the eardrum can also occur in chronic ear disease, threatening further ossicular disruption. The ear therefore needs to be carefully assessed before deciding between the different management options.

The two main options for treatment of the CHL in these cases are the use of a hearing aid or surgery in the form of ossiculoplasty. If there is a persistent marked CHL in an ear with a well-ventilated, stable tympanic membrane, surgical exploration can be considered. This may be part of a planned second procedure, in, for example, 'second look' surgery after canal wall-up mastoidectomy, or as a stand-alone procedure. The tympanic membrane is elevated and the middle ear visualised. Sometimes the cause of ossicular disruption is already known, for instance if the incus was removed when clearing a cholesteatoma, but if not, the ossicular chain is assessed for obvious damage and also gently probed using micro-instruments to ascertain if there is any fixation of the ossicles. Any procedure on the ossicles needs to be carried out with great care, as with excessive movements energy may be transferred to the cochlea causing sensorineural hearing loss.

Fixation of the malleus can be treated by clearing adhesions, or by removing bony overgrowth that has formed between the malleus and the attic wall. Care has to be taken when drilling bone around the malleus, that the ossicle itself is not touched by the drill, as this can cause a sensorineural hearing loss. Fixation of the incus can be treated by removing it and, after remodelling, placing it to lie between the malleus handle and stapes head as a 'strut' to conduct sound vibration. Fixation of the stapes is dealt with in the section on otosclerosis.

When there is *ossicular discontinuity* due to loss or erosion of one of the bones, there are a number of materials that can be used to reconstruct the ossicular chain. Autologous materials include remodelling the patient's own incus or using some cortical bone taken from the nearby mastoid cortex. Allografts (synthetic materials) are also used and include bone cement to bridge small gaps, and a variety of other bio-inert materials such as hydroxyapatite or titanium. The replacement ossicles are described as partial ossicular prostheses (PORPs) if they are used to bridge the gap between an intact stapes and either the incus, malleus handle or tympanic membrane, and total ossicular prostheses (TORPs) if there is no stapes superstructure and the prosthesis connects the stapes footplate to the other ossicles or drum (Figure 9.10). A large amount of research has looked at ossicular prostheses, and results seem to suggest that the mate-

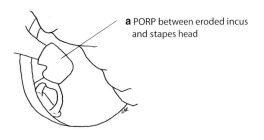

a PORP between eroded incus and stapes head

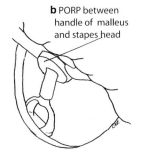

b PORP between handle of malleus and stapes head

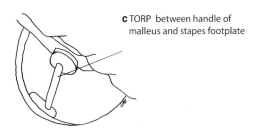

c TORP between handle of malleus and stapes footplate

Figure 9.10 Ossiculoplasty or repair of ossicular damage. **a**, a partial ossicular replacement prosthesis (PORP) bridging the gap between an eroded incus and the stapes; **b**, a PORP replacing the incus, positioned between the stapes head and handle of the malleus; **c**, a total ossicular replacement prosthesis (TORP) replacing the incus and stapes superstructure positioned between the stapes footplate and the handle of the malleus.

rial used needs to be as light and as stiff as possible to give the best outcome.

The results of ossicular reconstruction are variable, with some procedures giving complete closure of the audiological air–bone gap and normal hearing, and some giving no improvement in hearing at all. Approximately 50% of operations will lead to a good hearing improvement. The reasons for this low success rate are structural and functional. It must also be remembered that the natural arrangement of the ossicles gives a small degree of amplification of sound, and movement of the tympanic membrane produces a rocking movement at the stapes footplate. A new arrangement cannot often reproduce these natural effects entirely.

Any reconstruction relies on a structurally good contact between the ossicles, and excellent vibration conduction. Lifting and replacing the eardrum means that this may heal with lateralisation, moving the new ossicles apart, or medialisation, causing their alignment to change and alter their stability. It is difficult to predict this process. PORPs tend to give better results than TORPs, as balancing the prosthesis on the stapes head is more stable than placing it on the flat footplate (like balancing a drawing pin on a plate). Functionally, if there are persistent changes and poor ventilation of the middle cleft, this will impair the surgical outcome. Research continues to try and find the best material for ossicular reconstruction and also ways of stabilising the new ossicular chain postoperatively to give better results.

If there are ongoing problems with chronic changes in the middle ear, or Eustachian tube dysfunction, surgery is not always appropriate. The patient's age and also general medical health must also be considered. If the tympanic membrane or its grafted remnant is intact and the ear dry, an air-conduction hearing aid will give excellent amplification and hearing improvement. Occasionally, due to ongoing disease and poor healing, an ear may remain with a perforation or recurrent discharge. In this case, an aid in the canal will add to the problems as the mould will prevent much-needed ear ventilation. A bone-conduction aid, or BAHA can be very effective in these circumstances.

Otosclerosis

Aetiology and presentation

Otosclerosis is a hereditary disease of the petrous temporal bone. It is a form of osseous dysplasia where normal compact bone is replaced by vascular spongy bone. The French call the condition otospongiosis, which reflects the condition's histology. The cochlea in the embryo ossifies in cartilage. A small area of residual or degenerative cartilage just near the oval window, called the *fissula ante fenestram*, is the commonest site for otosclerosis to occur. This leads to new spongiotic bone formation and fixation of the stapes footplate causing a CHL. Otosclerosis can, less commonly, be more widespread in the petrous bone and, if this occurs around the cochlea, may result in a sensorineural hearing loss. This always needs to be considered when assessing a patient with otosclerosis.

The condition has an autosomal dominant type inheritance but not all patients with the disease will have clinical symptoms. Otosclerosis will normally present in the late 20- to 40-year age group, and in women may be exacerbated during pregnancy. There is a gradual hearing loss in one or both ears. Tinnitus is often noted by the patient. The tympanic membrane is normal to examination, except in the early stages of the disease when a red flush called 'Schwartze sign', caused by the increased vascularity of the otospongiotic bone, is sometimes seen through the drum. Tuning fork tests are very important to assess whether there is a true CHL, for, as mentioned above, a sensorineural loss may also be present. The usual audiological picture is of a CHL, often with an apparent sensorineural loss at 2000 Hz, described as a Cahart notch. Stapedial reflexes are usually absent.

The CHL caused by the slow fixation of the stapes footplate in otosclerosis can vary from a mild loss to a maximal 60 dB hearing change. Frequently, the audiogram will show a sensorineural dip at 2 kHz, the so-called Cahart notch, which is an apparent as opposed to a real sensorineural change. True sensorineural hearing loss due to otosclerotic (or 'otospongiotic') change around the cochlea can, however, co-exist with the conductive loss. It is important that the level of bone conduction hearing is assessed carefully, especially when considering surgery, as if this is severe, correction of a relatively small conductive component will achieve relatively little, while exposing the patient to risk. This assessment can be difficult in patients with bilateral otosclerosis, as masking the bone conduction of sound when there is a bilateral CHL can be inexact.

Management

The management of the CHL due to otosclerosis will depend on the degree of loss, and also whether this is unilateral or bilateral. The main treatment options are simple observation, provision of a hearing aid, or surgery. In the past, use of oral sodium fluoride has been tried, to replace the calcium ions laid down in the otosclerotic process with fluoride ions, in order to retard the progression of the disease. This was mainly used before the advent of general water fluoridation, and now is rarely used.

The hearing loss with otosclerosis does often worsen in women around the time of childbirth, probably due to the effects of the increased oestrogen on bone turnover. This has led to concerns about the use of hormone replacement therapy (HRT) in women with known otosclerosis. Studies, however, have not shown any proven increase in otosclerotic hearing loss with HRT, but it is probably prudent for such women who need to start hormone therapy to have regular audiograms to look for hearing deterioration.

Patients with a mild, especially unilateral, hearing loss, who are not troubled by their loss and who are managing well may not want any active intervention. They need a thorough explanation of the condition, and often it is useful to repeat their audiology after about a year to see if there is any obvious disease progression.

The majority of patients with otosclerosis will have an almost pure CHL until age or cochlear otosclerosis intervenes. This means that amplification with a hearing aid will usually give excellent hearing results. Even if there is a sensorineural loss, aiding can provide excellent access to sound and speech. For patients who have a symptomatic mild hearing loss, who

feel they are not managing, or for those with a greater hearing change, a trial of a hearing aid is the first line of management. Hearing aids can be uni- or bilateral, depending on audiological changes.

Many patients are greatly benefited by aiding and wish for no further treatment, but some may have problems with the hearing aids. This can be a physical issue – recurrent otitis externa, mould irritation, feedback and fullness – or it can be one of acceptance of the aid either cosmetically, or with the sound quality it gives in the different environments.

Surgery for otosclerosis can give excellent hearing results and correction of the CHL. Most surgeons would counsel their patients to try a hearing aid before embarking on the surgical route, as this can be a risk-free and well-tolerated treatment. Those patients who receive no benefit or have problems with an aid, as listed above, and who are fit enough for the operation, may be considered for surgery.

The underlying pathology in otosclerosis that leads to the CHL is fixation of the stapes footplate. Early ear surgeons found that physically mobilising this led to an improvement in hearing, but this unfortunately deteriorated quickly, as the footplate re-fixed. The operation evolved with a stapedectomy, where the whole stapes was removed and the oval window grafted with tissue. A piston attached to the long process of the incus was then placed on the graft to allow movement of the ossicles to be transmitted to the inner ear fluids. This operation was very successful, and is still carried out.

The surgery continues to evolve to try and minimise any trauma to the inner ear. Instead of removing the whole stapes, a small hole is made in the footplate: a stapedotomy procedure. The most widely used technique is to approach the stapes and oval window niche by means of a tympanomeatal flap. Under general or local anaesthesia, usually through the ear canal, a cut is made in the meatal skin, and this and the tympanic membrane are slowly elevated to expose the middle ear. The diagnosis is confirmed by testing the mobility or fixation of the stapes by palpation with micro-instruments. The stapes is exposed, the stapes tendon cut, and the body and crura (the suprastructure) are removed from the footplate with either a fine pick, microscissors or a laser. Care must be taken not to mobilise the footplate while doing this, or the operation may have to be abandoned. A stapedotomy, a tiny hole in the footplate, is made with either a fine drill or a laser, usually 0.4–0.8 mm in diameter. A Teflon or platinum piston is then attached to the incus and placed just into the stapedotomy (Figure 9.11). To try and prevent leakage of

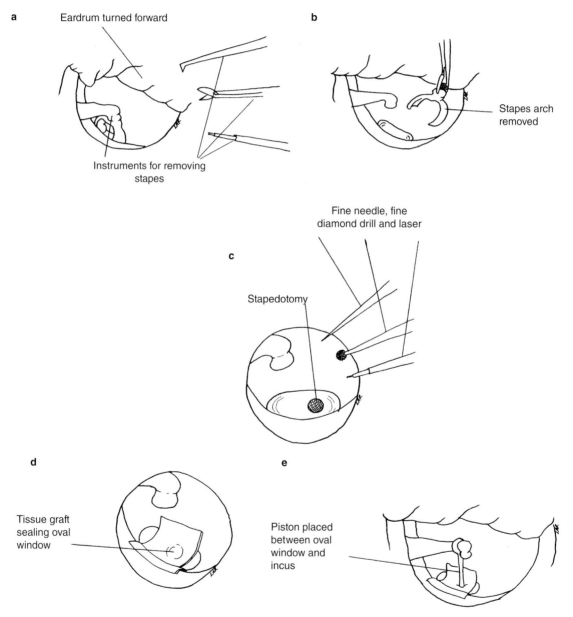

Figure 9.11 Surgery for otosclerosis. **a**, The tympanic membrane is elevated and the stapes and incus exposed. Micro-instruments are used; **b**, the crura of the stapes are divided and the superstructure removed with micro-forceps; **c**, a stapedotomy or small hole is drilled in the stapes footplate; **d**, a small graft such a piece of vein may be used to close the stapedotomy; **e**, a Teflon/platinum piston is placed into the stapedotomy on top of the graft and crimped to the long process of the incus.

the inner ear fluids from around the prosthesis, some surgeons use a small vein graft to cover the stapedotomy before placing the piston; some pack a little fat around the piston. The tympanic membrane is then returned to its original position.

The results of surgery in the hands of an experienced surgeon are excellent, with good improvement in the CHL and a good closure of the air–bone gap on audiological testing in 85–95% of cases. Patients report great satisfaction if the surgery goes well. Case selection is important, however, as those with a marked bilateral conductive loss will have more to gain from surgery, and less to lose, than those with an unilateral loss. A patient with a bilateral conductive loss, if one ear is improved, especially if the postoperative thresholds are better than 30 dB, will see a marked overall hearing improvement. A patient with a unilateral loss may only notice an overall improvement if the operated ear gains a hearing level of better than 20–25 dB HL (normal levels) or to within 15 dB of the other ear. This is described as the 'Belfast rule of thumb'. Some surgeons do not feel surgery is warranted in such unilateral cases, but, if successful, patients with unilateral otosclerosis do notice a definite overall improvement in hearing with surgery. There is a benefit from having symmetrical hearing in the ability to detect sound direction, with hearing in noise, and an overall binaural lift of 5–10 dB.

In some patients there can be dual pathology, with fixation of not only the stapes but also the malleus. This is uncommon, but may account for some cases where what seemed to be a very successful stapes operation did not resolve the CHL. In these ears, it is possible to divide the fixed head of the malleus, mobilise the malleus handle and attach a longer piston to this, which then is placed in the stapedotomy. This arrangement can be intrinsically less anatomically stable, and care is needed when considering this surgical variation.

The risks of stapes surgery are small, but the major risk is that of total sensorineural hearing loss, which can occur in 0.5–2% of cases. This can be due to inadvertent direct damage to the inner ear at surgery, but in some patients the cause is unknown, possibly due to an overly sensitive cochlear structure that is harmed purely by opening the inner ear. Vertigo or dizziness can occur after surgery. This is usually short-lived, but, rarely, can be persistent. Tinnitus may be a feature of otosclerosis, and, if the hearing is improved by surgery, often regresses or can disappear. Uncommonly, it can worsen after surgery and this tends to be the case if there is any worsening of the postoperative sensorineural hearing threshold.

The chorda tympani nerve, which supplies taste sensation to the anterior two-thirds of the tongue, travels across the middle ear, under the handle of the malleus, directly over the long process of the incus and stapes. During surgery this nerve can dry out, be bruised or, very occasionally, divided. Patients may describe alteration of taste after surgery, often a slightly metallic taste on the tongue on that side. This usually slowly settles after 2–6 months, but it is important to warn patients of this risk during counselling for surgery, especially if they are by profession a cook, sommelier or wine buyer!

There are differing opinions among surgeons as to whether a patient with bilateral otosclerosis should be offered surgery on the second ear after successful surgery on the first. There is a small risk of late-onset sensorineural loss after stapes surgery, and if this were to occur in both ears, it would be catastrophic for the patient. This is rare, however, and as stated above there is a definite benefit in binaural good hearing. As with all surgery, it is a question of careful discussion of the risks and benefits with the patient, and a sensible decision being made that takes all the individual's circumstances into account.

Acknowledgements

I am very grateful to James Robinson FRCS and his daughter Lucy Robinson for Figures 9.1, 9,3, 9.8, 9.9, 9.10 and 9.11, which were in the 6th edition of *Ballantyne's Deafness* and have been redrawn for this edition. Kate Lay at the UCL Ear Institute Department of Medical Illustration kindly helped with the preparation of the line drawings for publication.

Reference

Mehta (2006) Mehta RP, Rosowski JJ, Voss SE, O'Neil E, Merchant SN (2006) Determinants of hearing loss in perforations of the tympanic membrane. *Otology and Neuro-Otology* 27: 136–143.

Acquired sensorineural hearing loss

Martin Burton

10

Introduction

Sensorineural hearing loss occurs when there is damage to the hearing mechanism within the cochlea or abnormal function of the cochlear nerve (see Chapter 3). A small proportion of patients are born with such problems (see Chapters 11 and 24) but in the vast majority sensorineural deafness is acquired in adult life.

Features of acquired sensorineural hearing loss that should be looked for while taking a history from the patient

When first questioning a patient about their deafness the following list includes topics that may be relevant:

- age of the patient
- one or both ears affected
- duration of deafness
- progressive or sudden
- accompanied by:
  - ☐ tinnitus
  - ☐ vertigo
  - ☐ pain
  - ☐ discharge from the ear (otorrhoea)
- family history of hearing loss
- history of noise exposure, head trauma, medication
- other illnesses, past and present.

'Normal' deafness with ageing (presbyacusis)

Some cells in the body can be replaced when they die or degenerate. The highly differentiated cells of the auditory system and pathways do not belong to this group. The 'durability' of the auditory system depends on both genetic and environmental factors. With advancing age, it is normal for hearing to deteriorate and this is termed 'presbyacusis'; it is not a disease, rather the term acknowledges the association between ageing and hearing loss.

Presbyacusis presents in a variety of ways. The disability caused by the reduction in hearing thresholds varies considerably. Two patients with the same thresholds measured with pure tone audiometry may have quite different problems in terms of their abilities to communicate, hear in the presence of background noise, use the telephone, and so on. This may in part relate to differences in their ability to discriminate speech. But also, some patients develop better listening strategies. Those who have lost their hearing more slowly and gradually may compensate better than those who do so suddenly.

Several studies have looked, post-mortem, at the inner ears of elderly patients with 'presbyacusis', and the pathological findings have been correlated with the clinical features of the patients' deafness. As a result, several different 'types' of presbyacusis have been described. However, this classification is of limited clinical usefulness. Sometimes patients ask if their hearing is 'normal' for their age. Their thresholds may be compared with average values for people of different ages, produced from population-based studies.

Deafness due to other causes

Clues as to the cause of sensorineural deafness are obtained from the history of the deafness itself and from information about other symptoms of ear disease. The onset may be gradual or sudden. Both ears may be affected equally or one more than the other. These factors may help determine the nature of the underlying disorder. Most sensorineural deafness occurs gradually and equally in both ears, reflecting the fact that the underlying cause (such as the ageing process, industrial noise or an ototoxic drug): (a) is not directed specifically at one ear alone and (b) exerts its influence over an extended period of time. Patients who have a unilateral problem are more likely to have some localised disease. Some processes, such as trauma, may be directed at one ear only, or at both (a major head injury). Trauma is a good example of a process likely to result in sensorineural deafness of sudden or rapid onset. Fluctuating sensorineural deafness is unusual, but characteristic of Ménière's disease.

The other cardinal symptoms of ear disease are tinnitus, discharge (otorrhoea), pain (otalgia), vertigo and facial weakness. The presence or absence of these provides further clues to diag-

> **Box 10.1** Causes of acquired sensorineural deafness.
>
> *Progressive deafness with vertigo*
> - Ménière's disease
> - Syphilis
>
> *Progressive deafness without vertigo*
> - Ototoxic drugs
> - Vestibular schwannoma
> - Neurofibromatosis
> - Disorders of bone
>   - Otosclerosis
>   - Osteogenesis imperfecta
>   - Paget's disease
> - Chronic otitis media
> - Noise
> - 'Presbyacusis'
>
> *Sudden deafness with trauma*
> - Ear surgery
> - Head injury
> - Barotrauma
> - Blast injury
> - Perilymph fistula
>
> *Sudden deafness without trauma*
> - Infections
> - Idiopathic
> - Immunological

nosis. The various causes of sensorineural deafness will be considered on the basis of the characteristic history, as this is how the diagnosis is usually reached (Box 10.1). The headings serve as a broad outline only.

Progressive deafness with vertigo

Ménière's syndrome, Ménière's disease and endolymphatic hydrops

In 1861, Prosper Ménière published details of the disorder which bears his name. He recognised a condition characterised by episodic vertigo.

Although patients with the classical features of Ménière's disorder are readily identifiable, considerable problems have arisen surrounding the diagnosis of some patients and the terminology used to describe the disorder. Diagnosis is not straightforward, as no 'gold standard' diagnostic test exists. The Committee on Hearing and Equilibrium of the American Academy of Otolaryngology-Head and Neck Surgery (AAOHNS) has produced guidelines for the diagnosis of Ménière's and evaluation of therapy; these provide a useful starting point for improving diagnostic rigour. They propose that the only 'certain' cases of Ménière's are those in which a clinical diagnosis of 'definite' disease (as defined – see below) is accompanied by histopathological (post-mortem) confirmation. A distinction can be drawn between Ménière's *syndrome* and *disease*.

Ménière's syndrome consists of the following clinical features:

- recurrent episodes of spontaneous vertigo
- fluctuating hearing loss
- tinnitus
- a feeling of fullness in the ear.

Ménière's disease is the term used to describe *idiopathic* cases of *Ménière's syndrome*.

Apart from Ménière's disease itself, other causes of the syndrome are: trauma, infection, syphilis and classic or atypical Cogan's syndrome.

Some patients with Ménière's syndrome have specific histopathological findings in their inner ear: these findings are termed 'endolymphatic hydrops'. There has been a tendency to use the term endolymphatic hydrops interchangeably with Ménière's disease or syndrome. This is a mistake for several reasons. Endolymphatic hydrops is found in a wide range of disorders, to the extent that it is seen in about 1 in 20 of all human temporal bones with otological pathology. The proportion of patients with Ménière's syndrome who have the histological changes of endolymphatic hydrops is unknown. Conversely, however, only about one-third of patients with endolymphatic hydrops on histological examination are known to have had episodic vertigo in their life. The inference that some factor or factors produce endolymphatic hydrops, which in turn produce Ménière's syndrome, and that the syndrome can only occur by this mechanism, may be fallacious. Notwithstanding, the theory that hydrops is responsible for Ménière's syn-

drome is the dominant one in current thinking. Endolymphatic hydrops may turn out to be an epi-phenomenon simply indicating inner ear dysfunction. It is likely that Ménière's syndrome is multifactorial in origin, and hereditary elements may combine with a wide variety of external stimuli.

The natural history and clinical features of Ménière's disease are well documented, but the reader should bear in mind the caveat above about diagnostic 'accuracy'. The symptoms usually start in middle age (mean age 40–45 years). Men and women are probably affected equally, although women present slightly more often. There is a family history in about one patient in 20. Although there have been few formal studies of psychosocial factors, it is more common in the higher social classes and rare in developing countries. Patients are more commonly 'intelligent, introspective and somewhat obsessive'. Stress undoubtedly precipitates disease activity.

The 'classic' Ménière's attack consists of a feeling of fullness in the ear accompanied by increasing tinnitus, reduced hearing and the sudden onset of rotatory vertigo. This lasts from 20 minutes to several hours and may be accompanied by autonomic symptoms such as nausea, vomiting, sweating, diarrhoea, etc. The patient does not lose consciousness. The attack can come on at any time even when asleep. After the acute vertigo has stopped, the patients continue to feel unwell and their balance is poor, often for the rest of the day.

Between attacks it is not uncommon for patients to experience fullness in the ear, tinnitus or positional vertigo, or simply instability with quick movements, or they may be asymptomatic. There is great variability in the pattern of the disease. Some patients have only one or two attacks per year and their hearing remains relatively stable. Others have periods of frequent attacks for weeks or months, then periods of remission. Some are totally incapacitated by their disease, becoming housebound and unable to work.

The hearing loss of Ménière's begins with sound appearing distorted and having a 'tinny' quality. The audiogram shows a low-frequency sensorineural loss. Loudness recruitment is present so the patient may develop hyperacusis and be intolerant of loud noises. When the hearing drops during an attack, it will usually recover within a few hours in the early stages of the disease.

The AAOHNS criteria allow a diagnosis of 'definite' Ménière's disease to be made when two or more episodes of vertigo lasting more than 20 minutes are associated with audiometrically documented hearing loss and tinnitus or fullness in the affected ear. 'Probable' Ménière's disease requires all these features but only one attack of vertigo. Diagnostic difficulties may occur when the full set of symptoms does not develop at the same time.

The history is the most important factor in making the diagnosis of Ménière's disease. However, several diagnostic tests have been proposed and promoted by their enthusiasts, including electrocochleography (ECochG) and the glycerol dehydration test. These tests are of dubious value in establishing or refuting the diagnosis in patients with equivocal histories.

The aim of the medical treatment of Ménière's disease is to (a) reduce the number and severity of attacks and (b) limit the symptoms during an individual attack. The patient is encouraged to follow a low-salt diet, and betahistine hydrochloride (Serc®) is prescribed. A mild diuretic can also be added. The acute attacks may be aborted by the use of a vestibular sedative such as prochlorperazine; sublabial versions or suppositories are available, since tablets may be lost during vomiting. In some patients, oral steroids may have a role.

If this medical regimen fails to control the patient's symptoms, more invasive treatment may be considered. Ménière's disease is a disorder with a high natural resolution rate and this makes the evaluation of alternative therapies problematic.

Surgery for Ménière's disease may aim to preserve hearing, while modulating or abolishing vestibular function, or it may be destructive, destroying both hearing and balance in the affected ear. One of the least invasive surgical procedures is endolymphatic sac decompression. The procedure should not affect hearing. If an initial improvement is not maintained, it can be revised.

The vestibular nerve can be cut (preserving the cochlear nerve and hence the hearing), to prevent the vertiginous symptoms of Ménière's. There is an associated risk of hearing loss and facial weakness and if all the nerve fibres are not divided, the results may not be wholly satisfactory.

If hearing is poor and unserviceable, a formal labyrinthectomy may be performed, destroying the inner ear. All hearing is lost as a result. Currently, medical labyrinthectomy with hearing preservation is more popular. The tendency for some ototoxic antibiotics to be more vestibulotoxic than cochleotoxic (see below) has led to the use of intratympanic gentamicin to perform a 'medical labyrinthectomy'. A grommet or needle is placed in the tympanic membrane, and gentamicin introduced into the middle ear through it. This procedure has several advantages, including few side-effects and the avoidance of the risks associated with major ear surgery. Various timing and dosage regimens have been proposed. It is important to monitor hearing on a regular basis during treatment, as occasionally this is made worse. This technique has been shown to be both effective and safe if the appropriate precautions are followed.

Syphilis

Syphilis is an infectious disease caused by the spirochaete *Treponema pallidum*. For many years this sexually transmitted disease was in decline; its incidence has increased again recently. It is an extremely rare cause of hearing loss.

Progressive deafness without vertigo

Ototoxic drugs

Drugs that are toxic to the ear ('oto-') and impair auditory and vestibular function, affecting hearing and balance either temporarily or permanently, are 'ototoxic'. The commonest groups of compounds are shown in Box 10.2.

The aminoglycoside group contains some very useful, albeit potentially toxic, antibiotics. They

Box 10.2 Drugs affecting auditory and/or vestibular function.

Commonly:
- Aminoglycoside antibiotics (e.g. gentamicin, tobramycin)
- Quinine and related compounds
- Salicylates (aspirin)
- Loop diuretics

Occasionally:
- Erythromycin
- Cisplatin
- Nitrogen mustard
- Practolol
- Ampicillin
- Tetanus antitoxin
- Naproxen
- Potassium bromate

are normally only used in very serious infections. Some, such as streptomycin, dihydrostreptomycin and neomycin, are predominantly toxic to the cochlea rather than to the vestibular system. Other risk factors for influencing toxicity include:

- concomitant exposure to other ototoxic drugs
- noise exposure
- duration of therapy
- total dose, plasma level and level in the perilymph
- age
- sex
- liver or renal dysfunction
- bacteraemia
- dehydration
- hyperthermia.

To minimise the risk of developing ototoxicity, efforts are made to keep blood plasma levels within a 'safe' range. The fact that the drugs continue to be used at all reflects their usefulness in certain clinical situations when their potential life-saving properties have to be weighed carefully against the risk of side-effects. Prospective studies have demonstrated some degree of hearing loss in 7–15% of patients receiving 'safe' doses of gentamicin and tobramycin. The hearing loss may progress after the treatment has been discontinued. The loss is usually in the high frequencies and may be unilateral or bilateral. In about half the patients, hearing recovers.

Much attention has been focused on the possibility of hearing loss resulting from the use of ear drops which contain aminoglycoside antibiotics. There should be no problem in patients with an intact eardrum, as the drops will not reach the inner ear. The situation is different if there is a hole in the drum or a grommet in place, allowing the drops to enter the middle ear. In these circumstances, the drops may reach the round window niche, where the only barrier between them and the inner ear is the round window membrane itself. In theory at least, the aminoglycoside could diffuse through the membrane, enter the inner ear and have a toxic effect. The evidence that this occurs in practice is extremely limited, especially when one considers the vast number of patients worldwide who take potentially ototoxic ear drops of this type in this manner. In the presence of active middle ear infection or inflammation, when the mucosa is swollen and oedematous, the medication may have difficulty diffusing through the round window membrane. In any event, such patients run a risk of developing inner ear dysfunction as a result of the infective process itself, and so treating this with aminoglycoside may be the lesser of two evils.

Current recommendations by ENT-UK (the professional association of UK ear, nose and throat (ENT) surgeons) are that when treating a patient with a discharging ear, in whom there is a perforation or patent grommet:

- if a topical aminoglycoside is used, this should only be in the presence of obvious infection
- topical aminoglycosides should be used for no longer than 2 weeks
- the justification for using topical aminoglycosides should be explained to the patient
- baseline audiometry should be performed, if possible or practical, before treatment begins.

Before using aminoglycoside drops, the necessity for the combination of steroid and antibiotic should be reviewed: is the antibiotic component necessary? Is there a bacterial infection present? In some situations, drops containing steroid alone may be equally appropriate. When infection is present, the infecting organism is often *Pseudomonas*, and topical ciprofloxacin, available in the form of eye drops, may be a reasonable alternative although not currently licensed for this indication in the UK.

Quinine and related compounds are used to treat malaria and night cramps. Toxic doses may produce a syndrome known as cinchonism. This includes deafness, tinnitus, vertigo, headache, nausea and visual disturbance. The auditory disturbances are usually temporary but may be permanent.

The salicylate group includes acetylsalicylic acid – aspirin. In high doses, it can produce deafness, tinnitus and occasionally vertigo. These changes are reversible.

Furosemide (formerly frusemide) and ethacrynic acid are 'loop diuretics' used to increase fluid excretion from the body. They may produce permanent or temporary hearing loss, the latter being more common. Patients most at risk are those with impaired renal function, and premature infants.

Reversible hearing loss, tinnitus and vertigo have been described with large doses of the macrolide antibiotic erythromycin. Several antineoplastic agents (cytotoxic drugs used in treating cancer) are ototoxic. Cisplatin has been used to treat a variety of malignancies. It produces an irreversible, high-frequency hearing loss related to the dose of drug administered. Tinnitus may be a warning sign of impending hearing loss.

Vestibular schwannoma – 'acoustic neuroma'

Tumours of the ear and temporal bone are not common. They are extremely important because prompt diagnosis and treatment are likely to lead to more favourable outcomes. For many years, the commonest tumour of the temporal bone, and hence the commonest tumour diagnosed by otologists, was known as an 'acoustic neuroma'. This name is in fact a misnomer; the tumour in

question arises not from the acoustic (cochlear) nerve but from the schwann cells covering the superior or inferior vestibular nerves. The preferred name is *vestibular schwannoma*.

Vestibular schwannomas account for between 6% and 10% of all intracranial tumours and 80–90% of all tumours in the cerebellopontine angle. They occur in approximately two people per 100,000 population per year. The tumours arise in the internal auditory canal and are slow-growing, benign tumours that do not infiltrate local tissues or spread to distant sites in the body. However, as they grow they compress adjacent tissues and produce their clinical effects in this way. These pressure effects may be serious because of the inability of the bony cranial cavity to expand. While they lie within the internal auditory canal, the tumours only affect the vestibular and cochlear nerves (the facial nerve is extremely resistant to pressure). When the tumour starts to grow out of the internal canal, it may press on the brainstem, producing a rise in intracranial pressure and, ultimately, death.

The reason why patients develop vestibular schwannomas is unknown in most cases. Men and women are affected equally and the mean age at diagnosis is about 50 years. The advent of an accurate and efficient means of diagnosing these tumours (the magnetic resonance imaging (MRI) scan, discussed below) may be responsible for an apparent increase in the 'incidence' of tumours noted in recent years. It is probable that a large number of tumours are asymptomatic and remain undiagnosed during a patient's lifetime. In the past, histopathological studies of temporal bones have shown tumours to be present in a much larger proportion of such bones than expected from the number of tumours diagnosed in the general population. This may be because many stop growing, or shrink without producing symptoms.

The most common clinical presentation is progressive unilateral sensorineural deafness, due to slow compression on the cochlear nerve. However, the hearing loss may be sudden in 15–25% of cases. Other features include unilateral or asymmetric tinnitus (occasionally the only symptom) or balance disturbance. The latter is often not a prominent feature and the only sign may be a sense of imbalance when, for example, moving and turning quickly. If the tumour becomes large, more sinister symptoms can develop: cerebellar symptoms of motor incoordination, pain or numbness in the face, headaches, double vision and vomiting due to raised intracranial pressure.

The audiogram classically shows asymmetrical sensorineural hearing loss that is worse in the higher frequencies. Usually there is a difference of at least 15 dB between the thresholds of the two ears at 1, 2 and 4 kHz; sometimes the difference is much smaller. Speech discrimination is reduced to a greater degree than would be expected from the audiogram. Occasionally the audiogram appears normal. The 'gold standard' diagnostic test is an MRI scan. The test is non-invasive and regarded as risk free because it does not use x-rays. However, the widespread use of MRI scanning as a screening test in patients with ear symptoms may have unintended consequences. Such is the sensitivity of the scan that, not infrequently, abnormalities are detected within the brain; so-called 'incidental findings'. These may result in undue anxiety for the patient and doctor when a decision has to be made about whether or not they need further investigation or treatment.

In the past, a range of audiovestibular tests were used as a screening tool to select those patients in whom MRI scanning might be most appropriate. Nowadays, in the UK, almost everyone with unilateral sensorineural hearing loss or tinnitus, or a unilateral vestibular weakness on balance testing, is offered an MRI scan.

The management of a patient with a vestibular schwannoma depends on the size of the tumour and the patient's general medical condition. In some patients it may be appropriate to monitor the growth of the tumour with regular scans and defer treatment, potentially indefinitely. Many centres now use this 'watch, wait and rescan' policy for smaller tumours. The factors that influence the growth rate of tumours are not well understood. The 'average' tumour (if such a thing exists) grows at a rate of 0.1–0.2 cm diameter per year, but 10–15% of tumours grow at more than 1 cm per year. In contrast, growth may be self-limiting in some patients, and a tumour may

even shrink. The arguments for operating on these tumours once they have been diagnosed are: firstly, that the rate of growth can be unpredictable; secondly, that the risk of surgical complications increases as the tumour grows; and thirdly, that as the patient becomes older they may be less able to withstand major surgery.

Radiotherapy treatment with the 'gamma knife' is another non-surgical option. This non-invasive technique is popular with many patients, and its proponents argue that the long-term results are as good as, or better than, surgery.

Surgical treatment aims to remove the tumour and prevent the risks associated with continued tumour growth. If the patient still has serviceable hearing, a secondary aim of surgery may be preservation of this, by leaving the cochlear nerve intact. Similarly, whenever possible, the function of the facial nerve should be preserved. The proximity of the nerve to the tumour (it may be intimately applied to it, even stretched over it) puts it at risk during surgery. Several different surgical techniques are available and the use of one rather than another depends on several factors, including the size of the tumour, the desirability of trying to preserve hearing and the experience of the surgical team. A team approach involving otologists specialising in this type of surgery, neurosurgeons, neuro-anaesthetists and intra-operative neurophysiological monitoring personnel is desirable.

Neurofibromatosis

Two related genetic disorders, neurofibromatosis types 1 (NF1) and 2 (NF2) are associated with vestibular schwannomas. NF1 is inherited as an autosomal dominant disorder, but sporadic cases are common. The clinical manifestations are variable but characteristically consist of 'café-au-lait' spots on the skin and multiple neurofibromas on peripheral nerves. Unilateral involvement of the cochleo-vestibular nerve occurs in probably less than 2% of patients. In contrast, in NF2, bilateral vestibular schwannomas are common. This disorder is autosomal dominant and is associated with other neoplasms of the central nervous system (especially meningiomas). The tumours develop in childhood or early adult life and are more aggressive than other vestibular schwannomas, growing rapidly and eroding and enveloping local tissues. Management of an individual patient with NF2 may be extremely taxing and require a series of difficult decisions on the part of the surgical team and of the patient and his or her family. Apart from the risks to life and health associated with the growth of existing (and potential future) tumours in the skull and spinal cord, there are the risks of bilateral damage to facial nerve function and of damage to hear-ing. Acquired sensorineural hearing loss is associated both with the tumours themselves and with their surgical removal. Genetic counselling is an important part of management of the affected patient.

Disorders of bone

Otosclerosis

This is a hereditary disorder in which the bone of the otic capsule (the hard, compact bone surrounding the structures of the inner ear) is replaced by bone of greater cellularity and vascularity. The presence of this abnormal bone at the edge of the oval window results in fixation of the stapes footplate within the window, and consequently a conductive hearing loss. There is contradictory evidence about the damage that otosclerosis may cause to the inner ear, with the production of a sensorineural hearing loss. Some authors have suggested that the abnormal bone produces toxins, which damage the inner ear; others have disputed this, stating that the sensorineural loss observed is no greater than one would expect in unaffected patients of the same age, etc. There is particular disagreement about the entity known as 'cochlear otosclerosis' – otosclerosis affecting the inner ear without signs and symptoms of fixation of the stapes. While this is recognised by some clinicians, there is little pathological evidence to support its existence.

Surgery may correct the conductive deafness (see Chapter 9) but it will not improve any co-existing sensorineural deafness. Moreover, profound sensorineural deafness is a potential complication, either at the time of surgery or many years later. The surgical procedure for otosclerosis is stapedectomy. Stapedectomy carries

a small risk of sensorineural deafness, because opening into the inner ear may lead to damage to the delicate structures therein.

Sensorineural deafness may occur many years after stapedectomy. Sometimes there is a definite history of barotrauma (see below); on other occasions the loss is apparently spontaneous. Various factors have been implicated, including a perilymph fistula through an area of deficient graft or secondary endolymphatic hydrops. When a potential fistula is present, the middle ear may be explored.

It will be clear from the above comments that all patients undergoing stapes surgery should be aware of the possibility of total sensorineural hearing loss following the procedure, especially since it is a purely elective one. What is the risk of sensorineural deafness following stapedectomy? A figure of 1–2% is widely quoted, but for most patients this may not be an accurate assessment of the risk they themselves run, as it refers to the past results of those international authorities who have published their own series. Some surgeons will have better results, others worse.

Osteogenesis imperfecta

Osteogenesis imperfecta is a disorder characterised by fragile bones, blue sclera of the eyes and deafness. This condition is due to defects in the synthesis of type I collagen – an important component of bone. It is quite distinct from otosclerosis, although the two conditions could co-exist. The diseased bone may obliterate the oval and round windows. Sensorineural hearing loss may develop.

Paget's disease

Paget's disease is a disorder of bone; it often presents late in life. The cause may be hereditary, or a slow virus of the paramyxovirus group may be responsible. Classically, the patient has an enlarged skull and a progressive kyphosis (curvature of the spine) resulting in a loss of stature, but more often a subclinical form of the disease is present. It is estimated to occur in 3–4% of individuals over 40 years old. The skull is involved in about 70% of cases of Paget's disease, and hearing is affected in 50% of these. The hearing loss is of a mixed type and several patho-logical processes have been advanced as potential causes. Given that the disease is not uncommon, the otological diagnosis of deafness due to Paget's disease is made rather infrequently. The under-lying disorder can be diagnosed on the basis of a skull radiograph and blood tests for alkaline phosphatase and determination of the level of hydroxyproline in the urine. Other features of Paget's disease include pain and neurological symptoms. These can be treated with aspirin or non-steroidal anti-inflammatory medication. The use of calcitonin and disodium etidronate may stabilise hearing loss in the long term.

Chronic otitis media

It is now thought to be rare for sensorineural hearing loss to result from uncomplicated chronic otitis media. However, active squamous chronic otitis media (cholesteatoma) may produce sen-sorineural deafness if the cholesteatoma erodes the bone of the otic capsule. The most usual site for this is the horizontal semicircular canal. The expanding cholesteatoma may produce a fistula into the canal by pressure erosion, or as a result of an erosive osteitis. Vertigo is the usual initial symptom, but deafness may ensue.

Sudden deafness with trauma

Ear surgery

The deafness that may follow stapedectomy surgery for otosclerosis has been discussed above. Sensorineural deafness may arise following any otological procedure, and the patient should be warned of this preoperatively. For some proce-dures the risk is extremely small.

Very little has been published about the risk of deafness following the most minimally invasive of procedures – insertion of a grommet (ventilation tube). Sensorineural deafness and otitis media with effusion often co-exist in young children, and occasionally it is not possible to quantify the degree of sensorineural loss until the effusion has been treated. The proportion of patients in whom sensorineural deafness following grommet insertion occurs as a direct

result of this procedure is undoubtedly extremely small. This risk must be balanced against the risk of patients with otitis media with effusion and/or recurrent acute otitis media acquiring such deafness as a result of their underlying disease.

The risk of sensorineural deafness from other surgical procedures on the ear depends on the nature of the procedure, the underlying disease and the skill of the surgeon. It is likely that the appropriately trained otologist will expect sen-sorineural deafness following a straightforward myringoplasty in fewer than 1% of cases. The risks are greater in mastoid surgery. The com-monest injury resulting in deafness is inadvertent opening into the horizontal semicircular canal. This is more likely to occur if the bony covering has been eroded by cholesteatoma and a fistula is present (see above). Over-manipulation of the ossicular chain may result in dislocation of the ossicles or subluxation or fracture of the stapes footplate. If a rotating burr being used to drill the mastoid comes into contact with an intact ossicular chain, the vibrations transmitted to the inner ear may produce a high-frequency sensorineural hearing loss.

While the risk of sensorineural deafness must always be considered prior to ear surgery, it takes on particular importance when the ear to be operated on is either the better-hearing or the only hearing ear. The potential benefits of surgery must be balanced carefully against the risks to the patient's overall hearing ability.

Head injury

It has been estimated that trauma to the temporal bone occurs in between 30% and 75% of head injuries. The temporal bone is very hard and dense, and a large amount of force is required to fracture it. For this reason, the majority of such fractures are associated with multiple injuries at other sites and, as such, the temporal bone frac-ture can easily be overlooked. Blunt trauma is the usual cause. A blow to the head that is severe enough to cause a fracture will almost certainly result in a period of loss of consciousness. Traditionally, temporal bone fractures have been divided into two types depending on the direction in which the fracture runs through the temporal bone. However, very few fit neatly into a particular category and the majority could probably be categorised as 'mixed'. Temporal bone fractures are diagnosed on the basis of high-resolution computerised tomography (CT) scan images.

Longitudinal temporal bone fractures result from blows to the side of the head. Clinical features include a conductive hearing loss (due to dislocation of parts of the ossicular chain with or without a tympanic membrane perforation) and bleeding from the ear. In about 15% of cases, there is temporary weakness of the face due to facial nerve involvement. Leakage of cerebrospinal fluid (CSF) is common because the fracture crosses the roof of the middle ear, but often subsides spontaneously. Sensorineural hearing loss affecting the high frequencies, and most severe at 4 kHz, is common. Some improvement may occur in the first 3 weeks after injury.

A transverse fracture crosses the axis of the temporal bone. It usually results from a blow to the back of the head. Bleeding from the ear is not common, but bleeding into the middle ear produces a haemotympanum. The facial nerve is torn in 50% of cases and produces paralysis of immediate onset. Profound sensorineural hearing loss and vertigo are common since the fracture passes through the inner ear. These may also be due to a perilymph leak (see below).

A head injury may result in damage to the inner ear without producing a temporal bone fracture. Both sensorineural deafness and imbalance can occur. The cause may be damage to the central nervous system or the inner ear itself. Even a relatively moderate blow may produce sensorineural deafness. It has also been suggested that Ménière's disease may arise in some cases as a long-term consequence of head injury. Other injuries around the head and ear may damage the inner ear, producing sensorineural deafness – foreign bodies poked into the ear may lead to disruption of the tympanic membrane and ossicular chain, and may produce subluxation or fracture of the stapes footplate with consequent perilymph leakage from the oval window.

Barotrauma

Barotrauma may occur when the ear is exposed to sudden pressure changes, such as those experienced when flying or diving. At sea level the ambient pressure is one atmosphere. In flight, as one ascends the pressure falls, halving with each 18,000 feet (about 5500 m) of ascent. In 'pressurised' aircraft, the cabin is usually pressurised to 8000 feet. When diving, the pressure increases by one atmosphere for every 33 feet (about 10 m) of descent. As pressure decreases during ascent when flying or diving, the volume of gas in the middle ear and mastoid increases. The pressure will be dissipated by the release of gas down the Eustachian tube into the nasopharynx unless there is total tubal obstruction. During descent, however, the reverse occurs and the volume of air in the middle ear decreases. If the Eustachian tube does not open, intense negative pressure in the middle ear results in the tympanic membrane, round window membrane and stapes footplate being pulled into the middle ear; swelling of the middle ear mucosa with bleeding or tissue fluid leakage also occurs. The tympanic membrane may rupture. A forceful Valsalva's manoeuvre in these circumstances will lead to an increase in CSF and perilymph pressure, and the pressure differential between the inner and middle ears will become even greater. Whether or not a Valsalva's manoeuvre has been performed, the round window membrane may rupture in these circumstances, producing a perilymph leak. Inner ear decompression sickness is another possible cause of audiovestibular dysfunction following diving, if a diver rises to the surface too quickly. The damage may be related to gas-bubble formation or hypercoagulation within the inner ear.

Blast injury

A nearby explosion may produce a blast injury as a result of the high intensity of noise and the shock wave. The damage occurs as the pressure rises in the ear: the rapidity of this rise seems important. Pressure changes of less than one atmosphere may produce damage. Sensorineural deafness following blast injuries can range from total deafness in one or both ears, to a relatively minor high-frequency loss; some degree of spontaneous recovery may occur.

Perilymph fistula

A perilymph fistula is an abnormal communication between the perilymphatic space and the middle ear. The usual sites are (a) a defect in the round window membrane or (b) a breach in the ligament between the stapes footplate and the oval window itself. The leakage of perilymph (which may also be associated with the entry of air into the inner ear) is usually associated with sensorineural deafness and vestibular symptoms of sudden onset.

Fistulas are discussed in this section because there is little disagreement about their existence as a result of certain types of trauma. Postoperative fistulae have been discussed. Direct trauma to the ossicular chain (from a cotton bud poked into the ear canal for example), or indirect trauma to the head, may produce a fracture or dislocation of the stapes and consequent leak. There are patients with congenital abnormalities of the middle ear in whom recurrent meningitis arises as a consequence of a congenital fistula. In all these cases, exploration of the middle ear and the plugging of any defect with soft tissue are appropriate.

Controversy surrounds the concept that more minor trauma, such as mild barotrauma or the trauma associated with physical exertions such as straining, lifting, coughing, laughing, vomiting, etc, may produce a fistula. Still more controversial is the notion that a 'spontaneous perilymph fistula', unprecipitated by any stress, can be a cause of sudden sensorineural deafness. If there is a clear history of a sudden onset of sensorineural deafness and vertigo occurring synchronously with an episode of exertion, it seems reasonable to entertain the diagnosis. The author is much more sceptical about the concept of spontaneous fistulae. When the diagnosis is in doubt, a period of conservative treatment is advised. This should comprise bed rest with the head raised. A significant proportion of cases will settle spontaneously. Progression of symptoms or failure to improve should prompt consideration of surgical exploration.

Sudden deafness without trauma

Sudden sensorineural deafness is a medical emergency. Unfortunately this is not always appreciated, and patients often present late for specialist treatment. Patients who are suspected of suffering sudden sensorineural deafness, or in whom conductive deafness has been excluded by tuning fork tests, should be referred urgently to an otolaryngology clinic.

Sudden sensorineural hearing loss has been defined as 30 dB or more loss in three contiguous audiometric frequencies occurring within 3 days or less. A slower loss is termed 'rapidly progressive'. In some cases, the cause of the hearing loss is immediately apparent, such as those described above in association with trauma. The deafness may also be a presenting feature of an acoustic neuroma or may mark an initial attack of Ménière's disease. There are many case reports and short series describing sudden hearing loss in a variety of systemic disorders affecting the vascular, haematological, immune, metabolic and skeletal systems. The imputed cause of deafness is cochlear damage. Similarly, there is a long list of disorders of the peripheral and central nervous system in which sensorineural deafness has arisen. However, there remains a large group in whom no cause can be found, and this hearing loss is termed 'idiopathic' (see below). It will be appreciated that this is a diagnosis of exclusion and one that can only be reached after a comprehensive series of investigations has excluded other causes.

Infections

Bacterial infection of the inner ear (labyrinthitis) is an uncommon complication of acute otitis media when infection spreads into the labyrinth. In contrast, serous labyrinthitis occurs when bacterial toxins spread to the labyrinth. The characteristic clinical features are sensorineural hearing loss and vertigo, which recovers partially or completely as the infection subsides.

Bacterial meningitis may be a complication of otitis media or sinus disease, but in many cases the disease follows an upper respiratory tract infection and the mechanism by which the offending organism reaches the meninges is unknown. Meningitis can lead to sensorineural deafness when the labyrinth is infected. It is one of the commonest causes of severe or profound acquired deafness in infants and children. The pathway by which the infection spreads is usually via the cochlear aqueduct, but it may be through the internal auditory canal. The deafness is usually bilateral and may be associated with other problems, such as mental disability, blindness, epilepsy, spasticity and ataxia. In young children, the risk of developing these complications is greater *the younger the child*, and the more prolonged the delay in treatment. The prognosis is also dependent on the causative organism, *Meningococcus* and *Pneumococcus* infection having a particularly bad prognosis. The incidence of hearing impairment following meningitis has been estimated at between 4% and 40%. Ossification of the basal turn of the cochlea often follows meningitis, and in cochlear implant surgery will complicate insertion of the electrode into the cochlea. This process continues even after the hearing has been destroyed.

Many cases of acute deafness or vertigo or both cannot be attributed to a specific cause, and a viral infection is often implicated. This is partly because, on many occasions, upper respiratory symptoms or an influenzal type of illness are associated with the episode. When viral labyrinthitis does occur, it can involve the inner ear or the audiovestibular nerves. The symptoms and the resulting long-term deficits may affect the cochlea or labyrinth or both, producing deafness or vertigo alone or together.

The effects of some *viruses* have been more clearly defined. Herpes zoster oticus (Ramsay Hunt syndrome) is caused by the virus that also causes chickenpox. The main features are facial weakness on the same side as a severe pain in the ear. Vesicles can be seen in the ear canal. In the current context, this infection is important because sensorineural deafness, tinnitus and vestibular symptoms may also occur. The hearing loss is usually high frequency and, unless severe, some recovery is usual. Treatment is with appropriate antiviral agents such as acyclovir, with or without steroids.

Measles and mumps (childhood illnesses caused by paramyxoviruses) are both associated with sensorineural deafness. In measles, the loss is usually moderate to profound and bilateral. In mumps, bilateral loss is extremely uncommon, the patient usually developing a unilateral loss varying from a mild high-frequency loss to profound deafness. There does not appear to be a relationship between the severity of the mumps and the development of hearing loss. Encephalitis may complicate both measles and mumps. In the former, the chance of developing hearing loss is increased. The prognosis for the latter is better and carries no greater risk of deafness. There can be little doubt as to the cause of hearing loss or vertigo when these symptoms develop during the course of an infection, and the latter is confirmed by rising titres of antibodies in the bloodstream. However, it is not uncommon for a patient (often a child or teenager) to present with unilateral profound deafness and a past history of mumps. In these circumstances, it is difficult to be categorical about the cause of the deafness. Many other viruses have been implicated as causes of sensorineural deafness, including herpes simplex, Epstein–Barr virus, influenza and parainfluenza viruses.

There is a high prevalence of otological symptoms, including sensorineural hearing loss, vertigo, tinnitus and aural fullness, in patients with HIV infection and AIDS. These patients often receive multiple medical therapies, some of which may be ototoxic, and are also prone to opportunistic infections.

'Idiopathic sudden sensorineural hearing loss'

About half of the patients who experience sudden deafness, and in whom no cause is found, also experience some vestibular symptoms. In about one-third of patients, spontaneous recovery occurs. If this happens it normally does so in the first 2 weeks. One-third have a partial recovery and one-third have no recovery. Unfavourable prognostic features include a severe loss, a downwards sloping audiogram showing a high-frequency loss, and the presence of vertigo.

Several possible causes of idiopathic sudden sensorineural hearing loss (ISSNHL) have been suggested. A viral aetiology is near the top of the list. Reduced cochlear blood flow due to vascular spasm or micro-emboli is another popular hypothesis.

The patient with ISSNHL is often extremely distressed, particularly if the loss is severe. They are often worried that they may have some sinister intracranial problem and are anxious about the future, especially about losing their hearing altogether. The focus of any investigations is the exclusion of a treatable underlying cause. A number of blood tests are usually recommended, but the yield of these is not great. A 'standard' battery of tests might include a full blood count and erythrocyte sedimentation rate (ESR), syphilis serology, random glucose, thyroid function tests, serum lipids and possibly viral titres. An MRI scan should be obtained to exclude a vestibular schwannoma or the demyelination of nerve fibres that occurs in multiple sclerosis.

Treatment is often initiated before all the test results are available. There are no high-quality randomised controlled trials with conclusive results on which to base a rational treatment protocol. Many different regimens have been proposed. As the patient must implicitly accept any risks of the treatment proposed, the empirical nature of the treatment should be made clear during the process of obtaining consent to it. No matter which treatment strategy is followed, it is mandatory to follow the patient up and arrange the appropriate auditory rehabilitation for those whose hearing does not improve. The medical treatments with the greatest 'acceptance' in the UK, and which the author favours include:

- a short course of oral steroids (e.g. enteric-coated prednisolone 60 mg/day for 3 days, then 45 mg/day for 3 days, then 30 mg/day for 3 days, then 15 mg/day for 3 days, then stop)
- betahistine hydrochloride (Serc) 16 mg three times a day
- an antiviral agent such as acyclovir.

Treatment should be initiated as soon as possible after the hearing is lost, and certainly within 2–3 weeks. Treatment after this time is less likely to be rewarding.

Immunological hearing loss

There is still not widespread acceptance that immunological mechanisms are responsible for deafness, and the diagnosis of 'autoimmune inner ear disease' remains controversial. The term covers a variety of different clinical syndromes in which cell-mediated or humoral-mediated mechanisms produce inner ear dysfunction. Two distinct types are recognised: organ-specific and non-organ-specific. The former relies on establishing the presence of auto-antibodies or cell-mediated immune responses directed against inner ear antigens, resulting in inner ear disease. A clinical syndrome comprising rapidly progressive bilateral sensorineural deafness occasionally associated with dizziness has been described and attributed to such a process.

Non-organ-specific autoimmune inner ear disease is diagnosed in patients with a similar clinical presentation, but in whom a systemic immune disease co-exists. The disorders in question include polyarteritis nodosa, Wegener's granulomatosis, Behçet's syndrome, relapsing polychondritis, systemic lupus erythematosus and rheumatoid arthritis. Cogan's syndrome is a disorder of young adults characterised by interstitial keratitis and audiovestibular dysfunction. Acute episodes of hearing loss associated with tinnitus and vertigo progress over a period of a few months to total deafness. 'Atypical Cogan's syndrome' is a term used to describe similar audiovestibular symptoms but with ocular problems other than keratitis, such as episcleritis, uveitis or conjunctivitis. The importance of recognising cases of autoimmune inner ear disease lies in the possibility of treating those patients with immunosuppressive medication. In the future, the development of clear diagnostic criteria (in particular the advent of a simple serological test which is both sensitive and specific) may lead to the appropriate randomised controlled trials to determine the most effective treatment.

Summary

This chapter has provided an overview of the main causes of acquired sensorineural deafness.

In the future it is likely that both causes and treatments will change. Some infective causes will become less common because of immunisation. Traumatic causes should be reduced by the wearing of seat belts in cars and crash helmets on motor cycles. Some causes, like syphilis, may nearly disappear but then resurface. The aetiology of deafness is markedly different between developing countries and the developed ones. In the future it is likely that the use of drugs, stem cells and other techniques may be effective in repairing the damaged cochlear hair cells and their nerves. Much experimental work is taking place, and although many practical difficulties remain, these should eventually be overcome, to introduce major new therapies for those with acquired sensorineural deafness.

Genetic causes of hearing and balance disorders

11

Henry Pau and Sarah Healy

Introduction

With the exception of identical twins, no two people are exactly the same. Differences between individuals are determined by our genes, inherited from our parents, as well as our environment. Genes encode the entire repertoire of proteins needed for normal human development and function, with each cell containing the entire complement of genes.

Genetic material consists of the molecule DNA, deoxyribonucleic acid, which is a double helical molecule. The DNA is wound around histone proteins, and then coiled, supercoiled and condensed into chromosomes, which are visible using a conventional light microscope. An individual has two copies of every gene, one maternally and one paternally inherited, each situated on a pair of chromosomes. The only exception to this is genes on the sex chromosomes, where only a single copy of some genes exists in males.

Members of the same family will have a similar genetic makeup. This is because the parents will have passed some of their own genetic information down to their children. However, the combination of genes handed down, or 'inherited'

will vary, and so each of their children will be different. Genes are stored on long strands called *chromosomes* within body cells. Each chromosome will contain many genes along its length, made up of the nucleotide, DNA, the building blocks of all living things. The information contained in each gene is called the *genotype*, while the physical appearance such as eye colour is called the *phenotype*. Genes are very important, not only because they determine how we look, but also because they can increase the risk of being born with a disease, or developing an illness as we get older. Genetics are therefore critical for our future health and survival. We inherit 23 chromosomes from each parent, giving a total of 46 chromosomes paired together. The total number of human genes is between 20,000 and 25,000.

Genes can be faulty because of a mistake or 'mutation' in the genetic information. Mutations can occur as an error when cells divide and multiply in the growing foetus, or can be passed down in faulty genes from the parents. Mutations can have beneficial effects. For example, if a species of butterfly usually has green wings, a change in the genetic information could result in the offspring developing brown wings. This would provide better camouflage from predators and so would improve the butterfly's chance of survival, which is the basis of natural selection and evolution. Mutations of this kind may be beneficial for the individual and the species concerned, or may simply be neutral in this respect.

However, this is not always the case, and some mutations can be harmful. Genetic mutations are an important process in the aetiology of many medical conditions, such as cystic fibrosis and Down's syndrome. This can be illustrated by imagining genes as building bricks which, when stacked together, build a house that is strong and sturdy. A mutation or fault in one of the bricks making it a different shape will not only affect that brick, but may make the entire house less stable. In this way, faulty genes which alter the development of a particular organ or tissue can have dramatic effects on the person and their health.

In some cases, the defective gene causes such a major abnormality that the affected individual does not survive long enough to reproduce. In this case the mutation dies out. Other effects, such as deafness, do not affect survival and the ability to reproduce, so may be passed on to the next generation.

Deafness is a common childhood problem and affects 1:800 newborns (Fortnum *et al.*, 2001). Hereditary deafness occurs when defective genes responsible for the development of hearing are passed from parent to child. The child will then suffer from deafness due to the genetic mutation. If deafness is the only inherited abnormality, it may be called non-syndromic deafness. If other inherited conditions are found together with the hearing impairment, this is called syndromic deafness. Several distinct syndromes exist which include some form of deafness (Table 11.1) (Van Camp and Smith, 2008).

We have two of each chromosome in our cells, one from each parent, arranged in pairs, and, as mentioned above, genes are stored on the chromosomes. This means that for each gene, we will have two copies or *alleles*, one on each paired chromosome. Genes can be inherited in a variety of ways:

- if John, who has a gene resulting in deafness, marries Jane, who has normal hearing, their children will also be deaf if they inherit the faulty gene from their father. This will happen even although they inherit a normal gene from their mother. This is *autosomal dominant* inheritance and requires only one mutant gene to be passed to the offspring for the effect or disease to be seen. The odds of this happening are one in two

- Jack and Jill are both normal hearing adults. They have four children, one of whom is deaf. This is because both Jack and Jill have one faulty gene out of the pair of hearing genes. For one child to be deaf, they must inherit a faulty gene from each parent. This is an example of *autosomal recessive* inheritance. In this case a person needs to have two copies of the defective gene to inherit deafness. The odds of this happening are one in four. If a child inherits only one mutated gene they will not be deaf. They will be a *carrier* for the abnormality and could pass this gene on to their children. The odds of being a carrier are one in two when both parents have a copy of the defective gene

- there are particular chromosomes that code for our sex. These are paired, as are all chromosomes, one from each parent. Females have the genotype XX, while males are XY. Some abnormal genes are 'sex-linked' and are only found on the X chromosome. If, for example, Jenny carries an abnormal gene for deafness on one of her X chromosomes, she would not suffer from the disease because she has another 'normal' X chromosome. However, if she passes her affected X chromosome to her son Jake, he will be deaf.

Interestingly, genetic mutations can cause either 'congenital' deafness which is present from birth, or else predispose to progressive hearing loss with age (see below). Identifying these particular genes and their effects is important in understanding and managing genetic forms of deafness.

At present, 39 autosomal recessive genes, 51 autosomal dominant genes and 8 X-linked genes have been reported to cause deafness (Van Camp and Smith, 2008).

Table 11.1 Syndromes that include some form of deafness.

Syndrome	Causative genes	Clinical presentations
Alport syndrome	*COL4A5, COL4A3, COL4A4*	Sensorineural hearing loss, renal and eye disorders
Branchio-oto-renal syndrome	*EYA1*	Deafness and abnormal neck lumps/clefts, pinnae and renal function
Norrie syndrome	Norrin	Early blindness, progressive deafness, developmental delay and mental retardation
Pendred syndrome	*SLC26A4*	Goitre and abnormal thyroid function, deafness and large vestibular aqueduct
Stickler syndrome	*COL2A1, COL11A2, COL11A1*	Craniofacial abnormalities, small jaw, large tongue, eye abnormalities, deafness
Treacher Collins syndrome	*TCOF1*	Craniofacial abnormalities, conductive hearing loss, visual disorder
Usher syndrome	*MYO7A, USH1C, CDH23, PCDH15, USH2A, USH3*	Visual disorder/blindness, sensorineural hearing loss
Pfeiffer syndrome, Kallmann syndrome, craniosynostosis	*FGFR1*	Craniofacial abnormalities, deafness, dental problems, short fingers and toes
Waardenburg syndrome	*PAX3, MITF, SLUG, EDNRB, EDN3, SOX10*	Deafness, white forelock, different coloured eyes (irises)
Jervell and Lange-Nielsen syndrome	*KVLQT1, KCNE1 (IsK)*	Deafness and abnormal heart rhythm
Maternally inherited diabetes and deafness (MIDD)	*tRNALeu, tRNALys, tRNAGlu*	Deafness and diabetes
Mitochondrial encephalopathy, lactic acidosis and stroke-like episodes (MELAS)	*tRNALeu*	Muscle weakness, heart failure, deafness, visual disorder, sudden infant death syndrome, developmental delay
Myoclonic epilepsy and ragged red fibres (MERRF)	*tRNALys, tRNALeu*	Similar to MELAS
Kearns–Sayre syndrome (KSS)	Several tRNA genes	Neuromuscular disorder, deafness, heart block, ataxia
Progressive myoclonic epilepsy, ataxia and hearing impairment	*tRNASer*	Similar to KSS

Embryological development of the external, middle and inner ear

The ear is divided into the outer ear, comprising the pinna and external auditory canal, the middle ear extending from the tympanic membrane to include the ossicles, and the inner ear housing the cochlea and semicircular canals.

The outer ear

The pinna is formed by a gradual fusion of the first and second branchial arches, while a deep-ening groove between the arches gives rise to the external ear canal. The development of the outer ear is controlled by genes responsible for the specification of the first and second branchial arches. This process is mediated by the hindbrain. Therefore, mutations in genes that control the hindbrain can cause abnormalities in the normal development of the outer ear (Fekete and Wu, 2002).

The middle ear

The embryological origins of the middle ear are diverse. The tympanic membrane has three layers formed by the linings of the external ear canal and middle ear cavity, with a central fibrous layer between. A central role of the development of the tympanic membrane is played by the tympanic ring, which is a C-shaped membranous bone that develops from the midbrain and hindbrains and provides physical support to the tympanic membrane.

The ossicles – the malleus, incus and stapes – are small bones that conduct sound from the tympanic membrane across the middle ear and are derivatives of the neural crest cells of the hindbrain. The timing of migration of the neural crest cells that will form each of the different middle ear components follows a typical sequence. The first to migrate are those contributing to the head of the malleus, followed by those forming the body of the incus. The next to migrate are hindbrain crest cells, contributing to the stapedial footplate. The crest cells that make the tympanic ring and the handle of malleus start their migration shortly after this, followed by cells that form the stapedial arch and those contributing to the neck of the malleus. The last cells to migrate form the long process of the incus. This process involves more than just the formation of individual components. They have to be connected in a specific and orderly fashion so that the middle ear can function properly. The insertion of the handle of the malleus between the two epithelial layers of the tympanic membrane relies on the proper formation of the external ear canal. The handle of the malleus can be formed even in the absence of most of the malleus, provided that the external ear canal is present. Connections between these structures are reliant upon genetic information, and any mutations will affect the ability of the ossicles to function effectively, therefore impairing hearing (Mallo, 2001).

The inner ear

During embryonic development, the inner ear forms from a simple epithelium adjacent to the hindbrain called the otic placode. This then folds to form the otic cup, which gives rise to the cochlear and vestibular neurons. The otic cup then pinches off to form a hollow ball of cells called the otic vesicle or the otocyst. The inner ear then enlarges to assume its final shape.

The inner ear contains the cochlea, which develops from a portion of the otocyst. The cochlea reaches its final shape of two and a half turns by the twenty-fifth week of embryonic life in humans (Wright, 1997). The organ of Corti develops from the cochlear duct and contains the inner and outer hair cells, which are involved in the transmission of sound. The inner ear also houses the vestibular apparatus: the semicircular canals, which are important in the control of balance (Martin and Swanson, 1993). It has been demonstrated in humans that the lateral semicircular canal is the most commonly affected part of the vestibule in congenital abnormalities (Jackler *et al.*, 1987). A mouse model for this defect has been established recently for future research purposes, as outlined above (Pau *et al.*, 2004).

Types of deafness

Clinically, deafness is divided into conductive, sensorineural or mixed hearing loss. Conductive hearing loss is due to abnormalities of the outer or middle ear, which affect the conduction of sound to the inner ear. This can include wax or a foreign body in the external ear canal, a middle ear effusion and defects of the ossicles, for example ossicular discontinuity or otosclerosis. Most sensorineural hearing loss (SNHL) is due to abnormalities of the inner ear involving the organ of hearing, the cochlea, resulting in disruption of the transmission of sound to the brain. Mixed hearing loss, as the name suggests, has both sensorineural and conductive components.

Hereditary inner ear deafness can be further divided into three groups: morphogenetic, cochleosaccular and neuroepithelial. *Morphogenetic* deafness results from abnormal development of the ear, leading to an anatomical malformation, and only occurs in 15–29% of profoundly deaf humans (Steel, 1995). This is because the genes involved in the development of the ear are also important for many other areas of development in the foetus. Mutations in these genes are therefore likely to have such severe consequences that they result in antenatal death. *Cochleosaccular* deafness refers to abnormalities in the stria vascularis, a layer of cells which produce and regulate endolymph for the scala media, one of the three fluid-filled compartments of the cochlea. The third and probably most common type of inner ear deafness is *neuroepithelial*, which is caused by defects in the organ of Corti within the cochlea. This contains the hair cells responsible for the first step in the pathway to translate sound information into messages carried by nerve impulses.

Investigation of suspected genetic congenital deafness

The parents of a recently diagnosed congenitally deaf child are likely to want to know why their child is deaf. In some cases there is a clearly defined non-genetic reason, for example an intra-uterine infection such as rubella or cytomegalo-virus infection, meningitis soon after birth, or episodes of low oxygen in the blood associated with prematurity. In developed countries, such 'extrinsic' causes are relatively uncommon. When there is no obvious extrinsic reason for the child to be deaf, a genetic cause may well be likely. More than 50% of cases of early-onset, non-syndromic sensorineural hearing loss are attributable to genetic causes (Siemering *et al.*, 2006). www.hearing.screening.nhs.uk/getdata.php?id= 149 is a website that contains protocols for the aetiological investigation of a deaf child.

There are several other reasons for the parents' desire to know the cause of deafness:

- they will want to know the risks of deafness if they have more children
- if the deafness is not profound they will want to know the risks of it becoming worse
- they may want to know whether the child may have any other problems linked to the deafness, in other words if the child may have a syndrome linked to deafness
- a deaf child, at a later age, may want to know the risk of having deaf children.

Naturally the initial focus will be in defining the degree of hearing loss, but then the child should be examined to identify any other visible abnormalities. The parents should be asked whether they know of other family members with hearing problems, especially dating from childhood. The parents themselves will usually be offered hearing tests. Assuming that neither parent has a hearing loss, which would suggest an autosomal dominant inheritance of the deafness, further investigations will be arranged, particularly to exclude syndromes associated with deafness (see Table 11.1):

- an electrocardiogram, to exclude Jervell and Lange-Nielsen syndrome
- an ophthalmic appointment, to exclude syndromes associated with visual defects
- an electroretinogram in children who present with severe or profound deafness and delay in motor development, in order to make a presymptomatic diagnosis of type 1 Usher syndrome
- an ultrasound of the kidneys, in children with ear pits or other malformations, to exclude branchio-oto-renal syndrome
- imaging of the temporal bone, to identify morphogenic cochlear malformations, including widening of the vestibular aqueduct, which would suggest Pendred's syndrome (see Chapter 8).

An appointment with a clinical genetics department should be offered to discuss the above issues. In addition, the geneticist will ask about other conditions, including hearing loss in the extended family, and will draw the family tree.

- Here the child will be examined, to look for evidence of any syndrome. There are very many syndromes that include deafness. The commonest include abnormal pigmentation, cysts and sinuses in the neck, abnormalities in the shape of the external ears, and disorders of vision.
- The geneticist will be able to estimate the risk of deafness in subsequent pregnancies and will explain to the family how this risk is estimated (based on inheritance of a known

syndromic or non-syndromic cause of deafness, or based on empirical data where the cause is not known).

- Genetic testing will be performed. Blood samples are sent to a genetics laboratory to screen for known genetic abnormalities associated with deafness, where clinically indicated. Approximately 20% of cases of genetic deafness are attributable to an abnormal dominant gene and 80% to a recessive gene.

This will usually allow the risk of further pregnancies resulting in a deaf baby to be calculated. Clearly if the cause is a dominant gene, the risks, as shown above, will be 1 in 2 if one parent carries the affected gene. If a recessive form of inheritance is likely, the risk will be 1 in 4 of the child having the disease, and both parents will be 'carriers' of the genetic mutation which causes deafness.

The genetic basis of hearing loss

There are now a large number of genes known to cause deafness, although many of these cannot be routinely tested for on a diagnostic basis, unless they are a common cause of deafness. http://webh01.ua.ac.be/hhh is the homepage of the website of the Hereditary Hearing Loss, listing the currently known genes that cause recessive and dominant congenital deafness. The genes are usually listed by locus (position on the chromosome), then the name of the gene, then the protein, or other cell constituent the gene is normally responsible for. Loci of recessive genes are classified as DFNB, then a number, denoting the order in time in which they were discovered. Loci of dominant genes are classified as DFNA, followed by a comparable number. At present 21 dominant genes and 23 recessive ones that cause inherited deafness have been identified. Dominant genes are responsible for about 20% of cases of inherited deafness, recessive genes for about 80%.

The commonest gene responsible for recessive hearing loss, the connexin gene *GJB2*, is found at a locus named DBNB1 on chromosome 13

and is responsible for the creation of 'gap junctions' (hence 'GJ') between neighbouring cells, involving the protein Connexin 26. These gap junctions form channels that allow chemicals, such as potassium, to flow from one cell to another. If they are absent, because the connexin 26 gene is faulty (defects in this gene are responsible for 30–50% of cases of recessive deafness in Caucasians and some other populations), the gap junctions between the supporting cells, which lie next to the hair cells on the basilar membrane, do not form properly. This has a damaging effect on the chemical composition of endolymph, and so on the functioning of the cochlea. Other examples of recessive genes include the *OTOF* gene, which is responsible for the correct functioning of the synapse between the inner hair cells and the cochlear nerve, and the gene responsible for the protein Pendrin, in which mutations cause Pendred syndrome: deafness associated with widening of the vestibular aqueduct and thyroid malfunction.

The genetics of age-related hearing loss

The genetics of age-related hearing loss (ARHL) in humans are much more poorly defined than for congential deafness, and no associated genes or loci have yet been identified. The available data do, however, implicate genetic factors in ARHL. Evidence has been gleaned from a study of 557 male twin pairs aged 36–80 years, ascertained from the Swedish Twin Registry. Similarity in audiogram thresholds was consistently greater for monozygotic *versus* dizygotic twins in all age ranges, but particularly so in the youngest group. These findings were interpreted as showing that genetic and environmental factors are important sources of variation in hearing at all ages, with genetic factors being particularly important for the younger men (Karlsson *et al.*, 1997). Additionally a family-based case-control study examined members of the Framingham Heart Study and Framingham Offspring Study cohorts. The authors (Gates *et al.*, 1999) compared audiometric hearing threshold data from people who were genetically related (siblings or parent–child) with those who were not (spouse pairs). A familial aggregation of ARHL was demonstrated.

Mouse genetic studies strongly indicate that genetic factors can be important in ARHL. Many different inbred mouse strains show accelerated ARHL, and in at least 10 of these the gene involved is *ahl*, which maps to mouse chromosome 10. This gene is inherited in a recessive pattern. At least two other mouse age-related hearing loss loci, designated *ahl2* and *ahl3*, exist), with *alh2* mapped to mouse chromosome 5.

Using mouse mutant models in understanding human genetic deafness

In order to identify the gene that causes a particular type of deafness, you must first locate the mutation on the affected chromosome. This is the technique of 'genetic mapping'. In human populations, this is complicated by the fact that it is difficult to diagnose the cause in many types of deafness, especially non-syndromic deafness where there are no associated features. To minimise the grouping together of cases of deafness in which the causative gene may be different, genetic mapping must be done on 'isolated' populations where there has been no movement of people in or out of the group (Kiernan and Steel, 2000). This means that the variation in mutations found will be minimal, and so any genetic abnormalities can be attributed to a select few mutations. To a certain degree, this approach has been successful in that researchers have been able to localise over 100 non-syndromic forms of deafness (Van Camp and Smith, 2008). However, the step between locating a gene on a part of the chromosome and actually identifying the mutated gene is extremely difficult.

The mouse appears to be the best model for understanding genetic hearing and balance defects in humans, for several reasons. Firstly, because large numbers of mice can be produced which all carry the same mutation, it is easier to pinpoint the region of the chromosome where the mutation can be found. This makes the mouse a powerful tool for genetic identification. Due to genetic similarities between mice and humans,

the mutated genes can be positioned and identified in the mouse, and the corresponding human genes can be identified and checked for possible mutations. Secondly, the mouse cochlea is structurally very similar to that of humans. Both mice and humans have common inner ear disorders, and in some cases, the same gene is involved in causing deafness in both species, a so-called *orthologous* gene. As our understanding and ability to manipulate mouse genes has evolved, it has become the most appropriate specimen to use for identifying mutated genes and in the production of potential models for therapeutic interventions. Finally, the mouse is particularly useful in embryological and developmental studies. Physiological tests can be carried out on anaesthetised mice, which provide vital clues to the basis of dysfunction but could not ethically be carried out in humans.

Researchers in Munich have used a substance called *N*-ethyl-*N*-nitrosourea (ENU) (Hrabé de Angelis *et al.*, 2000) to produce mutations in mice. This allows scientists to study a gene's normal functions and the physiological consequences when mutated, making it ideal for modelling human diseases (Noveroske *et al.*, 2000). Two of these mouse mutants were called Flouncer and Hush Puppy. The flouncer mice were used to breed further animals which could be used to identify dominant and semi-dominant characteristics or 'phenotypic' traits.

So far, over 150 mouse mutants have been identified with auditory abnormalities, and the genes responsible for their mutations have been identified in less than half of them. Over 400 human syndromes are associated with some form of deafness, but the location of the mutation has only been found for about 200 syndromes (Online Mendelian Inheritance in Man (OMIM), 2003). To date, causative genes of only 17 syndromes have been identified (Van Camp and Smith, 2008).

The Flouncer mutation was produced by a large scale ENU mutagenesis programme and the flouncer mouse carrying this mutation was identified by its circling and hyperactivity behaviour. The circling behaviour is associated with constriction of the lateral semicircular canal, and the mutation is found on chromosome 4. Minor, variable anomalies of ossicles and hair cell numbers in parts of the cochlear duct were also observed, although these are unlikely to affect function significantly and the mice respond to sound, so are not deaf.

Embryonically, the first two semicircular canals to develop are the superior and posterior ones, whereas the lateral canal develops separately. Analysis of the inner ear of the Flouncer mutants revealed various degrees of abnormality of the lateral semicircular canal, ranging from pinching off to complete constriction. It has been suggested that in other mutants with a similar inner ear malformation, there is an error in the information determining the portion of the canal that should remain unfused, resulting in abnormal narrowing of the canal (Kiernan *et al.*, 2002). These mutations map to a region of mouse chromosome 4 that shows some correspondence with human chromosomes 6 and 8 (http://www.informatics.jax.org/).

The lateral semicircular canal has been described to be the most commonly affected part of the inner ear in humans (Jackler *et al.*, 1987), and Flouncer provides a mouse model for genetic analysis of such defects. It also raises the possibility that the same chromosomal location may be susceptible to mutation in humans and in the mouse. Once the gene carrying this mutation is identified, its human homologous counterpart can then be investigated.

A group of patients have been described that have 'Tumarkin falls' (sudden drop-attack falls secondary to vertigo spells) but with clinically normal hearing. They may have a similar phenotype (abnormal lateral semicircular canal) to the Flouncer mouse mutant, and in these cases it would be useful to perform three-dimensional high-resolution magnetic resonance imaging of their inner ears to investigate the morphology of the semicircular canals (Arnold *et al.*, 1996).

Balance disorders (see also Chapter 24)

Hereditary hearing disorders are often associated with vestibular, or balance problems. Unilateral

and bilateral vestibular dysfunction is found in over 30% of patients with congenital autosomal dominant hearing loss (Konigsmark and Gorlin, 1976; Huygen *et al.*, 1993). Thirty-one per cent of patients with congenital autosomal dominant unilateral deafness demonstrate ipsilateral vestibular dysfunction (Konigsmark and Gorlin, 1976). Autosomal recessive sensorineural hearing loss is also associated with unilateral vestibular abnormalities (Mengel *et al*, 1969; McLeod *et al*, 1973; Konigsmark and Gorlin, 1976; Huygen *et al.*, 1993). It has been reported that progressive mixed hearing loss is accompanied by unilateral or bilateral vestibular loss (Cremers and Huygen, 1983; Cremers *et al.*, 1985). Congenital and syndromic deafness including Waardenburg's syndrome, Pendred's syndrome, albinism deafness syndrome, congenital hearing loss with onychodystrophy, Klippel–Feil syndrome, Wildervanck syndrome, Albers-Schönberg disease, Usher syndrome, Wolfram syndrome, Alport syndrome, otosclerosis, osteogenesis imperfecta, progressive vestibulocochlear dysfunction with high-tone sensorineural deafness, hereditary sensory radicular neuropathy with sensorineural hearing loss, and familial acoustic neuroma have been reported to be associated with vestibular disorders (Phillips and Backous, 2002).

Combined hearing and vestibular dysfunction in a child may only be expressed in subtle disturbances of normal development. However, since the vestibular system is responsible for maintenance of visual acuity during movement, older children with combined hearing and vestibular loss can have significant visual impairment during normal daily activities (Demer *et al.*, 1988). They would also encounter motor incoordination and locomotor problems that could limit normal development (Admiraal and Huygen, 1997). Finally, the vestibular system is responsible for coordinating sensory inputs into a coherent modality by providing a head-centred reference to which other sensory signals can be aligned (Andersen, 1997). Vestibular loss can therefore impair the processing of sensory stimuli critical to development and perception of external and internal sensations.

Recent advances in genetic and stem cell therapy in hereditary deafness

Deaf communities in the United Kingdom and other developed countries are very advanced and have their own culture. There has been anecdotal evidence that deaf couples do not necessarily want their children to be able to hear if it means that they will be excluded from the deaf community to which their parents belong. Some in the deaf community believe that deafness is not a 'disease' and therefore does not need to be 'treated'. Clinicians dealing with deaf children will certainly respect the views of parents with this opinion. However, the majority of parents of deaf children are normally hearing and in most cases express the desire that they would prefer their congenitally deaf child to be able to hear, by whatever methods are currently available.

As described above, work is continuing to identify the individual genes responsible for the early development of the ear. This would be the first step towards correcting the various developmental abnormalities that lead to deafness.

The hope is that it may one day be possible to identify all the abnormal genes responsible for abnormalities of hearing development, so that we may be able to correct them. Genetic screening programmes will need to be implemented for early and accurate diagnosis, to give us the best chance of treatment in order to preserve some hearing (Smith *et al.*, 1998, Steel, 2000).

Gene transfer

One method of trying to correct a mutated gene is by putting a normal gene in its place. This is the basis of *gene transfer*. If you think about a chromosome as a necklace, you can imagine a mutated gene as a broken link in the chain. Although only one link is damaged, the rest of the chain cannot be worn. Using our genetic map we should be able to find this faulty gene and replace it with a new link so that the necklace is repaired. In this way the new gene should be able

to function normally, and the individual will no longer suffer the effects of the damaged gene.

For this process to work there must be some way of transporting the new gene into the cell to replace the gene that doesn't work. This is done by a *vector* which acts like a vehicle to carry the new gene into the cell and deposit it into the chromosome. Vectors used in medicine include viruses such as adenovirus and herpes simplex virus (Lalwani *et al.*, 2002). These vectors can be used in two ways. They can be applied directly into the affected organ, such as into the cochlea in hereditary deafness. This allows a high dose to be given straight to the area that is not working. A vector can also be given systemically, such as in tablet form or injection. However, this means that more of the body's cells will be exposed and there may be side-effects from the effect of the vector on other body tissues (Lalwani AK *et al.*, 1998).

Stem cell therapy

Stem cells are very special cells that have the ability to develop into any body cell such as skin cells or nerve cells. Scientists can use these cells to grow new tissue in a laboratory. This new tissue can then be introduced into a person to replace damaged cells or tissues that are not working properly.

This may be of value in treating deafness. The cochlea contains the inner and outer hair cells that are responsible for our ability to hear. These hair cells are very sensitive to any changes in their environment, especially the composition of the endolymph that surrounds them, and will die if they cannot function properly. Once dead, hair cells are not naturally replaced. One idea is to try to trigger the hair cells to regrow. However, if the hair cells were faulty because of a genetic mutation, any new cells would have the same defect and so would also die. The obvious answer to the problem is to use stem cells to grow normal hair cells which can be injected into the cochlea to improve hearing (Steel, 1999). A recent study on dissection of temporal bones has shown that it is possible to enter the endolymphatic compartment of the cochlea by a simple mastoid-ectomy approach (Pau *et al.*, 2006). Scientists have been successful so far in growing new skin for skin grafts, and with time they should be able to grow more and more complex tissues to treat a vast range of conditions, including deafness.

The timing of intervention

In humans, the organ of hearing, the cochlea and the balance system are fully formed by the 25th week of gestation. The pinna has developed by the fourth month but continues to grow during childhood (Wright, 1997). This is important to know if we want to try to change or correct a genetic mutation before the baby is born. Surgical procedures on the unborn child or foetus can now be carried out for life-threatening abnormalities, and there is now a movement towards operating on less severe conditions before the baby is delivered (Farmer, 2003; Shirose *et al.*, 2003).

If genetic transfer techniques and stem cell therapy become a reality for treatment, then it is not ridiculous to propose that surgery could be carried out on human embryos to correct the damaged gene or tissue before the child is born. At present, doing an operation to fix the genetic makeup of an embryo to prevent deafness sounds like something out of a science fiction film, but as the technology and our understanding of the genes involved develop, this may one day become a possibility.

Drug therapy

Medical treatment often involves the use of drugs. Drugs come in various forms but are essentially substances that enter the body and have an effect on a particular tissue. The way in which many drugs work is clearly understood; however, new drugs are constantly being trialled to provide alternative ways of treating disease. It may be possible to develop a drug that can enter a cell and repair the defect in a gene caused by a mutation. This is an exciting area for future research.

Conclusion

Genetic testing for deafness is now a reality. It has dramatically changed the way we can assess and manage deaf patients, and will provide a useful tool for surgeons and physicians investigating their patient's deafness. If we can find the mutated genes responsible for causing the deafness, new methods such as gene therapy offer exciting possibilities for curing these patients in the future. Genetic testing and counselling will also have a place in reproductive planning and antenatal diagnosis of deafness, and will enable us to provide more information to our patients. With the increasing success of the universal newborn hearing screening programme in the United Kingdom and other developed countries, the demand on genetic services is set to undergo considerable expansion over the coming years. It is therefore essential that otolaryngologists and associated professionals have an understanding of the role of genetics in deafness. It is also paramount that we make ourselves aware of new discoveries and protocols for genetic testing and develop links with clinical genetics departments if our patients are to benefit from this ever-developing field.

References

Admiraal RJ and Huygen PL (1997) Vestibular areflexia as a cause of delayed motor skill development in children with the CHARGE association. *International Journal of Pediatric Otorhinolaryngology* 39:205–222.

Andersen RA (1997) Multimodal integration for the representation of space in the posterior parietal cortex. *Philosophical Transactions of the Royal Society of London Series B, Biological Sciences* 352(1360):1421–1428.

Arnold B, Jager L, Grevers G (1996) Visualization of inner ear structures by three-dimensional high-resolution magnetic resonance imaging. *American Journal of Otolaryngology* 17:480–485.

Cremers CW, Hombergen GC, Scaf JJ *et al.* (1985) X-linked progressive mixed deafness with perilymphatic gusher during stapes surgery. *Archives of Otolaryngology – Head and Neck Surgery* 111:249–254.

Cremers CW, Huygen PL (1983) Clinical features of female heterozygotes in the X-linked mixed deafness syndrome (with perilymphatic gusher during stapes surgery). *International Journal of Pediatric Otorhinolaryngology* 6:179–185.

Demer JL, Porter FI, Goldberg J, Jenkins HA, Schmidt K (1988) Dynamic visual acuity with telescopic spectacles: improvement with adaptation. *Investigative Ophthalmology and Visual Science* 29:1184–1189.

Farmer D (2003) Fetal surgery. *British Medical Journal* 326:461–462.

Fekete D, Wu DK (2002) Revisiting cell fate specification in the inner ear. *Current Opinion in Neurobiology* 12:35–42.

Fortnum HM, Summerfield AQ, Marshall DH, Davis AC, Bamford JM (2001) Prevalence of permanent childhood hearing impairment in the United Kingdom and implications for universal neonatal hearing screening: questionnaire based ascertainment study. *British Medical Journal* 323:536–540.

Gates GA, Couropmitree NN, Myers RH (1999) Genetic associations in age related hearing thresholds. *Archives of Otolaryngology – Head and Neck Surgery* 125:654–659.

Greenspan SI (1989) The development of the ego: biological and environmental specificity in the psychopathological developmental process and the selection and construction of ego defences. *Journal of the American Psychoanalytic Association* 37:605–638.

Hrabé de Angelis MH, Flaswinkel H, Fuchs H et al. (2000) Genome-wide, large-scale production of mutant mice by ENU mutagenesis. *Nature Genetics* 25:444–447.

Huygen PL, van Rijn PM, Cremers CW, Theunissen EJ (1993) The vestibulo-ocular reflex in pupils at a Dutch school for the hearing impaired; findings relating to acquired causes. *International Journal of Pediatric Otorhinolaryngology* 25(1–3):39–47.

Jackler RK, Luxford WM, House WF (1987) Congenital malformations of the inner ear: classification based on embryogenesis. *Laryngoscope* 97:2–14.

Karlsson KK, Harris JR, Svartengren M (1997) Description and preliminary results from an audiometric study of male twins. *Ear and Hearing* 18:114–120.

Kiernan AE, Erven A, Voegeling S et al. (2002) ENU mutagenesis reveals a highly mutable locus on mouse Chromosome 4 that affects ear morphogenesis. *Nature Genetics* 13:142–148.

Kiernan A, Steel K (2000) Mouse homologues for human deafness. In: Kitamura K, Steel K, eds. *Genetics in Otorhinolaryngology. Advances in otorhinolaryngology*, vol 56, pp 233–243. Basel: Karger.

Kho SP, Pettis RM, Mhatre AN, Lalwani AK (2000) Safety of adeno-associated virus as cochlear gene transfer vector: Analysis of distant spread beyond injected cochleae. *Molecular Therapy* 2:368–373.

Konigsmark B, Gorlin R (1976) *Genetic and Metabolic Deafness*. Philadelphia: WB Saunders.

Lalwani AK, Jero J, Mhatre AN (2002) Current issues in cochlear gene transfer. *Audiology and Neuro-otology* 7:146–151.

Lalwani AK, Walsh BJ, Carvalo GJ, Muzyczka N, Mhatre AN (1998) Expression of adeno-associated virus integrated transgene within the mammalian vestibular organs. *American Journal of Otology* 19:390–395.

Mallo M (2001) Formation of the middle ear: a recent progress on the developmental and molecular mechanisms. *Developmental Biology* 231:410–419.

Martin P, Swanson GJ (1993) Descriptive and experimental analysis of the epithelial re-modellings that control semi-circular canal formation in the developing mouse inner ear. *Developmental Biology* 159:549–558.

McLeod AC, Sweeney A, McConnell FE et al. (1973) Autosomal recessive sensorineural deafness: a comparison of two kindreds. *Southern Medical Journal* 66:141–152.

Mengel, MC, Konigsmark BW, McKusick VA (1969) Two types of congenital recessive deafness. *Eye Ear Nose Throat Monthly* 48:301–305.

Noveroske JK, Weber JS, Justice MJ (2000) The mutagenic action of N-ethyl-N-nitrosourea in the mouse. *Mammalian Genome* 11:478–483.

Online Mendelian Inheritance in Man (OMIM) (2003) www.ncbi.nlm.nih.gov/sites/entrez?db=omim (accessed 13 November 2008).

Pau H, Fagan P, Oleskevich S (2006) Locating the scala media in fixed human temporal bone for therapeutic access – a preliminary study. *Journal of Laryngology and Otology* 120:914–915.

Pau H, Hawker K, Fuchs H *et al.* (2004) Characterisation of a new mouse mutant, flouncer, with a balance defect and inner ear malformation. *Otology and Neurootology* 25:707–713.

Phillips JO, Backous DD (2002) Evaluation of vestibular function in young children. *Otolaryngologic Clinics of North America* 35:765–790.

Siemering K, Manji SSM, Hutchison WM *et al.* (2006) Detection of mutations in genes associated with hearing loss using a microarray-based approach. *Journal of Molecular Diagnostics* 8:483–489.

Shirose S, Sydorak RM, Tsao K *et al.* (2003) Spectrum of intrapartum management strategies for giant fetal cervical teratoma. *Journal of Paediatric Surgery* 38:446–450.

Smith SD, Kimberling WJ, Schaefer GB, Horton MB, Tinley ST (1998) Medical genetic evaluation for the etiology of hearing loss in children. *Journal of Communication Disorders* 31:371–388.

Steel KP (1995) Inherited hearing defects in mice. *Annual Review of Genetics* 29:675–701.

Steel KP (1999) Perspectives: biomedicine. The benefits of recycling. *Science* 285:1363–1364.

Steel KP (2000) Science, medicine, and the future: new interventions in hearing impairment. *British Medical Journal* 320:622–625.

Van Camp G, Smith R (2008) Hereditary Hearing Loss homepage (see Table 050.1). http://webh01.ua.ac.be/hhh

Wright A (1997) Anatomy and ultra-structure of the human ear. In: Kerr A, ed. *Scott-Brown's Otolaryngology*, vol 1, pp 1 and 6–8. Oxford: Butterworth Heinemann.

The causes, identification and confirmation of sensorineural hearing loss in children

12

Shakeel Saeed, Rachel Booth and
Penny Hill

Introduction

The prevalence (number of affected individuals at a given point in time per population figure) of hearing loss in children is dependent on the age group studied. In their regional and UK national studies, Fortnum and colleagues estimated that the prevalence of moderate to profound bilateral deafness at birth was 1.12 per 1000 live births, rising to 1.65 per 1000 for a 9-year-old cohort of children, with the increase in part at least being attributed to hitherto under-recognised permanent hearing loss occurring later in childhood (Fortnum and Davis, 1997; Fortnum *et al.*, 2001). The scope of this chapter is to provide the reader with an overview of the causes of such permanent sensorineural deafness in children and to detail how the hearing loss is identified and subsequently confirmed.

The traditional classification of hearing loss as congenital (present at birth) or acquired (as a consequence of events in infancy or childhood) is helpful in structuring the management of the deaf child and his or her family. Congenital deafness is further considered as having a genetic (inherited) basis or as a consequence of acquired prenatal or immediate perinatal events such as maternal rubella or birth hypoxia. Parents understandably will have concerns regarding the implications for the child's general health and development, as well as the risk to subsequent children if the basis for the hearing loss is genetic. The last decade has witnessed a tremendous increase in interest in congenital deafness, primarily for three reasons: neonatal hearing screening, advances in genetic and molecular biological techniques and the impact of cochlear implantation. The subsequent discussion combines the traditional classification of hearing loss with the enhanced (but still incomplete) understanding of deafness based on the advances described above.

Congenital hearing loss

Genetic congenital hearing loss

Around 60% of all permanent childhood hearing impairment has a genetic basis, of which 70% is described clinically as non-syndromic (NSHL), where the hearing loss is an isolated abnormality, and 30% is syndromic (SHL), in which the hearing loss is part of a clinical picture that includes symptoms and signs attributable to abnormalities affecting other organs (Marazita *et al.*, 1993). In genetic terms, both groups may exhibit the various modes of inheritance as described in Chapter 11. What has become apparent over the last decade is the large number (several hundred) of genetic loci that are implicated in congenital deafness. The genes within these loci are continuously being identified, characterised and then mapped, in an attempt to enhance our understanding of genetic deafness and how a particular gene affects the function of the inner ear. The ultimate aim is to identify new therapies to reverse the effects of a defective gene and hence modify or even reverse the hearing loss. Chapter 11 gives a detailed discussion of genetic deafness.

Acquired congenital hearing loss

By definition, this implies that a prenatal or perinatal event has led to deafness as an isolated finding or as part of a more generalised illness. Such events are traditionally classified as infective and non-infective.

Infective

Historically, maternal infection during pregnancy, particularly viral infections, was a common cause of newborn deafness. Up to 40 years ago it was postulated that up to one-third of cases of newborn deafness were due to such infections. There was some debate around the relationship between non-specific viral infections and deafness, but the causal link between either maternal rubella (German measles) or maternal cytomegalovirus (CMV) infection and congenital deafness was robust. This observation prompted universal rubella immunisation in the developed world, and in the last three decades the incidence of congenital rubella deafness has markedly reduced. Despite this, cases still arise, either as a consequence of maternal re-infection but, more recently, due to increasing movement of people from areas of the world without universal immunisation.

CMV is a herpes virus which, as a primary infection, causes a mild systemic viral illness. The virus, however, remains *in situ*, and re-activation may result in foetal infection. The effects on the unborn child are variable, but primary infection of the mother during pregnancy may cause significant central nervous system damage, including severe or progressive deafness.

Non-infective

Perinatal events, particularly prematurity, have historically been implicated in a significant proportion of neonatal deafness. As the intensive care of pre-term infants has improved, the prognosis for even very low birth weight infants is favourable, and currently the incidence of sensorineural deafness is less than 1%. Two specific inter-related factors are recognised, birth hypoxia or asphyxia and intrauterine/neonatal jaundice.

The blood supply to the cochlea is via a single artery, and therefore reduction of blood flow or hypoxia makes the cochlea vulnerable to irreversible damage, resulting in deafness in the absence of other neurological injury. More profound hypoxia leading to central nervous system injury may be associated with both central and cochlear deafness. Such hypoxia may also occur as a consequence of intrauterine placental compromise or complications of birth in an otherwise healthy full-term child. The risks are compounded in the pre-term infant due to the reduced efficiency of pulmonary function that characterises such infants. Prior to universal neonatal hearing screening, prematurity was one of the risk factors warranting formal hearing assessment in the neonatal period.

Physiological jaundice is common in neonates and is self-limiting in most instances. Pathological jaundice occurs if the mother is rhesus blood group negative and the baby is rhesus positive. In this instance, the maternal rhesus antibodies break down the child's blood cells, giving rise to haemolytic disease of the newborn. Aside from anaemia, with its associated hypoxia, the massive bilirubin load in the neonate's bloodstream (hyperbilirubinaemia) overwhelms its capacity to detoxify and excrete it, and the excess bilirubin is deposited in various body tissues including the cochlear nuclei and basal ganglia. Progressive bilirubin deposition in the brain leads to kernicterus, which is characterised by seizures and may be fatal. Two measures have lead to a dramatic reduction in deafness due to hyperbilirubinaemia: immunisation of all rhesus-negative mothers with antirhesus antibody, and the utilisation of exchange blood transfusions in neonates that are at risk from haemolytic disease. Nevertheless, sporadic instances of deafness due to jaundice are still seen in paediatric audiology and cochlear implant clinics.

Acquired hearing loss

The causes of acquired sensorineural deafness in early childhood are numerous and varied. The majority are uncommon when compared to conductive hearing impairment due to otitis media with effusion. However, significant morbidity still arises from infective causes, with bacterial meningitis being the single most common cause of sensorineural deafness. The causative organisms include *Haemophilus influenzae*, *Streptococcus pneumoniae* and *Neisseria meningitides*. The severity and temporal progression of the deafness is variable but all cochlear implant programmes have a steady throughput of infants and children rendered profoundly deaf by meningitis, despite more recent national haemophilus and meningitis C vaccination programmes.

Historically, viral infections such as measles and mumps have been associated with varying degrees of sensorineural deafness. The prevalence of such hearing loss was reduced by universal measles, mumps and rubella (MMR) vaccination. More recently, as a consequence of the now discredited 'scare' linking the MMR vaccine and autism, there was a reduction in the MMR vaccination uptake. Current estimates suggest as many as one million children in the UK are potentially at risk of these infections, although it remains to be seen whether there will be an

increase in such illnesses and in associated hearing loss.

The less common causes of early childhood deafness constitute a disparate group including head injury and drug ototoxicity. The latter is of interest because the long-established observation that aminoglycoside antibiotics may cause sensorineural deafness has been further characterised at a molecular genetic level. The greater susceptibility of some families to this cause of deafness has been found to be as a result of a mutation in a mitochondrial gene (*MTRNR1*), which renders the individual susceptible to ototoxicity at plasma levels within the therapeutic range.

Newborn hearing screening

Historically there have been two hearing screens in the UK to identify children with hearing loss. The first was the Health Visitor Distraction Test (HVDT) carried out at around 7 months of age, followed by a school entry screen at age 5 years. The HVDT screen was used as a screening test to identify those infants requiring further investigation for hearing loss. However, the age at which it could be carried out meant that the age of identification of hearing loss was often over 1 year and there were reports of low yields, with poor coverage, sensitivity and specificity (Robertson *et al.*, 1995; Wood *et al.*, 1997). This is now considered to be unacceptable in light of clear evidence that early identification and intervention in hearing loss is in the best interest of a child's development (Yoshinaga-Itano, 2000).

To address these concerns, some centres in the UK devised local newborn screening programmes, targeting infants thought to be at high risk of a hearing impairment. At the same time in other countries, such as the USA, certain states were developing universal screening programmes. Screening programmes around the world all differ slightly in terms of the screening tests used, referral criteria for further diagnostic investigations and the target population to be identified by the screen. Here, we will concentrate on the nationally managed screening programme introduced in England in 2002. This aims to detect hearing loss that will significantly affect language development.

The technology used within screening programmes is based on tests including otoacoustic emissions (OAEs) and automated auditory brainstem responses (ABRs), that have long been used in diagnostic assessments (see Chapter 7). It should be mentioned that the screening versions of these tests give a 'pass' or 'refer' response. A 'refer' indicates the need for further testing at the audiology clinic, where diagnostic ABR testing is used to identify the nature and configuration of any hearing loss. In cases of profound bilateral hearing loss, and in conjunction with the parent's wishes, this can lead to a very early referral for a cochlear implant.

Additionally, infants who are thought to have a risk for progressive hearing loss but pass the hearing screen, enter a targeted surveillance programme. Currently in the UK, children still also receive a screen at school entry, although this may be stopped in the future when more information is obtained about the yield from the newborn hearing screen and the surveillance programme.

Diagnostic objective assessments

The aim of diagnostic audiological testing is to gain as much information as possible about a person's hearing across a range of frequencies. Audiological tests can be classified in two ways: (1) objective, where a measure of hearing level is made or inferred without a person needing to respond or (2) behavioural, where a person is asked to indicate in some way when a sound has been heard.

This section discusses objective tests that are commonly used when testing infants, highlighting their strengths, weaknesses and clinical application.

The auditory brainstem response

The auditory brainstem response (ABR) is an auditory evoked potential that can be used to estimate the hearing thresholds in babies and infants (Figure 12.1). It is ideal for application in a paediatric population because it can be recorded under natural sleep, although sedation can be used for slightly older children. The generation,

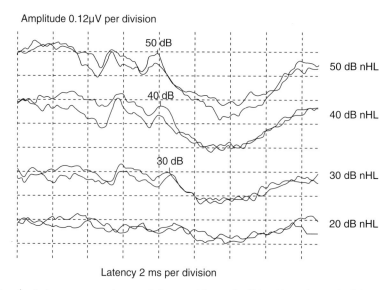

Amplitude 0.12μV per division

50 dB — 50 dB nHL

40 dB — 40 dB nHL

30 dB — 30 dB nHL

— 20 dB nHL

Latency 2 ms per division

Figure 12.1 Auditory brainstem responses from an infant aged 2 months. Wave V can be tracked down to threshold of 30 dB nHL. No response is present for a stimulus of 20 dB nHL. As the stimulus level reduces, latency of wave V increases and the amplitude of the response decreases. A threshold of 30 dB nHL is equivalent to a predicted threshold of 25 dB EHL. Horizontal axis: milliseconds; vertical axis: microvolts.

morphology and maturation of the response are described in detail in Chapter 7. We concentrate here on the factors particular to its use in identification of hearing loss in babies.

Traditionally electrophysiological thresholds have been reported in dB nHL (normal hearing level) to represent the fact that reference threshold data from normally hearing adults are used to calibrate equipment (ISO 389-6, 2007; IEC 60645-3, 2007). However, using dB nHL for paediatric testing is problematic, as the calibration values are still derived from adult data. To circumvent this, correction factors can be applied to convert dB nHL thresholds to 'dB EHL' or 'estimated hearing level'. This is an estimate of the infants' hearing level in dB HL that would be obtained if they developed to adulthood with the same level of hearing loss. These correction factors are based on meta-analysis studies (Stapells, 2000), and have been formalised for use in the clinic. For further technical information on these topics, readers are referred to the BC Early Hearing Program (2007) and the Newborn Hearing Screening Programme (NHSP Clinical Group, 2007).

Hearing thresholds (converted to dB EHL) are estimated from the lowest stimulus level at which there is a clear and repeatable wave V. To obtain a complete set of threshold information as quickly as possible before the child wakes, modifications of the amplifier and recording parameters are used to increase the speed of testing. The robust wave V is preserved, but the morphology of the other waves is reduced. Air- and bone-conduction ABR testing can be performed using both click and tone pip stimuli to help ascertain if a hearing loss is sensorineural or conductive.

Click ABR testing has traditionally been used in preference to tone pip ABR testing to give an overall measure of hearing level. This may be because click stimuli activate a wide region of the cochlea, dominated by the 2–4 kHz region, producing large-amplitude waveforms with clear morphology. In comparison, tone pip ABRs can be much harder to interpret, with much smaller amplitude waveforms. However, in the light of mounting evidence showing that it is in the child's best interest to provide amplification as soon as a hearing loss is identified (Yoshinaga-Itano, 2000), it is now no longer acceptable to identify

a hearing loss with a click ABR and then to wait several months to collect frequency-specific information using behavioural testing. Additionally, using click ABR testing alone may result in some configurations of hearing loss being missed. Therefore, tone pip ABR testing is now considered by many to be the clinical 'gold standard' for estimating elevated hearing thresholds in infants (Small and Stapells, 2006; American Speech Language Hearing Association (ASHA), 2004). This frequency-specific information can be used to predict hearing thresholds, and so be used to provide appropriate amplification if necessary until behavioural data are available (NHSP Clinical Group, 2007). For tone pip stimuli under good recording conditions, ABR thresholds are within 10 dB of behavioural audiometric thresholds (Stapells, 2002).

The interpretation of all ABR traces depends on the skilled subjective assessment of the waveforms by experienced clinicians. This is particularly important in paediatric testing, where latency and morphology of the waveform alter with age. Mistakes may result in hearing losses being missed in early infancy, which has been shown to have grave consequences on language development (Moeller, 2000). To address this, some hearing screening programmes are developing guidelines to bring more structure and quality to the marking of ABR traces (NHSP Clinical Group, 2007). Similarly, expert reviews of testing are being introduced to ensure high-quality assessments become standard.

Auditory steady-state response

A new electrophysiological technique that may soon be used routinely in clinical practice is auditory steady-state response (ASSR) testing. This uses amplitude and/or frequency-modulated sounds to evoke responses that are phase-locked to the stimuli (see Chapter 7). The 80 Hz modulation response, generated by the brainstem, is particularly promising for hearing threshold testing in infants and children. Like the ABR, ASSR tests can be performed using both air and bone conduction (Small and Stapells, 2006) and there is good agreement between thresholds measured behaviourally and with ASSRs (Stapells *et al.*, 2004). There are also a number of potential advantages of the ASSR over the ABR. Firstly, ASSRs can theoretically measure responses to up to four different frequencies in both ears simultaneously. This is considerably quicker than measuring several thresholds using ABRs. Secondly, unlike the ABR, it appears that the 80 Hz ASSR can be reliably measured whether a listener is awake or asleep (Picton *et al.*, 2003). Finally, ASSR detection is based on statistical tests rather than subjective interpretation (Stapells *et al.*, 2004), which may address some of the concerns with interpretation that are present with ABR testing.

Despite the clear research-based evidence for ASSR, there are a number of issues surrounding its clinical use. For example, there is little standardisation between different ASSR measurement systems, which could lead to disparity of results between clinics, and at present there have been few studies in babies and infants, especially those with hearing loss (Stapells *et al.*, 2004). Therefore, at the current time it is not recommended that ASSR alone should be used for fre-quency-specific assessment of hearing in infants (NHSP Clinical Group, 2007). However, we predict that as these issues are resolved, ASSRs will be an invaluable tool in the identification and confirmation of hearing loss in infants.

Otoacoustic emissions

Otoacoustic emissions (OAEs) are tiny sounds generated by cochlear outer hair cells (Figure 12.2). These outer hair cells do not themselves activate primary auditory nerve fibres. Nevertheless, if a robust OAE is present, this is taken to indicate good function in both the middle ear and cochlea (Kemp, 2002). The generation and measurement of OAEs are described in detail in Chapter 7. Therefore, we concentrate here on their application in the identification of hearing loss in babies.

Both transient evoked (TE) and distortion product (DP) OAE measurements provide a quick, simple and efficient method of inferring the presence of cochlear function, with some degree of frequency specificity (Kemp, 2002). It

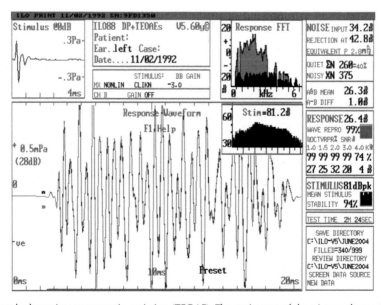

Figure 12.2   Click-evoked transient otoacoustic emission (TEOAE). The main part of the picture shows the positive response. The upper small box labelled 'Response FTT' compares the response (upper, grey area) with the noise level (lower black area).

is important to understand that the presence of OAEs means that there is outer hair cell function in the cochlea. However, their presence is not dependent on inner hair cell function, which can, uncommonly, be absent even although transient otoacoustic emissions (TEOAEs) are present, in which case the child will have a hearing loss.

One drawback of OAE testing is that conductive hearing losses will prevent OAEs being recorded. Therefore it is important that middle ear function is always assessed using tympanometry when using OAEs. High-frequency tympanometry is essential when testing infants under 6 months of age (NHSP Clinical Group, 2008a). However, OAEs also have a key role in the diagnosis of 'auditory neuropathy', where there is a pattern of results showing the presence of OAEs (and/or cochlear microphonics) but with absent or disordered ABRs (see also Chapter 13).

Behavioural hearing assessments

Behavioural tests of hearing have been developed to take into account the developmental level and listening skills of infants and young children, to ensure an appropriate and accurate response to auditory stimuli. In this chapter we cannot describe in detail how each of these tests of hearing should be carried out, and readers are referred to comprehensive books on paediatric testing (for example, McCormick, 1988; Newton, 2009). Here we describe the main principles of the tests and how they are used.

Role of behavioural hearing assessment

Behavioural assessment continues to be vital in the identification and confirmation of childhood hearing loss. Clinicians should strive to confirm any previously obtained electrophysiological test results with behavioural test techniques as soon as the infant is developmentally ready. Behavioural testing must be focused to determine the nature, degree and configuration of hearing loss in each ear from as early an age as possible. This

information provides an important baseline for comparison at all future assessments and helps establish appropriate management options and optimisation of any amplification.

It is important to reiterate that there are certain types of hearing losses that will not be detected by newborn hearing screening programmes. The prevalence of permanent childhood hearing loss at birth is around 1 per 1000 births, with an almost doubling of this by the age of 9 years due to late-onset and progressive hearing losses (Fortnum *et al.*, 2001). Other groups that might be missed are those with mild hearing losses, which may not be detected by the screen, and babies who wrongly pass the screen. Acquired hearing losses may occur and there is also the significant effect of temporary conductive problems on a child's hearing and development that must be identified (Gravel and Wallace, 2000). Behavioural testing is therefore invaluable in identifying these infants.

Choice of behavioural hearing assessment techniques

Early techniques of behavioural hearing assessment relied on unconditioned responses and observation of an infant's response to sound. Techniques using this strategy, such as BOA (behavioural observation audiometry) and distraction testing (developed from the 'distracting test' described by Ewing and Ewing in Manchester in 1944) have been long recognised as unreliable (Weber, 1969; Bench *et al.*, 1976; Wilson and Thompson, 1984), with large variations in judgements of responses between testers (Moncur, 1968). These tests rely on broad-band and high-intensity stimuli to elicit the unconditioned responses in young children. Unfortunately this means that the assessments are not frequency specific and they give unreliable estimates of hearing thresholds. Although in the UK the distraction test has been considered the test of choice for young infants who are considered not to be developmentally ready for other techniques, there is now clear evidence that infants as young as 6 months can be conditioned to respond to frequency-specific acoustic stimuli (Moore *et al.*, 1977; Wilson, 1978; Thompson and Wilson, 1984; Primus and Thompson, 1985; Widen, 1993). Therefore, test methods have been developed that adopt a conditioned response to sound, overcoming many of the criticisms and concerns regarding the reliability of BOA and distraction testing. It is also important that paediatric test techniques are able to determine frequency-specific, ear-specific and bone-conduction hearing levels from an early age.

The two main tests discussed below, when applied at the appropriate developmental level of the child, allow the clinician to meet the goals of behavioural testing.

Visual reinforcement audiometry

Visual reinforcement audiometry (VRA) is widely recognised as the test of choice for the early assessments of hearing. The test relies on the ability of the child to be conditioned to turn to a sound stimulus, or in some cases a tactile stimulus, and this motor response is reinforced by a visual reward (Figure 12.3). The aim of the test is to determine the minimum response level rather than the ability to localise the sound. Auditory

stimuli can be presented through speakers, headphones, insert earphones and bone conductors. In cases of suspected asymmetry, careful masking can be carried out. The test is applicable from an age of 6 months up to 2 or 3 years, at which point children quickly inhibit their responses (Primus and Thompson, 1985; Thompson *et al.*, 1992).

VRA is most commonly performed using a clinician (often in an observation room) who controls the test and presentation of the sounds, and an assistant who controls the attention of the child. The first stage of the test is to condition the child to turn to a visual reward when the sound is heard. During conditioning, the sound and visual reward are initially introduced together, with the assistant pointing out the reinforcer, if necessary. Once the child has associated the sound with the visual reward, the sound can be introduced alone and an appropriate turning response is rewarded by illuminating a toy in a box, or by an image appearing on a television screen. The quietest sound level at which the child reliably responds is recorded as the minimum response level. This should be obtained for as many frequencies in each ear as possible. Modifica-tions to the technique and reward are possible for those with additional difficulties. Technical details of the test procedure are widely available (Widen, 1993; NHSP Clinical Group, 2008b).

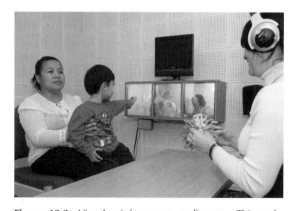

Figure 12.3 Visual reinforcement audiometry. This technique is more reliable than distraction testing and allows the two ears to be tested separately. The child hears the sound, from a loudspeaker, ear insert or bone-conduction transducer, and is rewarded by illumination and movement of a toy animal in a box, or by an image appearing on a screen.

Performance and play audiometry

The terms *performance test* and *play audiometry* are often used interchangeably to describe active listening tasks where the child gives a voluntary conditioned play response to a sound stimulus. Theoretically, the performance test refers to sound field stimuli, such as a voiced /go/, a sibilant /s/ and other consonants (Ewing and Ewing, 1944), although frequency-specific tones are now usually presented. In play audiometry, a range of transducers such as headphones and bone conductors are used. Given the increased auditory information gained from play audiometry, this is the test of choice.

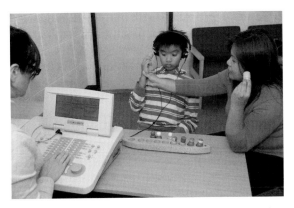

Figure 12.4 Play audiometry. The child is conditioned to wait for a sound, and to respond by some 'play' action, such as putting a wooden man into a boat.

Play audiometry is appropriate for assessing hearing in children with a developmental age of around two and a half years upwards, until cooperation with pure tone audiometry is achieved. Each time a sound is heard, the child performs a simple action, such as putting a man in a boat, a peg on a board or a similar simple action (Figure 12.4). During conditioning, the child is shown what to do and therefore does not require receptive language skills to learn the 'game'. Success of the test relies on the child's ability to inhibit his or her response until the stimulus has been detected. Often it is a younger child's inability to wait for the stimulus that pre-

vents the test being used, rather than their inability to respond when the sound is heard.

As this is an active listening task, responses can be elicited closer to threshold than in tests of hearing in younger children. Play audiometry can be used to obtain a full audiogram, including masked air and bone thresholds.

Speech discrimination testing

Speech discrimination tests can be useful in demonstrating the functional effects of a hearing loss. Some speech discrimination tests are described here in brief but again, for more information, readers are directed to Newton (2009) or McCormick (1988). However, it is important to emphasise that speech discrimination tests cannot be used alone to identify or confirm a hearing loss and should only be used as part of a test battery.

One of the most commonly used speech discrimination tests in the UK is the McCormick Toy Test (MTT; McCormick, 1977) which is suitable for typically developing children aged between 18 months and 5 years. This test measures the quietest level of speech needed to correctly identify similar-sounding toys such as 'cup' and 'duck' or 'tree' and 'key' without using lip reading (Figure 12.5). Initially, the MTT used live voice presentation, which requires great skill

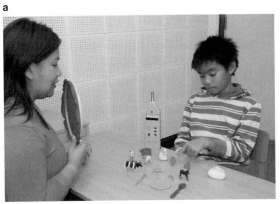

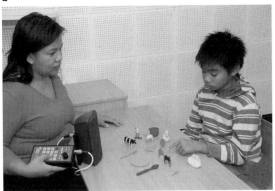

Figure 12.5 Speech discrimination tests. **a**, The McCormick Toy Test. The tester names one of the set of toys (keeping her mouth concealed) and the child responds by pointing to the toy. The intensity of the tester's voice, in dB(A), is measured by a sound level meter and the mouth of the tester is concealed from the child. **b**, The automated toy test (ATT). The tester has a control unit in her right hand and uses it to choose the name of the toy and the intensity of the pre-recorded voice coming from the loudspeaker.

in being able to reliably modulate the intensity of speech without whispering. However, new versions of the MTT are now available with digitised pre-recorded speech stimuli presented via a loudspeaker (commonly known as the automated toy test or ATT). Word discrimination thresholds measured with these automated tests also allow the prediction of the average pure tone threshold in the better hearing ear, which can be useful if the child will not cooperate for other types of audiometry (Ousey *et al.*, 1989; Palmer *et al.*, 1991).

Summary

Sensorineural hearing loss in children remains a significant cause of morbidity, with a potential lifelong adverse effect in terms of speech and language development and communication. Consequent to this is the effect on health and well-being, as well as educational and employment opportunities. The last decade has seen an explosion in our understanding of the molecular and genetic basis of such deafness but much work remains before we are able to redress the pathological effects on the function of the inner ear. In the meantime, the identification and confirmation of the hearing loss in a child is of paramount importance as part of the investigative process. There are a range of tests that can be used to identify and confirm hearing loss in children. Both objective and behavioural tests have important roles, provided that they are used appropriately. All diagnostic assessments used must be able to provide information about the configuration and nature of any hearing loss, as they form the basis for appropriate aiding and, if indicated, cochlear implantation. For this reason, all professionals in contact with children need to be vigilant to refer children for testing if there are concerns, regardless of the outcome of any hearing screening.

Acknowledgement

The authors are very grateful for the photographs in this chapter, which were prepared by Vicki Holmes BSc, MIMI, RMIP and Milanka Drenovak MSc, AudD at the Royal National Throat, Nose and Ear Hospital, London.

References

American Speech Language Hearing Association (ASHA) (2004) *Guidelines for the Audiologic Assessment of Children from Birth to 5 Years of Age.* http://www.asha.org/NR/rdonlyres/0BB7C840-27D2-4DC6-861B-1709ADD-78BAF/0/v2GLAudAssessChild.pdf (accessed 1 December 2008).

BC Early Hearing Program (2007) *Diagnostic Audiology Protocol DX100–1100.* www.audiospeech.ubc.ca/haplab/BCEHP_DiagnosticAudiologyProtocolsDec2007.pdf (accessed 13 November 2008).

Bench J, Collyer Y, Mentz L, Wilson I (1976) Studies in infant behavioural audiometry II: Six-week-old infants. *Audiology* 15:302–314.

Ewing IR, Ewing AWG (1944) The ascertainment of deafness in infancy and early childhood. *Journal of Laryngology and Otology* 59:309–338.

Fortnum H, Davis A (1997) Epidemiology of permanent hearing impairment in Trent region, 1985–1993. *British Journal of Audiology* 31:409–446.

Fortnum HM, Summerfield AQ, Marshall DH, Davis AC, Bamford JM (2001) Prevalence of permanent childhood hearing impairment in the United Kingdom and implications for universal neonatal hearing screening: questionnaire based ascertainment study. *British Medical Journal* 323:536–539.

Gravel JS, Wallace IF (2000) Effects of otitis media with effusion on hearing in the first 3 years of life. *Journal of Speech Language and Hearing Research* 43:631–644.

IEC 60645-3 (2007) *Electroacoustics – Audiometric Equipment – Part 3: Test signals of short duration.* Geneva: International Electrotechnical Commission.

ISO 389-6 (2007) *Acoustics – Reference Zero for the Calibration of Audiometric Equipment – Part 6: Reference threshold of hearing for test signals of short duration.* Geneva: International Organization for Standardization.

Kemp D (2002) Otoacoustic emissions, their origin in cochlear function, and use. *British Medical Bulletin* 63:223–224.

Marazita ML, Ploughman LM, Rawlings B *et al.* (1993) Genetic epidemiological studies of early onset deafness in the US school-age population. *American Journal of Medical Genetics* 46:486–491.

McCormick B (1977) The Toy Discrimination Test: an aid for screening the hearing of children above a mental age of 2 years. *Public Health* 91:67–69.

McCormick B, ed. (1988) *Paediatric Audiology: 0–5 years.* London: Taylor and Francis.

Moeller MP (2000) Early intervention and language development in children who are deaf and hard of hearing. *Pediatrics* 106:E43.

Moncur JP (1968) Judgement reliability in infant testing. *Journal of Speech and Hearing Research* 11:348–357.

Moore JM, Wilson WR, Thompson G (1977) Visual reinforcement of head turn in infants under twelve months of age. *Journal of Speech and Hearing Disorders* 42:328–334.

Newton VE, ed. (2009) *Paediatric Audiological Medicine,* 2nd edn. London: Whurr Publishers.

NHSP Clinical Group, Stevens J, Sutton G, Wood S, Mason S (2007) *Guidelines for the Early Audiological Assessment and Management of Babies Referred from the Newborn Hearing Screening Programme.* http://hearing.screening. nhs.uk/protocols_audioassess (accessed 13 November 2008).

NHSP Clinical Group, Baldwin M, Sutton G, Gravel J, Low R (2008a) *Tympanometry in Babies under 6 Months. A recommended test protocol.* http://hearing.screening.nhs.uk/ protocols_audioassess (accessed 1 December 2008).

NHSP Clinical Group, Day J, Green R, Munro K *et al.* (2008b). *Visual Reinforcement Audiometry Testing of Infants. A recommended test protocol.* http://hearing.screening.nhs.uk/ protocols_audioassess (accessed 13 November 2008).

Ousey J, Sheppard S, Twomey T, Palmer AR (1989) The IHR-McCormick Toy Discrimination Test – description and initial evaluation. *British Journal of Audiology* 23:245–249.

Palmer AR, Sheppard S, Marshall DH (1991) Prediction of hearing thresholds in children using an automated toy discrimination test. *British Journal of Audiology* 25:351–356.

Picton J, Dimitrijevic A, Purcell DW (2003) Human auditory steady-state responses. *International Journal of Audiology* 42:177–219.

Primus M, Thompson G (1985) Response strength of young children in operant audiometry. *Journal of Speech and Hearing Research* 28:539–547.

Robertson C, Aldridge S, Jarman F *et al.* (1995). Late diagnosis of congenital sensorineural hearing impairment: why are detection methods failing. *Archives of Disease in Childhood* 72:11–15.

Small SA, Stapells DR (2006) Multiple auditory steady-state response thresholds to bone-conduction stimuli in young infants with normal hearing. *Ear and Hearing* 27:219–228.

Stapells DR (2000) Threshold estimation by the tone-evoked auditory brainstem response: a literature meta-analysis. *Journal of Speech-Language Pathology and Audiology* 24:74–83.

Stapells DR (2002) The tone-evoked ABR: why it's the measure of choice for young infants. *The Hearing Journal* 55:14–18.

Stapells DR, Herdman A, Small SA, Dimitrijevic A, Hatton J (2004) Current status of the auditory steady-state responses for estimating an infant's audiogram. In: Seewald RC, Bamford JM, eds. *A Sound Foundation Through Early Amplification,* pp 43–59. Basel: Phonak AG.

Thompson G, Thompson M, McCall A (1992) Strategies for increasing response behaviour of 1-and 2-year old children during visual reinforcement audiology. *Ear and Hearing* 13:236–240.

Thompson G, Wilson W (1984) Clinical application of visual reinforcement audiometry. *Seminars in Hearing* 5:85–99.

Weber BA (1969) Validation of observer judgements in behaviour observation audiometry. *Journal of Speech and Hearing Disorders* 34:350–354.

Widen J (1993) Adding objectivity to infant behavioural audiometry. *Ear and Hearing* 14:49–57.

Wilson WR (1978) Behavioral assessment of auditory function in infants. In: Minifie FD, Lloyd LL, eds. *Communicative and Cognitive Abilities – Early Behavioural Assessment*, pp 37–59. Baltimore, MD: University Park Press.

Wilson WR, Thompson G (1984) Behavioral audiometry. In: Jerger J, ed. *Pediatric Audiology*, pp 1–44. San Diego, CA: College-Hill Press.

Wood S, Davis A, McCormick B (1997) Changing yield of the health visitor distraction test when targeted neonatal screening is introduced into a health district. *British Journal of Audiology* 31:55–61.

Yoshinaga-Itano C (2000) From screening to early identification and intervention: discovering predictors to successful outcomes for children with significant hearing loss. *Journal of Deaf Studies and Deaf Education* 8:11–30.

Habilitation of children with permanent hearing impairment

Josephine Marriage

13

Introduction

Early identification of hearing loss

The past decade has seen major changes in the management of permanent hearing loss in children, prompted by the implementation of neonatal hearing screening programmes (NHSPs) in developed countries to identify hearing-impaired children in very early life. There is the potential for improved speech communication and, ultimately, life choices, if auditory stimulation and learning are supported through the natural periods of neural development. Conversely, it is also recognised that there are risks to the emotional wellbeing of a family group, which may arise from the diagnosis of impairment so early in the life of a child. However, the potential benefit from early intervention may outweigh the negative impact of a devastating diagnosis in the neonatal stage if audiological management is competent, sensitive and orientated to the needs of the individual family. Before NHSPs, it was not uncommon for children with moderate and even severe hearing loss to be identified as late as $3^{1}/_{2}$ years of age. This is now much less common.

There are four main components for cohesive early intervention. The first is the early identification and definition of the extent of hearing impairment. This is followed by the provision and verification of an effective intervention, which is usually hearing aid amplification but may be cochlear implantation. The third factor requires full definition of the site of impairment within the hearing system, specifying middle ear, cochlear or neural components of hearing loss, and full information on the possible aetiology of the hearing loss. The fourth, and perhaps most important factor, is the opportunity to assimilate meaning to auditory and visual information, designed around the needs of the individual child within his or her own family. This evolves through developing parent–child interaction from early life. Some of the early programmes that had neonatal screening in place, but less-developed auditory management, showed limited benefit for hearing-impaired individuals, despite the early identification of hearing loss (Kennedy et al., 2005). A NHSP therefore should provide access to audiological management in the first year of life, but is not an end in itself.

As NHSPs have come on stream, professionals have needed to acquire a number of new skills and training in audiological management, communication and liaison strategies, appropriate for supporting an infant within a vulnerable family dynamic. This is a very different scenario from diagnosis of hearing loss in a child of one year of age or more. Luterman (Kurtzer-White and Luterman, 2003) states that 'Screening endeavours have far out-stripped our habilitation effort, leaving parents with a diagnosis but without support', and emphasises the need for parents to be given time and counselling following diagnosis of deafness, as fundamental to the process of coping with the hearing loss. By undertaking a NHSP we are relying on the main caregivers (the parents) to carry out much of the practical part of intervention, in addition to all the normal challenges of parenthood. This gives rise to the *family-centred* approach to habilitation. Thus, since the 1970s, paediatric audiology has evolved from being largely disease focused, to becoming more orientated to the needs of the patient, through the 1990s. With the implementation of a NHSP there is now the need to support the infant or child within the family. In this new perspective, the role of professionals is to support the *family*, allowing the parents to make their own informed choices about communication options. The subsequent development and communication profile for the child can be viewed as the *product* of that habilitation process for the family (Kurtzer-White and Luterman, 2003). As new procedures are integrated into clinical practice, and as early diagnosis encourages professionals to raise expectations for hearing-impaired children, the provision of services for these children must continuously be evaluated. This will underpin the continued development of better practice.

Plasticity and developmental processes in the human sensory system

There has been a huge increase in research around the neural mechanisms that underlie sensory perception in early life. The child's perceptual system initially develops in response to sensory stimulation from the environment. This phase is followed by episodes of neural retraction, or pruning, in neural networks that have low levels of excitation. Meanwhile, the functional pathways are consolidated by top-down learning effects as the cortical arousal mechanism applies attention to stimulation patterns, giving rise to recognition of visual and auditory patterns, or objects, within the first year of life (Moore and Linthicum, 2007).

The human auditory system develops from the peripheral to cortical levels, laying down myelination for the synchronous transmission of neural stimulation. Fundamental to the development of a sensory system is the concept of plasticity, whereby neural function is changed by previous experience. Plasticity allows the sensory organisation to be tailored, not only to the sounds encountered in the environment but also to the most salient or relevant information for the organism's needs and survival. Neural plasticity is recognised to be greatest during early development and is limited in time to 'sensitive' or 'critical' periods (Lorenz, 1958), during which the neural activity is either more susceptible to sensory experience, or is reliant on having specific types of stimulation to fulfil the sensory potential. Lack of auditory stimulation over early periods of life has been shown to constrain the development of the auditory system, and cannot be reversed by later amplification or electrical stimulation (Sharma *et al.*, 2005).

Between one and two children per thousand are born in the UK with a permanent hearing loss that will impact on the quality of life for that child (Fortnum *et al.*, 2001). If a hearing impairment can be identified and effectively managed from early life, the longer-term outcomes can be improved by giving sensory input and meaning to auditory signals during the natural periods of neural development.

Early identification of hearing impairment

Role of neonatal hearing screening

Neonatal hearing screening is available in many regions of the world with developed and integrated healthcare systems. Country- and state-wide screening programmes, using otoacoustic emissions (OAEs) or automated auditory brainstem response (AABR) techniques, have been shown to achieve screening rates of 85–95% of the newborn population. Screening identifies a group of children for whom further diagnostic tests are needed to fully define the extent and type of hearing impairment. This has proved to be more challenging than the logistics exercise that largely underpins a successful NHSP. There may be input from a number of professionals, with the family needs at the centre of management. For this, cohesive information and planning strategies need to be in place.

Management of hearing impairment in the first six months of life

The first priority for the audiological team is to define hearing levels as closely as possible, to fit hearing aids when necessary, and meet the communication needs of the child. Meanwhile, the role of the habilitation key worker, who may be a teacher of the hearing-impaired, a speech and language therapist, or auditory-verbal therapist (all will be referred to as 'hearing support teacher/therapist (HST)' in subsequent text) is to understand and support the family priorities and their evolving needs from the time of identification of a hearing loss. This is a very broad remit, requiring sensitivity to individual members of the family unit, often at a time of devastating loss and grief, occurring at a turbulent time for any family with a new baby. In the past, the role of the HST has been initiated around the fitting of hearing aids, but at this much earlier stage of the infant life, the focus should be on supporting the family. The aim is to embed the habilitation approach into the communication dynamic between family members and the hearing-impaired child, from infancy. The family needs to have impartial information to explore their own preferred choices for communication strategies, as a foundation for their child's future development.

Clearly the process of supporting early communication is heavily influenced by the extent of the hearing loss that a child has. The HST and the family require accurate information about the extent of hearing impairment, in order to develop a communication framework suitable to the child's needs.

Objective test techniques for defining hearing levels in the first months of life (see also Chapter 7)

In order for the child to benefit from the early identification of a hearing impairment, assessment should be completed by 3 months of age, and the fitting of hearing aids is usually undertaken within the first 6 months of life. When a child is under 6 months, the audiologist is reliant on using evoked potentials (EPs) to derive objective hearing results, as the young infant is not sufficiently consistent in making responses to sound. Evoked potentials can be recorded at different levels of the auditory pathways (see Chapter 7). At present, the auditory brainstem response (ABR) is the most widely used method of threshold definition, although there is a good deal of research being done into other techniques (Stapells *et al.*, 1984). Important supplementary information is given by recording of OAEs and acoustic reflex thresholds (ARTs) for cochlear status, with high-frequency tympanometry for the middle ear status. As with all audiological diagnostic strategies, the principle of a test battery approach is required to differentiate the site and extent of the hearing impairment, as no single test gives sufficient information in isolation. In order for audiologists to fit safe and effective levels of amplification, they need a high level of audiometric reliability, with consistency in results across several test techniques. An example for a 5-month-old baby might be responses at 80 dB for a 1000 Hz tone-burst ABR with air conduction and 75 dB with bone conduction, absent OAE, but normal tympanometry traces. These objective measures are compared to subjectively observed responses, such as the child stilling to a raised voice level at close range when not wearing hearing aids, but alerting to the speaker using a conversational voice level at a metre's distance when wearing hearing aids. Thus the profile of results, across both objective and subjective measures, is constantly cross-checked, to build up a picture of audiological certainty. For parents, the objective hearing results presented on a computer screen have much less relevance than seeing their child respond to a sound, so both objective and subjective testing have great importance.

If a child has a profound hearing loss or insufficient hearing aid amplification to make speech fully audible, there are still important benefits gained by early diagnosis of deafness. Early assessment leads to consideration of alternative strategies for communication, perhaps with increased reliance on vision, changes in hearing aid amplification, or assessment for cochlear implantation, while the child is still within the first year of life. Most cochlear implant programmes encourage referral of a child likely to need an implant by the sixth month of age, or earlier if possible.

Behavioural hearing tests

Behavioural testing in the clinic provides more information about hearing status and gives increased accuracy about hearing thresholds over time. In the first months of life, consistent changes in an infant's behaviour in response to different sounds indicate developing hearing responses in the suprathreshold audible range. However, ultimately, the absolute threshold for detecting a sound needs to be acquired for each ear separately. There is no longer a role for distraction testing in defining the child's absolute hearing levels (audiogram) for the fitting of hearing aids. Dr Jerry Northern, a pioneer in paediatric audiology in the US, notes that the use of 'distraction testing in the UK has stopped progress in applying modern methods of hearing assessment' (J Northern, personal communication), notably the competent use of visual reinforcement audiometry (VRA) (see Chapter 12). Many babies can be tested using VRA from 4 or 5 months' developmental age, and by 7 months' developmental age most babies can be tested using air-conduction and bone-conduction signals. By about 2 years'

developmental age, children are able to make conditioned responses, whereby they wait for a signal before responding by putting a bead on a stick or a peg in a board, using play audiometry. Both VRA and conditioned play audiometry can be used to fully define hearing thresholds when used in competent, child-focused situations. For children with developmental delay, it is important to use tests that are appropriate to their developmental, rather than chronological age.

Behavioural observation and early monitoring

There are important behavioural indications that an infant is detecting sounds in his or her environment during the periods when he or she is awake and responsive. Although these indications may be subtle, the importance of parents observing the child reacting to sounds, and responding to the child's rudimentary communication attempts, cannot be over-emphasised. By developing the parent's observation and reciprocation skills, the HST can help support them by building their confidence in communicating with the hearing-impaired child. Early support protocols (ESPs) empower parents and carers to observe and document changes in the child's awareness and understanding of sounds, in a clear and graded way.

Many parents benefit from meeting other families and hearing-impaired children in informal group settings. Parents have access to diverse sources of information from the internet, their own and other social groups, charities, and mandatory and independent support agencies. The information they find may give polarised views on aspects of communication management, and have variable relevance for their specific situation. The HST should be able to explore all of these options, allowing parents to make informed choices, without pre-judging the needs of the family and child. Thus, professionals who have high expectations for hearing-impaired children, updating their own skills and knowledge into individualised, flexible practice, are best placed to provide the framework for successful intervention.

Effective amplification

Fitting of hearing aids in the first months of life

The fitting of wearable hearing aids to give appropriate amplification is the second component of effective management. The audiogram has been derived through a combination of behavioural and objective hearing tests to specify hearing thresholds across speech frequencies in each ear.

Hearing aids are available in a range of models and sizes. Most infants can be fitted with behind-the-ear (BTE) devices (Figure 13.1), which can provide effective amplification for almost all extents of hearing loss. The benefit of BTE over body-worn devices is that spatial information about the direction and distance of sound sources is partly maintained, and the devices are usually more acceptable to parents. This is an important consideration, as establish-

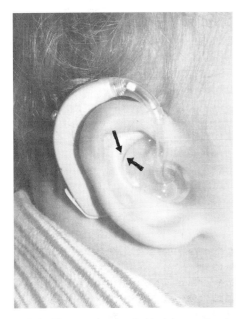

Figure 13.1 Photograph of a behind-the-ear hearing aid taken by parents and sent to audiology, to indicate where the earmould is not fitting well in the soft pinna (arrows), so that the impression can be modified to create a closer fit.

ing hearing aid use relies on parental perseverance and their understanding of the potential benefits from amplification. Choice of colours for the hearing aid casings and earmoulds may also help smooth acceptance, and increase use of the hearing aids.

The major practical factor in establishing hearing aid use is the provision of good earmoulds. Audiologists need to take deep, closely fitting earmould impressions at frequent intervals, possibly even monthly, to keep up with growth of the soft external ear structures. This can be helped by training of non-audiologists to take impressions, for example the child's HST, who will typically be visiting the family on a weekly basis. Earmoulds are usually made up of soft silicone, linked to the hearing aid with double-bend tubing so that the coupling between the earmould and the hearing aid has some flexibility. In hot weather stay-dry or anti-condensation tubing reduces susceptibility to moisture, which reduces high-frequency sound transmission. Parents need to be shown how to 'wind', or rotate the earmould into and out of the concha, so that the air seal between the earmould and canal wall is broken before the earmould is extracted. This avoids creating a vacuum in the ear canal and stretching the eardrum.

Hearing aids are held in position behind the pinna by well-adjusted tubing and, if necessary, with double-sided sticky (toupee) tape or 'huggies' that loop around the pinna. Hearing aids that fall forward or to the side of the pinna are unlikely to be used consistently. For very small children, a custom-made net bonnet can help retain the hearing aid in place. In general, if a child is determined to remove the hearing aids, no type of retainers will keep them in place. It is important to recognise that if a child is persistent in removing hearing aids or is very unsettled when they are worn, this is a strong indication that the acoustics of the hearing aids are not optimal, and the amplification should be reviewed. When hearing aid use is established in the first 6 months, it is generally much easier to maintain it as the child becomes mobile and able to exercise his or her own choice of activities.

Hearing aid prescriptions

The amount of gain given by the hearing aid is based on published rationales for amplified sound derived from the child's hearing levels. This emphasises the critical importance of having accurate hearing levels for each ear (audiogram) derived using objective and behavioural test techniques. There are two main prescription methods, which have been developed and verified for children; the NAL prescription, developed in at the National Acoustics Laboratory in Australia, and the desired sensation level (DSL) prescription developed in Canada, both of which have had updated prescription versions over time (Dillon, 1999; Seewald *et al.*, 2005). The NAL and DSL prescriptions apply rules, not only for amplification levels, but also for compression characteristics. Compression is the process of applying more gain to low-level sounds to make them audible, but less gain to high-level sounds, to prevent them from becoming uncomfortably loud. Therefore, in order to verify hearing aid amplification characteristics, the hearing aid output needs to be checked using different levels and types of input signals.

Use of aided thresholds to verify hearing aid amplification

The main focus of interest for audiologists is that speech should be made audible for the child, whether being spoken to at close range, for example when a child is being carried, or from a distance. The unamplified long-term average speech spectrum (LTASS), with a presentation level of 65 dB, is characterised as having a dynamic range of 30 dB, with absolute levels ranging from less than 20 dB to 65 dB across the speech frequencies 125–8000 Hz (Figure 13.2).

In the past, analogue hearing aids were set to give the same amount of gain to all incoming sounds, regardless of the level of input (linear amplification). In order to verify a linear hearing aid fitting for a child, clinicians relied largely on the use of aided thresholds (the lowest detectable signal through the hearing aid). Aided thresholds

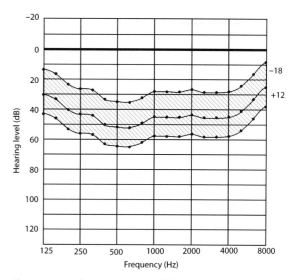

Figure 13.2 The minimum audible field binaural speech spectrum for combined male and female talkers with a presentation level of 65 dB. Note that 65 dB is the peak of the output with a 30 dB dynamic range and levels of less than 20 dB in some frequencies. (Derived from *Byrne et al.*, 1994.)

are now recognised to be wholly inadequate in assessing the amplification characteristics for the range of environmental sounds and speech that a child needs to hear. A common finding for analogue hearing aid fittings that were made using aided thresholds is that there is too much low-frequency gain relative to mid- and high-frequency gain, causing vowel sounds to mask out perception of consonants in speech.

With the era of digital hearing aids, aids are programmed through software and a computer interface, which gives fine control over many parameters of the hearing aid output.

Verifying the acoustic output of hearing aids in children

There are several methods for recording the real-ear-measurement (REM) response of the hearing aid output in the ear, which require the wearer to sit quietly in a specific position during the procedure. An alternative approach, which is useful for verifying the hearing aid output in children, is the SPL-o-gram. This has been developed by the DSL group as a way of assessing the acoustic characteristics of speech once it has been amplified by a hearing aid. The child's hearing levels are converted from decibels hearing level (dB HL) to dB SPL (sound pressure level), so that thresholds are directly comparable with the measured hearing aid output. The SPL-o-gram has the same frequency scale as the audiogram, and increasing dB SPL on the *y* axis (in the opposite direction to the audiogram). The acoustic characteristics of the child's own external ear structure with an earmould or insert can be included in the analysis, by recording the child's real ear-to-coupler difference (RECD). This is particularly important in babies and young children, as the small ear canal structure can give rise to very high levels of sound (Figure 13.3).

In Figure 13.3, the hearing thresholds are shown by the crossed line (left ear) and open circle line (right ear). Note that hearing levels for the left ear are poorer than for the right ear. The unamplified speech spectrum is shown by the dotted area towards the bottom of the graph and is inaudible without amplification for this patient. Once the speech spectrum has been amplified, as shown by the lined area, the speech is more compressed, so that it is largely above the hearing thresholds and therefore audible, but not uncomfortably loud. The predicted uncomfortable loudness levels (ULLs) are indicated by the asterisks, with maximum power output (MPO) for the aid shown by the uppermost line matching plus (+) symbols.

The hearing aid output can be viewed for different types and levels of speech input, for

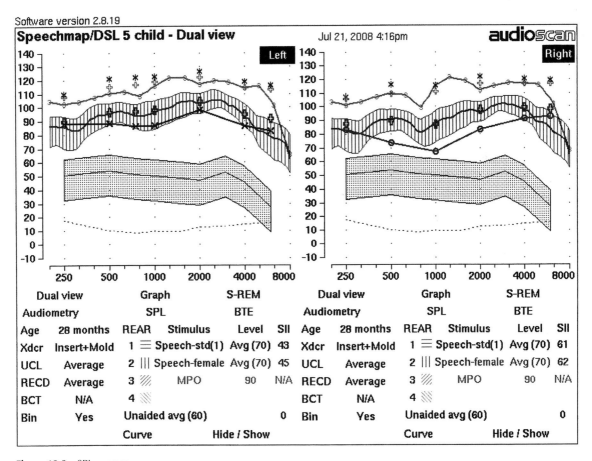

Figure 13.3 SPL-o-gram.

recording the maximum output of the hearing aid and the amount of compression that the hearing aid is applying to typical speech. Most hearing aids now incorporate some form of compression, to increase audibility of low-level signals while preventing high-level signals from being made uncomfortably loud for the wearer. Compression has been shown by several studies to be beneficial for speech discrimination in children with all extents of hearing loss, including severe and profound hearing loss (e.g. Marriage *et al.*, 2005). Information on compression characteristics, audibility of speech and the maximum output of the hearing aid is therefore represented in the SPL-o-gram. Using the SPL-o-gram, one can therefore infer the potential audibility of speech information.

There is less need for compression in amplification for conductive hearing loss. The use of a bone-conduction hearing aid on a soft headband may be a more practical approach for some types of conductive hearing loss, particularly if associated with pinna and ear canal abnormalities or chronic infection (see Chapter 21).

Parental reaction to the hearing loss

The coping strategy for parents in the face of an unexpected and devastating diagnosis of hearing loss within the first few weeks of life of their new baby varies widely. Some parents want to start hearing aid use as soon as possible, while others find the prospect of managing hearing aid use hard to contemplate, while struggling with the grieving process. However, with close, practical support, the first time that parents see their baby show awareness of sounds through hearing aids can be enormously motivating. Although there is an emphasis on early emotional support from the HST, for parents who wish to develop listening in their child there must be a parallel focus on the wearing of hearing aids, allowing observation of the child with amplification. In many cases these early responses to sounds can be seen and celebrated, when the hearing aid amplification is appropriately set. If no observable changes in behaviour can be seen, despite careful presentation of salient sounds and observation in a

range of situations, it is vital that the HST, in discussion with parents, feeds this information back to the audiologist for review of hearing levels and amplification. Although the introduction and use of technology can help parents through the grieving process, early intervention does not replace or avoid this painful process. Indeed it may defer acknowledgement of loss to a later time in the child's life.

Types of hearing loss

When diagnosis of a hearing loss is made in early life, the subsequent tests aim to identify the extent of the hearing loss and whether it is conductive (CHL) (due to outer or middle ear factors) or sensorineural (SNHL) (due to cochlear or neural factors). This is done by comparing results for air-conduction sounds, delivered via headphones or inserts, with results obtained by bone-conduction stimulation. The differentiation of type of hearing loss (conductive, sensory, neural, or a mixture) has important implications for: the information given to the parents, the likelihood that the condition is temporary or surgically correctable (some CHL), the amount of amplification required for each decibel of hearing loss and the predicted distortion that there will be for the child when listening to speech through hearing aids. In general, hearing aids fitted to match prescription targets for the audiogram will give rise to clearer speech with CHL than an equivalent SNHL. This is because there are recognised sources of distortion associated with cochlear or neural impairments, which means that no hearing aids will give 'normal' discrimination ability. It should be noted that children with SNHL are equally susceptible to an overlying CHL as children with typically developing hearing. It is recognised that early middle ear disease in otherwise normally hearing children can delay the maturation of listening skills (Hogan and Moore, 2003) and may have a greater impact for children with SNHL.

In SNHL, distortions associated with impaired function of the outer hair cell (OHC) mechanism in the cochlea (sensory impairment) include all of the following effects: loss of sensitivity to low-level sounds, abnormal growth of loudness with increased sound levels ('recruitment'), and poorer resolution of frequency and timing information. In addition, areas of the audiogram that appear to have some good residual function may be 'dead regions' (Moore, 2001). 'Dead' regions are parts of the cochlea that have no functioning inner hair cells (IHCs). Neighbouring hair cells respond to the frequencies normally transduced by the absent hair cell, but the benefit of amplification in these frequency regions will be limited. These effects of cochlear distortion increase with the severity of the hearing loss, so that although well-fitted hearing aids may make speech audible, discrimination of speech continues to be difficult. It is because the child's perception of speech is distorted, especially when in noisy situations, that a child's listening skills need to be underpinned by an effective habilitation programme, which should fall within the remit of the HST.

'Auditory neuropathy'

This was a term invented to describe the situation in infants who are found to have OEA present, often rather larger than normal, but with a hearing loss and absent evoked potentials such as ABR. It was originally thought that because the otoacoustic emissions were present but ABR was absent, the deafness was caused by damage of some kind to the cochlear nerve, or lack of synchronous firing of its fibres ('dys-synchrony').

Now it is recognised that this pattern of results can arise from damage to the IHC in the cochlea (e.g. following anoxia in premature babies), or loss of normal transmission between IHC and afferent dendrites of the cochlear nerve (e.g. OTOF syndrome), as well as asynchrony in neural firing in auditory neurones (McMahon *et al.*, 2008). However, all these groups have complex profiles of auditory awareness. Some children, for example, show awareness of simple tones, but very limited recognition of complex sounds and speech, which may be heard as noise-like. It is difficult to make predictions about how these children will progress with hearing aids:

their aided performance is markedly poorer than seen in more typical OHC cochlear impairment. This can lead to increased confusion and frustration for parents trying to support the audiological management of children with this profile of hearing results.

It is important that as much information as possible is obtained about the site of lesion in hearing losses with intact OAEs. In cases of 'auditory neuropathy', the criteria for referral for a cochlear implant assessment are not based on the audiometric thresholds, but on the functional hearing ability of the child, both with and without hearing aids. This highlights the importance of correctly identifying the site of lesion for all hearing losses, if children are to benefit from appropriate intervention in the first year of life.

These children have OAEs present around the time of birth and therefore may 'pass' the OAE hearing screening test. However, the ABR, which represents neural transmission, is likely to be absent or atypical, whether the site of lesion is due to IHC loss or asynchrony in neural firing. This underlies the importance of ABR as the appropriate screening technique for graduates of neonatal intensive care units. There is a specific ABR protocol which records the early component of the ABR generated by the cochlear microphonic (CM), to differentiate the diagnosis of cochlear-based IHC/neural asynchrony from OHC hearing loss.

Late-onset and progressive hearing loss

It is important to be aware that a NHSP cannot be 100% effective in identifying all cases of hearing loss in childhood. There will be a number of progressive or late-onset hearing losses, possibly related to intra-uterine infections, or genetic causes. Children with 'auditory neuropathy' will pass OAE screening but fail automated ABR, which is the screening technique of choice for premature or high-risk populations. In addition, there will be a proportion of cases of temporary conductive hearing loss, which are not the primary focus of hearing screening programmes, but may cause individual cases of significant disability and speech delay. Thus there is a need for audiology services to be responsive to cases of parental or professional concern about a child, even if the child passed the NHSP screen in early life. It is widely held that when a parent is specifically concerned about a child's hearing, there is very likely to be some sort of impairment.

Additional information is given by a battery of investigations focusing on known aetiologies of congenital hearing loss. The point at which parents wish to prioritise these investigations will vary considerably between different families. Aetiology investigations are usually arranged by the paediatric medical consultant and are based on rapidly evolving fields in genetics and including ophthalmology and radiology (see also Chapters 8, 11 and 12). Positive identification of a cause for hearing loss may well bring additional information about the likely site of impairment in the auditory system, and implications for management strategies. It is very important that families have as much information as they require about the potential cause of their child's hearing loss, to inform decision making for the future.

Effective team habilitation

The purpose of the NHSP is to enhance early auditory development through peripheral stimulation of the impaired hearing mechanism via hearing aids. However, there is an equally important component of habilitation, which develops the recognition and understanding of sounds through top-down processing. The structured process of auditory learning draws the child's attention to different sounds in the environment and associates meaning to the sound source. The impaired cochlear mechanism is unable to encode many of the subtle acoustic cues that are available to normally hearing children. By drawing the child's attention and awareness to sound sources although exploration and play, the auditory brain can lay down categories of auditory objects, developed around the auditory cues that the child is able to discriminate. Parents are 'empowered' by being encouraged to participate in auditory interaction with their children, introducing audible sounds to the environment of the

baby from an early age. Early sound types are graduated from simple, high-level alerting sounds, through to awareness of the parent's voice, to the child copying intonation contours on open-vowel voicing. This progression can enable parents to see the potential of their child, rather than solely the deficits in sensory perception.

Thus, the early identification and definition of hearing loss and provision of hearing aids puts in place the basic potential for auditory function. But it is the structured approach to exploring the soundscape that the child is surrounded by that enables the child to derive meaning from the sounds he or she hears.

The hearing-impaired child is reviewed in audiology every 2 or 3 months in the early stages of hearing aid management. However, the insight and observations made by parents and habilitation professionals, who are likely to be visiting weekly, will be a powerful indication of whether a child is hearing speech and other sounds through their hearing aids. Over the course of the first year, there is a combination of clinical hearing test results, hearing aid verification measures backed up by observations on the responsiveness of the child, and vocalisation development through structured monitoring. It will be apparent to the cohesive habilitation team which children may have better access to sound through a cochlear implant (CI). Although the prescription of acoustic hearing aids gives some stimulation of the neural pathways, the early referral and assessment for CI will maintain auditory potential if undertaken early in the first year of life. Decisions on supplementing auditory with visual information will be made with the family in the context of the child's developing language dynamic.

Continuing habilitation support through childhood

The achievements of individual hearing-impaired children who have had an early diagnosis and coherent management are startlingly different from outcomes typically seen 5 or 10 years ago. It would be easy to conclude that the impact of the hearing loss is lessened by the early intervention and improvements in technology. However, although hearing-impaired children may have evolved abilities in recognising spoken and visual information, the quality of the auditory signal that they perceive through the impaired cochlea or the electrodes of a cochlear implant can be rudimentary and distorted. The child may have learned to use this information more effectively, but the signal is still degraded. The hearing-impaired child has to apply cognitive effort throughout the listening day, to access meaning from the environment, and does not have access to the multiple acoustic cues that normally hearing individuals use in difficult listening conditions. Hearing-impaired children continue, therefore, to be reliant on the best technology for their hearing aids, radio aids, telephones and acoustic systems in the classroom.

Educational placement

As children approach school entry, they will be assessed for their educational needs by a multi-disciplinary team including representatives from education, health and social services. Each local authority for education will have policies outlining the communication strategies, provision of radio aids and other support provision available for the hearing-impaired children in their authority. The educational provision needs to be tailored around the learning outcomes for each child. Enlightened educational services are not constrained to the traditional list of school placements offered for hearing-impaired children, but are able to incorporate family, social and educational priorities for the benefit of the child. There may be a statement of special educational needs with specified support, or an individual education plan for the child. There is a risk that early-identified hearing-impaired pre-school children may be perceived to be only slightly delayed in communication compared to their normal hearing peers, and that appropriate educational support provision can therefore be reduced. This fails to recognise the input of the child, family and habilitation team in maintaining pre-school progress, the difficulties of hearing in noise, at a distance

and in groups, and the subtle disruptions of social interaction caused by hearing loss. Once the child enters full-time education, the initial input from family and the HST should be continued by the education service.

Past editions of this book have detailed the range of educational provision that hearing-impaired children attend. With improvements in spoken language outcomes, the numbers of children needing a residential school with signing or total communication are reducing. Children with profound deafness and cochlear implantation may function more similarly to children with severe hearing loss and hearing aids. However, a proportion of hearing-impaired children have additional complex needs and there continues to be a requirement for specialist education facilities. Many families support their hearing-impaired children in establishing strong and creative links with social groups of deaf culture, building in a sense of belonging and inclusion, but not to the exclusion of spoken language potential. In this way the family is maintaining choice for their child in the future.

Wider support agencies and technology considerations

As the child grows, the support he/she requires to help fulfil his/her social, language and academic potential will change. While technology continues to improve and miniaturise, there are points at which a high level of social and emotional support may be needed. It is not unusual for a hearing-impaired child or adolescent with age-appropriate language abilities to have a restricted group of friends and to be socially isolated at times. It may be, after seeing the child in his/her peer group, that family members reach a point of recognising the extent of their child's social disability, prompting a new period of loss and grieving (see Chapter 15). Some audiology departments have specific programmes of support which acknowledge differing needs of teenage and adolescent years. While new developments in technology will not reduce the devastating impact of a diagnosis of hearing loss for families, no one could doubt the social opportunities that mobile phones, texting, blue tooth receivers in hearing aids, webcams and email have opened up for hearing-impaired youngsters and their families.

Conclusion

The early identification of hearing loss in the neonatal stage has opened a new horizon for potential choices and achievements for hearing-impaired youngsters. It has also challenged professionals to develop new skills and training if they are to be able to provide effective habilitation for the children in their care.

References

Byrne D, Dillon H, Tran K *et al.* (1994) An international comparison of long-term average speech spectra. *Journal of the Acoustical Society of America* 96:2108–2120.

Dillon H (1999) NAL-NL1: A new prescriptive fitting procedure for non-linear hearing aids. *Hearing Journal* 52(4):10–16.

Fortnum, HM, Summerfield AQ, Marshall DH, Davis AC, Bamford JM (2001) Prevalence of permanent childhood hearing impairment in the UK and the implications for universal neonatal hearing screening: questionnaire-based ascertainment study. *British Medical Journal* 323:535–545.

Hogan SC, Moore DR (2003) Impaired binaural hearing in children produced by a threshold level of middle ear disease. *Journal of the Association for Research in Otolaryngology* 4:123–129.

Kennedy CM, Campbell MJ, Kimm L, Thornton R (2005) Universal newborn screening for permanent childhood hearing impairment: an 8-year follow-up of a controlled trial. *Lancet* 366(9486):660–662.

Kurtzer-White E, Luterman D (2003) Families and children with hearing loss: grief and coping. *Mental Retardation and Developmental Disabilities Research Reviews* 9:232–235.

Lorenz KZ (1958) The evolution of behaviour. *Scientific American* 1958:67–78.

Marriage JE, Moore BCJ, Stone MA, Baer T (2005) Effects of three amplification strategies on speech perception by children with severe and profound hearing loss. *Ear and Hearing* 26:35–47.

McMahon CM, Patuzzi R, Gibson WPR, Souli H (2008) Frequency specific electrodes indicate that pre synaptic and post synaptic mechanisms of auditory neuropathy exist. *Ear and Hearing* 29:314–325.

Moore BCJM (2001) Dead regions in the cochlea: diagnosis, perceptual consequences and implications for the fitting of hearing aids. *Trends in Amplification* 5:1–34.

Moore JK, Linthicum FH (2007) The human auditory system: a timeline of development. *International Journal of Audiology* 46:460–478.

Seewald R, Moodie S, Scollie S, Bagatto M (2005) The DSL method for paediatric hearing instrument fittings: historical perspective and current issues. *Trends in Amplification* 9:145–157.

Sharma A, Dorman MF, Kral A (2005) The influence of a sensitive period on central auditory development in children with unilateral and bilateral cochlear implants. *Hearing Research* 203:134–143.

Stapells DR, Linden D, Suffield JB, Hamel G, Picton TW (1984) Human auditory steady state potentials. *Ear and Hearing* 5:105–113.

Noise and hearing

Mark Lutman

14

Introduction

The first controlled epidemiological study to establish that noise at work caused damage to hearing was published at the end of the 19th century. Since then, noise-induced hearing loss (NIHL) accrued in industry has become the most common preventable form of hearing impairment, accounting for at least one-third but maybe up to half of hearing impairments in people under 50 years old. According to population studies carried out by the Medical Research Council's Institute of Hearing Research, 11% of men and 3% of women in the UK in the early 1980s had already accrued sufficient cumulative noise exposure to constitute a risk to hearing. Noise from gunfire, particularly during military training or combat, is an additional source of exposure that has become less common in the UK since the Second World War, but is prevalent in other countries experiencing conflict. Increasing social noise exposure, particularly from amplified music, affecting large sections of the younger population, has offset this decline.

Noise and its measurement

For the purposes of assessing risk to hearing, large population studies have shown that the appropriate way to measure noise levels is using the A-weighting scale, which emphasises frequencies according to the sensitivity of the human ear. Sound pressure levels measured using A-weighting are given units of dB(A). Virtually all sound level meters incorporate the A-weighting setting.

For steady noises, a simple sound level meter is sufficient to measure the noise level by sampling over a period of a few seconds. However, most noises fluctuate and a longer period of sampling is required to obtain a representative reading. This requires the use of an integrating sound levels meter, which accumulates noise energy over the sampling period and divides by time, in order to give the average level in energy terms. This averaged level is referred to as the equivalent continuous sound level, generally abbreviated L_{eq}.

Personnel may be exposed to noise during only a part of the day, or only a part of the week, thereby reducing the risk of hearing damage. Risk has been shown to depend on the total A-weighted energy reaching the ear, and therefore daily risk can be characterised by the level of a noise that, if present for a nominal working day of 8 h, would contain the same energy as the actual pattern of noise exposure. This equivalent daily noise level is symbolised by $L_{EP,d}$. Guidance documents for permissible noise exposures are usually phrased in terms of $L_{EP,d}$.

Cumulative risk from noise exposure is assessed by further integration of noise energy over the lifetime of an individual. This can be achieved by multiplication in energy terms of $L_{EP,d}$ by the number of days per week, weeks per year and number of years of exposure to derive the noise immission level (NIL). As an example, a person exposed at an $L_{EP,d}$ of 90 dB(A) for 10 years of normal full-time work will accrue an NIL of 100 dB(A). NIL is an important measure of cumulative exposure in epidemiological studies and for the diagnosis of noise-induced hearing loss (see below).

Noise surveys typically entail measurement of noise levels in the vicinity of the exposed person, with the aim of estimating the level occurring at the expected position of the person's head. However, when personnel move around during their work, that approach is problematic and resort is made to noise dosimetry using what is in effect a wearable integrating sound level meter. Small portable devices are available that can be attached to the lapel or to protective equipment such as a hard hat. They usually log parameters of the noise-exposure history over a period of several hours in a way that can be read out on a master display unit afterwards. In this way, it is possible to estimate L_{eq} for the period of measurement, and hence estimate $L_{EP,d}$.

Impulsive noise from gunfire is not amenable to measurement in the same way. Instantaneous sound pressure levels close to weapons may reach 180–190 dB but last only a few milliseconds. Risk to hearing from gunfire is therefore often characterised simply in terms of the number of rounds of exposure.

How noise affects the ear

NIHL develops insidiously until it has reached a certain degree. The main site of damage is the outer hair cells of the cochlea, where the damage is irreversible. Very high levels of noise exposure can lead to acute mechanical damage to inner and outer hair cells, but this form of damage is rare. More commonly, there is chronic damage that builds up slowly over time. Current scientific knowledge suggests that the main mechanism is *excitotoxicity*. Excessive exposure to sound creates a build-up of the metabolic products of normal outer hair cell activity, at a rate that exceeds the capability of the cell to neutralise those products. These by-products of cell function are toxic to the cell and may either damage the cell structures themselves, or damage the DNA of the cell. In the first case, the cell dies as a consequence of critical damage (necrosis), and in the second case the DNA damage triggers a process of 'programmed cell death' (apoptosis). Both processes cause the cell to die and be replaced by scar tissue. Hence, NIHL is irreversible, and the main form of treatment is prevention.

Minor loss of outer hair cells can occur without any audiometric change or functional consequences for hearing. However, more substantial outer hair cell loss leads to a reduction in the normal amplification process occurring in the cochlea, which in turn leads to a loss of sensitivity to quiet sounds at frequencies associated with the region of damaged hair cells. NIHL is evident on the audiogram as mild or moderate bilateral sensory (cochlear) hearing loss, predominantly at high frequencies. The greatest hearing loss is commonly at 4 kHz, giving rise to the typical 4 kHz notch in the audiogram pattern. This loss of sensitivity for quiet sounds is accompanied by a loss of frequency resolution ability, which means that sounds at the affected frequencies are more easily masked by sounds at other frequencies, especially lower frequencies. This phenomenon in referred to as increased upward spread of masking and has the consequence of making speech less clear. When listening to speech in quiet, increased upward spread of masking tends to mean that low-intensity higher-frequency consonant sounds in speech are masked by the more intense vowel sounds. This effect is exacerbated by reverberation in the environment. The result is reduced accuracy of speech recognition, especially confusion of words that are distinguished by weak high-frequency consonant sounds (e.g. bat *versus* back). Loss of frequency resolution ability also impairs ability to recognise speech in noisy backgrounds, as important speech sounds are masked by noise at adjacent frequencies. Typically, people with NIHL complain of loss of perceived clarity of speech and greater difficulty than normal following speech in a background of noise. They often require the television to be turned up louder than suits unaffected members of their family, which can cause discord at home. Loss of frequency resolution ability is most evident when hearing threshold levels exceed approximately 30 dB. Damage to the outer hair cell amplification mechanism, which predominantly increases sensitivity to low intensities but does not affect response to high intensities, leads to the phenomenon known as recruitment, which is defined as abnormally steep growth of loudness with increasing sound intensity.

Hearing aids primarily work by amplifying sound selectively as a function of frequency, according to the hearing loss of the recipient. Modern hearing aids are non-linear and amplify low-intensity sounds more than high-intensity sounds; in other words they compress the dynamic range of input sounds to compensate for recruitment. Non-linear amplification can compensate to an extent for loss of sensitivity to quiet sounds and may help to restore normal loudness. However, hearing aids cannot compensate for loss of frequency resolution ability and they do not restore speech recognition in noise to normal levels. Typically, people with mild-to-moderate sensorineural hearing loss require speech to be 5–10 dB more intense, relative to background noise, for recognition scores equal to those of normal listeners.

NIHL is commonly, but not universally, accompanied by tinnitus. In many cases, noise-induced tinnitus is not particularly troublesome but in some cases it is the most problematic consequence of noise exposure. The character of noise-induced tinnitus is commonly described as ringing or whistling, which is consistent with the high-frequency locus of noise damage.

Audiometric characteristics of noise-induced hearing loss

The audiometric pattern of NIHL is a symmetrical bilateral sensorineural hearing loss affecting predominantly the high frequencies. The characteristics are of a sensory, or cochlear, type of hearing loss displaying loudness recruitment. There is typically a dip or notch in the audiogram in the vicinity of 4 kHz. Figure 14.1 shows an example audiogram from a case of NIHL.

The symmetrical pattern of hearing loss assumes that both ears are exposed equally, which is normally the case, and that both ears are equally sensitive to noise. However, in some instances noise exposure is asymmetrical; for example, firing a rifle from the right shoulder causes the left ear to be more exposed, while communication headsets may deliver sound to only one ear. Nonetheless, in most cases of NIHL the audiometric pattern is fairly symmetrical, and substantial asymmetry would suggest an alternative or an additional cause of hearing loss, at least on the more affected side.

Although noise does not cause conductive hearing loss, there may be an overlay of conductive hearing loss on NIHL. In that case, the audiometric pattern of the bone-conduction thresholds is relevant. However, note that conductive hearing loss concurrent with noise exposure will attenuate sound reaching the cochlea and therefore have a protective effect, similar to wearing an earplug.

Harmful levels of noise

People vary substantially in terms of susceptibility to NIHL. Some people have been exposed

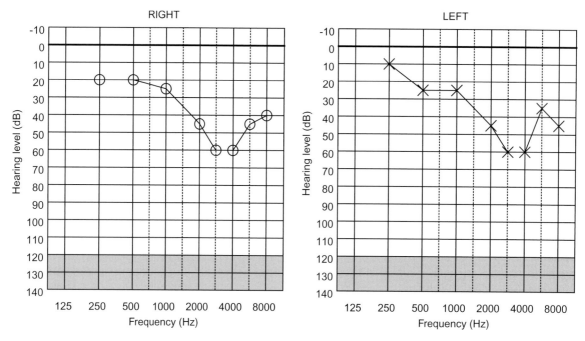

Figure 14.1 Typical noise-induced hearing loss, from a man aged 65 years who has worked in a metal casting factory for 13 years without hearing protection.

habitually to high levels of noise for many years yet show little evidence of any damage, at least insofar as damage is evident on the audiogram. Other people experience NIHL from short periods of relatively moderate levels of noise, or even from isolated instances such as attending a nightclub or exposure to a single impulsive sound. Therefore, the distinction between safe and hazardous noise levels is statistical rather than definitive. Over the years, governments and bodies responsible for safety at work have set guideline levels that attempt to balance safety of the vast majority of the workforce against practicality and cost to industry of implementing lower noise levels.

In the UK, it was considered by medical and scientific experts at least by the early 1960s that noise levels of 90 dB(A) and above were harmful to many people and that there was a residual risk at lower levels for more susceptible individuals. Publication by the Ministry of Labour of the leaflet *Noise and the Worker* in 1963 disseminated this knowledge widely to employers over

the next decade. More recently, European agreement to common standards of safety at work recognised the need to address risk of NIHL at levels of 85 dB(A) and above, which led to the Noise at Work Regulations of 1989 in the UK. This trend has continued, and further European agreement has reduced the level at which employers must take action on noise down to 80 dB(A). The corresponding UK legislation is contained in the Control of Noise at Work Regulations of 2005 (HSE, 2005). It is unlikely that there will be any further reductions of this type in the foreseeable future.

Statement of harmful levels of noise can therefore be summarised as follows. Daily exposure to noise levels, expressed as $L_{EP,d}$, of 90 dB(A) and above constitutes a definite risk to hearing that affects many people. At noise levels between 85 and 90 dB(A), some people will experience some NIHL. There is a residual risk to hearing for the most susceptible individuals at noise levels between 80 and 85 dB(A). Below 80 dB(A), risk of NIHL becomes so small that it can be ignored.

Further quantitative examination of the relationship between noise exposure and hearing loss is explored in the next section.

Relationship between hearing threshold level, age and noise exposure

The gradual onset of NIHL over a long period of time in most cases means that NIHL is confounded by age-associated hearing loss. Therefore, studies of NIHL must attempt to separate the effects of noise and age. As the two effects cannot be distinguished with any certainty within individuals, the separation of effects is inevitably statistical.

Knowledge concerning the relationship between noise exposure and NIHL is based on cross-sectional studies of people exposed to noise, much of which was conducted several decades ago and which concentrated on people exposed continuously to high levels of noise that were more common in the 1950s and 1960s. This knowledge is far from complete. Most studies have suffered from lack of appropriate non-exposed control subjects, and longitudinal studies are almost entirely lacking. Authoritative studies have involved large primary studies or synthesis of data from several large primary studies. The seminal study of Burns and Robinson (1970) has been influential in the UK and elsewhere. It formed the basis of the first edition of the international standard ISO 1999 in 1975, which quantified the expected effects of noise on hearing. The study has been embodied in the National Physical Laboratory tables that are still used widely for prediction of NIHL in populations exposed to noise. The later version of ISO 1999 in 1990 synthesised data from studies in the US, as well as from Burns and Robinson's study, to derive formulae for predicting NIHL. An advantage of ISO 1999 is that it allows the user to insert different values to account for the effects of age-associated hearing loss. This facility has enabled ISO 1999 to keep up with developing understanding of the effects of age on hearing and the recognition that there

are important socioeconomic factors governing hearing acuity. This is important because the non-exposed controls used in many studies of NIHL have been drawn from socioeconomic groups (e.g. office worker, researchers, university staff) that are different from those of the exposed participants.

The above methods account for the combined effects of age and noise exposure by simple addition of the hearing losses from the two effects, or a slight modification of simple addition. The modified addition incorporated in ISO 1999 slightly reduces the resultant hearing loss compared to simple addition. However, this effect is negligible for combined hearing loss lower than 40 dB, and for most practical purposes can be ignored.

ISO 1999 allows prediction of the distribution of NIHL to be expected from any cumulative amount of noise exposure. This is combined with (in most cases simply added to) the distribution of age-associated hearing loss appropriate to the population in question. The resulting distribution allows estimation of the probability that any given magnitude of overall hearing loss will be exceeded. Based on ISO 1999, Table 14.1 shows the extent of NIHL to be expected from a working lifetime of 45 years at daily continuous noise levels of 80, 85, 90 and 95 dB(A). The values are for NIHL at 4 kHz, which is the frequency predicted to give the greatest hearing loss. Values are given for the median and the fifth centile (hearing loss exceeded by 5% of population). These data constitute the

Table 14.1 NIHL predicted from ISO 1999 as a function of noise level for 45 years.

HTL at 4 kHz in dB	Daily noise level in dB(A)			
	80	85	90	95
Median	1.7	6.6	14.9	26.5
5th centile	2.2	8.8	19.6	35.1

noise-induced component of hearing loss alone. Note that hearing loss is minimal for exposures at 80 dB(A), even at the fifth centile, and increases at higher levels.

As indicated above, NIHL is nearly always accompanied by age-associated hearing loss, so that the audiogram reflects the combined effect of both. Hearing ability deteriorates with increasing age in virtually all members of human populations. Numerous studies have quantified this phenomenon, to the extent that it is characterised in international standard ISO 7029 (2000). The standard models the distribution of hearing threshold levels in males and females separately, in terms of deviations from a baseline set at the age of 18 years. The distributions are semi-normal, defined by mean values and standard deviations representing the upper and lower parts of the distribution. The mean (equal to median) values rise gradually with age at first, then accelerate for older people. The standard deviations also increase with age, giving a wide spread for older people. Hearing deteriorates more with age in men than in women, as defined in the standard. The standard only specifies the distributions up to the age of 70 years, due to limitations in the source data.

There has been substantial debate about the baseline value used to represent hearing threshold level for 18 year olds. The original standard implied that a value of 0 dB should be assumed based on numerous studies of highly screened populations of young adults. However, those studies involved participants who were not representative of the population at large and had thresholds that are slightly better than the whole population. More recent population studies have shown that a baseline in the range 2–7 dB is more representative of the otologically normal UK population (Lutman and Davis, 1994).

Figure 14.2a shows a case of NIHL for a man aged 52 years who has been exposed to noise at a level of 90 dB(A) for 30 years. This is compared with the expected combined effects of age for a man of the same age and with the same noise exposure on hearing threshold levels. The shaded area represents the interquartile range so that one-quarter of the population are expected to have better thresholds than the top of the shaded area, and one-quarter worse than the bottom. The white line in the centre of the shaded area represents the median. Figure 14.2b shows the effect of age alone in a similar format. In both figures, age-associated hearing loss is from ISO 7029 with the baseline set in accordance with the UK National Study of Hearing (Lutman and Davis, 1994).

Examination of Figure 14.2a shows that this case of NIHL follows the expected range fairly well. Most thresholds are within the interquartile range. In the crucial frequency range from 2 to 6 kHz, the thresholds are towards the better end of the interquartile range. Examination of Figure 14.2b shows that the expected range of thresholds for age alone is somewhat better in the range 2–6 kHz, compared to Figure 14.2a, although the difference is only approximately 5–10 dB. This small difference reflects the moderate level of noise exposure and demonstrates the fact that NIHL does not generally cause much hearing loss. Comparison of the measured thresholds with the range of age-associated hearing loss in Figure 14.2b shows that the thresholds are now worse than the median at 3 kHz and 4 kHz, exceeding the upper quartile on the left ear at 3 kHz.

Interaction of noise and other noxious agents

Hearing has been shown to be susceptible to exposure to organic solvents, such as toluene, that are used in several industrial processes. Studies in laboratory animals using high concentrations of solvents have shown an interaction between noise and solvent exposure, whereby the combination has greater effects than the sum of the separate effects. However, data from humans exposed to lower concentrations of solvents, which would be representative of industrial exposures, are limited. The available evidence suggests that interaction of solvent and noise exposure is unlikely to be a substantial issue for concentrations experienced in industries in developed countries.

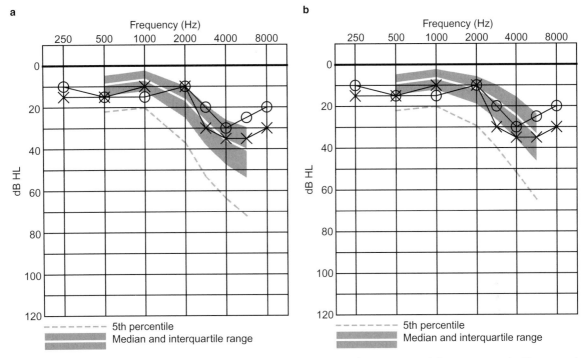

Figure 14.2 Audiograms for case of noise-induced hearing loss (circles, right ear; crosses, left ear) compared with expected range of thresholds. **a**, expected combination of effects of age and of noise at 90 dB(A) for 30 years, for a man of 52 years, in terms of quartiles and 5th percentile; **b**, expected effect of age alone.

Diagnosis of noise-induced hearing loss

Diagnosis of NIHL depends on establishing that there has been sufficient noise exposure, demonstration of an audiometric pattern that is consistent with NIHL, and exclusion of, or allowance for, other identifiable causes. Coles *et al.* (2000) have published guidelines for diagnosis, which are widely used in medico-legal cases. The guidelines describe three main requirements that should be met for a diagnosis of NIHL. Estimated cumulative noise exposure should generally exceed a noise immission level of 100 dB(A) after allowance for effective use of hearing protection, although 90 dB(A) may be sufficient when there is a very clear audiometric pattern. The hearing loss should be predominantly at high frequencies and be of the sensorineural type, usually having a fairly symmetrical pattern. There

should be a dip in the audiogram in the frequency region of 3–6 kHz amounting to at least 10 dB. In addition to the three main requirements, the magnitude of the noise-induced component of hearing loss should be commensurate with the amount of noise exposure, and other potential causes should be accounted for.

Because many patients with NIHL will also have a component of age-associated hearing loss, assessment of the high-frequency hearing loss and dip in the audiogram must take into account the expected age-associated hearing loss for a person of the same age and sex. The formula in ISO 7029 is suitable for estimating the shifts in hearing threshold level as a function of age. Coles *et al.* (2000) tabulate suitable values for men and women using a baseline for young adults that is representative of the otologically normal population in the UK (see above). Determination of any noise-induced dip entails looking for hearing thresholds that fall below the expected values for age in the key frequency range of 3–6 kHz. Figure 14.2b shows an example of a dip in the audiogram around 4 kHz, compared to the expected range of age-associated hearing loss.

It is worth re-iterating that diagnosis of NIHL in this way is merely statistical. Dips in the audiogram satisfying the above requirements can occur in people who have not been exposed to noise. Unpublished data from the UK National Study of Hearing show that in men with audiometric dips at 3 or 4 kHz in both ears, amounting to 15 dB relative to the average of the thresholds at 1 and 8 kHz, approximately two-thirds have been exposed to noise (NIL of 97 dB(A) or more). This implies that the odds of audiometric dips thus defined being actually caused by noise exposure are approximately 2:1 in cases with noise exposure, which is hardly definitive.

Diagnosis of noise-induced tinnitus

NIHL is commonly associated with tinnitus, as indicated above, and typically has a description that suggests involvement of damage at high frequencies, such as ringing or whistling. However, tinnitus is also common in the general population and, like hearing impairment, tends to increase with increasing age. The challenge of diagnosis of noise-induced tinnitus is to distinguish between tinnitus that has been caused by noise exposure and tinnitus that would have occurred anyway, without noise exposure. In some cases, there may be a clear temporal relationship to help with diagnosis, for example when a sudden high-intensity noise causes immediate onset of tinnitus. However, in most cases, tinnitus comes on insidiously and diagnosis becomes statistical rather than definitive.

As for NIHL, it is a requirement for diagnosis that there has been material noise exposure. A commonly used rule-of-thumb is that when a diagnosis of NIHL can be made, accompanying tinnitus is probably also noise induced, in the absence of evidence to the contrary. Tinnitus usually appears to be triggered by peripheral damage occurring in the cochlea, and so whatever causes peripheral damage is likely to be the diagnostic factor. There has been much debate whether noise exposure can have a delayed effect, causing tinnitus that has its onset long after cessation of noise exposure. While experimental evidence to confirm or deny this possibility is unlikely to become available from any feasible human or animal studies, expert opinion has expressed the view that delayed-onset tinnitus with a latency of years is improbable.

Audiological tests to characterise tinnitus, such as pitch and loudness matching or masking, are not useful for diagnosis of noise-induced tinnitus. Classification based on patient report of interference with everyday life is sufficient, usually on a scale of slight, mild, moderate or severe. Many patients report perception of tinnitus but they are seldom bothered by it, which would be classified as slight. Frequent interference with getting to sleep because of tinnitus merits a classification of moderate.

Prognosis for tinnitus, including noise-induced tinnitus, is that many patients experience a lessening of disturbance from tinnitus over time without treatment. This may be due to improved coping techniques or neurophysiological suppression. Counselling and treatment of patients with noise-induced tinnitus are no different from those for patients having tinnitus with other causes (see Chapter 16).

Prevention of noise-induced hearing loss

NIHL is preventable in virtually all situations by taking one or more of three steps, as advised in the Control of Noise at Work Regulations 2005. First, noise reduction should be implemented wherever possible to achieve the lowest levels that are reasonably practicable. Reduction to 80 dB(A) should be sufficient for the purposes of hearing conservation for virtually all personnel, but further reduction is desirable if it is reasonably practical to improve comfort and performance and to safeguard the minority of people who may be very susceptible to noise. Second, sound exposure received by personnel should be reduced as far as reasonably possible by enclosing noise sources or placing barriers in the transmission path, or by reducing the duration of exposure to noise. As a final resort, personal hearing protection can be used to reduce the sound energy reaching the ears of exposed people.

Hearing protectors vary in their attenuation characteristics. This variation is a function of the materials used to construct the device and how well the device conforms to the ear, thus preventing sound leakage past the device. For earmuffs, sound may leak between the soft plastic sealing cushion and the skin. For earplugs, sound may leak between the plug and the skin of the ear canal. For earplugs, the attenuation may vary according to how deeply the plug is inserted. The effectiveness of hearing protectors is quantified in terms of sound attenuation in decibels at a number of preferred frequencies. The sound attenuation is the amount by which the sound level is reduced when travelling from outside the protector to the eardrum.

Attenuation by hearing protectors is greater at high frequencies (above 1 kHz) than at lower frequencies, simply due to the physics of sound transmission. Foam earplugs and earmuffs are generally more effective than other forms of earplug. Attenuation values published by manufacturers are derived by testing volunteers, who perform sound field audiometry with and without protection. The volunteers are usually trained to fit the hearing protectors, and supervised to ensure a good fit. There is ample evidence to show that the real-world attenuation of hearing protectors is substantially lower than published by the manufacturers. Table 14.2 contrasts attenuation values from laboratory studies with the real-world values obtained from a variety of studies.

It can be seen that the real-world values are much lower than the laboratory values. Note that the values in the table are mean attenuation minus one standard deviation, which is the standard way to represent hearing protector performance and is an estimate of the attenuation exceeded in 84% of users.

Table 14.2 shows that the protection actually occurring when employees wear hearing protec-

Table 14.2 Real-world and laboratory attenuation of typical hearing protectors.

Protector type	Average real-world (dB)	Average laboratory (dB)
Foam earplug	13.4	29.0
Pre-moulded earplugs	3.9	24.0
Fibreglass down	5.3	21.0
Earmuffs	14.8	23.2

tion may be quite low for a fraction of the population. This is especially so for pre-moulded earplugs and fibreglass down products. The low protection arises from poor fitting of the protectors, and it follows that instruction on the use and fitting of ear protectors is of paramount importance in a hearing conservation programme. It is not sufficient to simply supply the protectors. This is especially important for pre-moulded earplugs and fibreglass down.

It is obvious that hearing protectors can only be effective while they are worn. Risk to hearing is governed by the total sound energy reaching the ear during the whole day, and the effective attenuation reduces rapidly if hearing protection is not worn for even a small part of the day. Therefore it is important to wear hearing protection throughout periods when noise levels are high. This applies to those working in an environment of industrial noise, but also to some musicians and to those working in the field of amplified recreational music.

Regulation and legislation

Current regulation of occupational noise exposure in the UK is through the Health and Safety at Work Act. More specific regulation is under Control of Noise at Work Regulations 2005, which came into force in April 2006. There are specific numbered regulations, the most important of which are as follows. Regulation 4 specifies the lower action level of 80 dB(A), upper action level of 85 dB(A) and exposure limit of 87 dB(A) at the ear, all expressed as $L_{EP,d}$. There are corresponding peak values of 135, 137 and 140 dB(C). Regulation 5 requires the employer to perform risk assessments regarding noise. Regulation 6 requires the employer to control noise, and reduce the risk of damage to the hearing of employees from exposure to noise, to the lowest level reasonably practicable. Regulation 7 requires the employer to ensure that employees exposed at the upper action level are provided with hearing protection that will keep the risk of hearing damage to below the exposure limit value. Furthermore, the employer must make hearing protection available on request to employees exposed at the lower action level. Regulation 8 concerns maintenance and use of hearing protection. Regulation 9 governs the need for health surveillance, involving monitoring audiometry. Regulation 10 requires the employer to provide information, instruction and training. The guidance notes lay emphasis on the need to pursue a systematic programme to encourage use of hearing protectors, recognising that people are often reluctant to use them.

The above regulations place statutory duties on employers, which are monitored via inspections by the Health and Safety Executive. Employers found not to be implementing the regulations may be served with an improvement notice. If they do not comply, there are further steps that can be taken to enforce compliance.

In addition to statutory regulation, there are two statutory compensation schemes for those who have suffered noise-induced hearing loss in noisy industries and in the armed forces. Both schemes apply the same definition of disablement, for which a pension may be payable. The least hearing impairment that qualifies for compensation is an average hearing threshold level of 50 dB, averaged over the frequencies of 1, 2 and 3 kHz, and based predominantly on the better-hearing ear. Reference to the sections above shows that this is a very severe NIHL, even when combined with the effects of age, and the vast majority of occurrences of NIHL will not qualify for statutory compensation. However, if the criterion for hearing loss is met, the claimant does not have to prove fault by the employer, and regular pension payments are ensured.

While few cases of NIHL will qualify for statutory compensation, any person may sue an employer under common law. Claims are generally based on negligence by the employer and are mainly for loss of amenity due to NIHL, with possible further claims for loss of earnings, and special damages to pay for equipment such as hearing aids. A successful claim must prove that the employer has been negligent (liability), that there have been actual harmful consequences and that these have been caused by the negligence of the employer (causation). Claims may relate to noise-induced tinnitus as well as NIHL. The onus is on the claimant to prove his case on the balance of probability. The notion of negligence is judged against the expected conduct of a reasonable and prudent employer informed by what he knew, or what he ought to have known. The regulations outlined above and the prior guidance and information contribute to the state of knowledge expected of employers. However, other information in medical, scientific and trade publications may be relevant, and large employers with corporate medical and safety departments may be expected to have greater knowledge of risks of noise exposure, particularly at levels of 85 dB(A) and below. Claimants also have a duty to initiate legal action within three years of knowing that they may have reason to claim.

References

Burns W, Robinson DW (1970) *Hearing and Noise in Industry*. London: HMSO.

Coles RRA, Lutman ME, Buffin JT (2000) Guidelines on the diagnosis of noise-induced hearing loss for medicolegal purposes. *Clinical Otolaryngology* 25:264–273.

Health and Safety Executive (2005) *Control of Noise at Work Regulations 2005*. Sudbury: HSE Books.

ISO 1999 (1990) *Acoustics. Determination of occupational noise exposure and estimation of noise-induced hearing impairment.* Geneva: International Organization for Standardization.

ISO 7029 (2000) *Acoustics. Statistical distribution of hearing thresholds as a function of age.* Geneva: International Organization for Standardization.

Lutman ME, Davis AC (1994) The distribution of hearing threshold levels in the general population aged 18–30 years. *Audiology* 33:327–350.

Non-organic hearing loss

15

Catherine Lynch and
Sally Austen

Introduction

> Responding to non-organic behaviour is unlike any other consultation (Feldman *et al.*, 1993).

Non-organic hearing loss (NOHL) provides a fascinating variant on routine clinician–patient interaction. Here defined as 'responses to a hearing test indicating a greater deficit than can be explained by organic (physical) pathology', such occurrences have been documented from the beginning of audiometric testing itself. The very existence of NOHL violates the expectation that a patient will be innately motivated to cooperate with their own testing and diagnosis.

NOHL requires detection, resolution of true hearing levels and appropriate patient management, all of which may present considerable challenges. Equally challenging may be the emotional response of the clinician, which can range from puzzlement through concern to intense frustration. There may also be medico-legal consequences, if, for example, residual hearing is lost through the fitting of over-powerful hearing aids or inappropriate surgery. Balko

et al. (2003) report an unnecessary cochlear implantation (CI) carried out on a patient with NOHL.

Negotiating NOHL to a satisfactory outcome is therefore an important component of audiological competency. NOHL is a topic with many dimensions, and at times requires input from mental health professionals. In this chapter we aim to unravel the threads of this subject and develop a framework of understanding to assist the audiology and ear, nose and throat (ENT) team. We consider the different subcategories of NOHL and their implications. These include extreme types of factitious NOHL involving deliberate self-injury of the ear.

What non-organic hearing loss is not

NOHL applies when no organic reason for the hearing loss can be found, and this designation should be used only after thorough consideration of all physically based possibilities, including investigations of the entire hearing pathway where necessary.

NOHL specifically requires that the patient is *driven by a motivation* (be it intentional or not) to affect the *hearing test itself*, in order to portray a greater degree of deafness than is actual. It is not simply a label for any hearing difficulty with a psychological dimension.

Inaccurate hearing tests may be the result of *test-taking difficulties* rather than NOHL. For example, cognitive impairment may prevent full compliance with test instructions, extreme tinnitus may affect the consistency of responses, and patients who are clinically depressed may lack the motivation to engage with testing.

Incidence of non-organic hearing loss

NOHL is not uncommon, especially in certain groups of patients. Jerger and Jerger (1981) suggest that although NOHL incidence is less than 2% in the general population, it can rise to 7% in children aged 6–17 years, and up to 50% in adults seeking compensation for workplace injuries, etc. Females aged 20–40 years, employed in medically associated fields and having experienced neglect or abandonment in childhood are thought to be prone to factitious conditions in general (Feldman *et al.*, 1993). Given the numbers assessed in a typical busy audiology setting, if clinicians are vigilant, NOHL will be found on a fairly regular basis.

Although NOHL can be superimposed on entirely normal underlying hearing, more usually it augments a genuine underlying organic hearing loss. The portion of the hearing loss attributed to NOHL is termed the *non-organic element, overlay or component.*

Detection and resolution of true hearing levels

Initial suspicions

Even before commencing testing, an experienced clinician may have suspicions of NOHL. The nature of the referral (medico-legal context; teenager under stress; young child with a deaf sibling) may alert the clinician. Routinely exchanging social pleasantries while performing tympanometry or examining an ear canal enables valuable assessment of the patient's reliance on lip-reading. As clinical experience develops, a sensitivity to when this informal assessment fails to correspond to audiometric results is formed. Additionally, an expectation of typical patient behaviour also develops with experience, and can alert the clinician to possible NOHL. For example, an overly cooperative patient who appears to be unusually keen to discuss the social impact of their deafness, one who appears particularly stressed, or one applying unusual levels of concentration during testing will raise suspicion with the experienced audiologist.

During the audiometric test itself, several additional indicators of NOHL may arise. These include:

- unusual lack of precision regarding threshold
- unwillingness to offer the normal occasional 'guessed' response, even when the tester leaves lengthy intervals without a stimulus
- a tendency to respond to a stimulus only if the stimulus duration is greatly lengthened
- in unilateral NOHL, the failure to obtain the expected shadow response. Audiological science dictates that once a sound is intense enough to pass across the cranial structures it will be detected by the contralateral cochlea. Therefore, even when testing a supposedly totally deaf ear, if the opposite cochlea is functioning, a response to a stimulus presented to the deaf side is expected at higher stimulus levels. Known as a shadow response, as it is not related to the ear supposedly being tested, NOHL patients are often unaware of this phenomenon and therefore do not feign it
- again with unilateral NOHL, gross differences in the unmasked bone-conducted (BC) response may be apparent, depending on whether the BC transducer is placed on the 'non-NOHL' ear or the 'NOHL' ear. The location of the transducer is in fact of little physical consequence, as the stimulating vibration travels almost equally to both cochleae regardless of side of placement. This fact is not intuitive to the NOHL patient who

will frequently provide different BC detection thresholds, depending on whether they think their 'good' or 'NOHL' ear is being tested.

Determining true hearing levels

There is a variety of behavioural tests that can be applied by the audiologist to explore the extent of the NOHL, including the delayed auditory feedback test, the Doerfler–Stewart test, and using Bekesey audiometry. See Gelfand (2001) for a comprehensive review of these techniques. Additionally, using standard speech perception tests, discrepancies between speech scores and the audiogram can be a clue to NOHL. Specific errors may relate to semantic category rather than auditory similarity, e.g. responding with 'dog' when presented with the target word 'cat'.

Such approaches have, however, been largely superseded by frequency-specific electrophysiological tests, which offer reasonably accurate frequency-by-frequency determination of true levels. Despite this, it should be remembered that as NOHL will often arise in busy audiometric clinics, it is important that the most effective behavioural methods are retained. Not having to reschedule every NOHL patient for full electrophysiological testing should be the goal, not just to save clinical resources but also to help bring the NOHL to a quicker conclusion, which could be psychologically advantageous. Many authors have recommended that NOHL should be resolved as swiftly as possible so that the patient does not realise the full advantages that might accrue – particularly pertinent advice for children.

For this reason we recommend that audiologists retain familiarity with at least two of the more valuable behavioural methods: (a) the ascending-descending gap test (Gelfand, 2001) and (b) the Stenger test (Altschuler, 1970).

Behavioural tests

The *ascending-descending gap test* exploits the fact that a person who is manufacturing a level of hearing loss in a test context will often set for themselves an 'internal loudness criterion', with the intention of refusing to respond at quieter levels (Ventry, 1976; Gelfand, 2001). They attempt to maintain their 'internal criterion' throughout the threshold evaluation, whether their artificial threshold is approached from an inaudible stimulus upwards in intensity or, alternatively, downwards in intensity from much louder stimuli. It is genuinely harder to hear a tone when threshold is approached in an 'upwards' manner, compared to tracking a previously heard tone 'down' to lower levels of intensity. Even normally responding (non-NOHL) patients will show some threshold variability depending on the direction of presentation, and there is an expected 5 dB or so difference between the two threshold measures known as the *hysteresis effect* or *gap*. With NOHL, however, the inability to accurately maintain the imaginary criterion typically produces a much larger gap, often rising to 15 dB or more.

Once the larger gap has been identified, the tester can then assume a strong possibility of NOHL and proceed to take the lower (better) estimated threshold as a marker. New threshold responses can be sought around this level and below, taking care not to present stimuli much above the marker. When a response is forthcoming, the intensity of the next stimuli may be dropped by more than the customary 10 dB. In this way, the audiologist can aim to disrupt the internal frame of reference for the patient and bring their 'internal criterion' steadily down to more accurate levels.

Although only applicable to cases suspected of unilateral NOHL, the *Stenger test* can resolve true thresholds with good accuracy. It exploits the non-intuitive psychophysical fact that when simultaneously presented with binaural stimuli of the same frequency, a person is only aware of hearing one sound, and will localise this to the ear perceiving the sound more loudly.

Using such binaural presentation, if unilateral NOHL is suspected the audiologist can test the veracity of a patient's responses. A quick calculation can determine a faint-but-audible stimulus for the good ear (by adding 5 dB to threshold, as the audiogram can be presumed to be accurate on this side). For the suspected NOHL ear, a level is chosen that ought to be inaudible (by subtracting 5dB from the threshold). If NOHL is present, however, this stimulus will in fact be heard clearly. Following similar instructions to conventional audiometry, the patient is instructed to respond when a signal is detected. Upon binaural presentation, therefore, if the patient is aware of the stimulus in the suspected NOHL ear, the faint contralateral stimulus will not be perceived. Failure to press the response button strongly indicates NOHL. Moreover, as the stimulus presented to the NOHL ear is progressively reduced in intensity (in 5 dB steps), there will come a point at which it is genuinely not heard. The simultaneous faint sound in the non-NOHL ear will then be apparent to the patient for the first time, causing the patient to respond. In this way, true threshold levels for the NOHL ear can be charted, frequency by frequency.

Non-behavioural (objective) tests

Despite the application of such methods, it is unlikely that the more psychologically resistant occurrences of bilateral NOHL will be resolved with behavioural testing alone. Such cases will therefore require referral for in-depth non-behavioural testing. There are historically intriguing tests such as electrodermal audiology, which relied on associating sound with mild electric shocks: once conditioned, the anticipation of the shock resulted in a measurable change in skin resistance, thus proving the sound had been perceived. These tests no longer have a place in the modern audiological setting, but see Gelfand (2001) for a review. When obtainable, analysis of stapedial reflexes can be useful; although it is difficult to accurately resolve true thresholds, particularly when there is a significant genuine hearing loss underlying the NOHL. Fortunately, the emergence of frequency-specific electrophysiological testing generally allows for straightforward resolution of true hearing levels. Methods developed for assessing frequency-specific sensitivity of young infants can be adapted for resolving suspected NOHL in children and adults alike.

Such tests include auditory brainstem responses (ABRs) and cortical electric response audiometry (CERA; see Sohmer *et al.*, 1977 and Coles and Mason, 1984). It is generally accepted that in skilled hands CERA is the favoured non-

behavioural test for resolving NOHL, as the hearing pathway is assessed to the level of the auditory cortex, thus ruling out more of the (rare) organic central causes of hearing loss.

The auditory steady-state response (ASSR), reviewed by Picton *et al.* (2003), also shows promise and has been used by one of the authors to successfully fit a hearing aid to a patient with a significant NOHL overlay. Where the clinical stakes are high, and undetected NOHL could pose a significant risk, one or more of these non-behavioural tests should be applied routinely in the assessment process, for instance before cochlear implantation. Spraggs *et al.* (1994) describe referrals for cochlear implantation that were found to have significant NOHL.

When the patient suspected of having NOHL is indefinitely resistant to providing accurate audiometric responses, or if subsequent audiometry cannot be shown to correlate with electrophysiological tests, radiological investigations should always be considered, to rule out central lesions.

Towards an improved understanding of NOHL

The existence of NOHL is uncontested. As outlined above, resolving true hearing levels is also no longer highly problematic. What remains confusing is the array of possible descriptions and explanations for the behaviour and how clinicians should interact with the individuals who behave in this way. Put simply: why do patients do it and how should we manage the consequences?

A model for understanding NOHL

There has long been an appreciation that all manifestations of NOHL do not arise from the same motivational source (Glorig, 1954; Williamson 1974; Sohmer *et al.*, 1977; Martin, 2002). Perhaps because of this, there is a confusing array of terms evident in the literature, including *functional deafness, hysterical deafness, psychogenic deafness, conversion deafness, pseudohypoacusis* and *malingering*. A review by Austen and Lynch (2004) of the concepts underpinning these terms reveals unhelpful inconsistencies in the use of terminology and implied causes of NOHL. Previous literature seemed to portray a crude dichotomy suggesting that non-organic behaviour was determined by a single construct: that it is either *conscious* (faking; malingering) or *unconscious* (hysterical; conversion; psychogenic).

Austen and Lynch (2004) found it more productive to categorise NOHL behaviour along two dimensions. Working to ensure compatibility with a well-known manual for diagnosing psychiatric conditions, the *Diagnostic and Statistical Manual of Mental Disorders*, (DSM-IV; American Psychiatric Association, 1994), a model incorporating the dimensions of *nature of gain* and *degree of intentionality* was devised.

The first dimension is the *nature of the gain* driving the behaviour. It may not be immediately obvious, but the experience of most illnesses and disabilities brings with it associated advantages. These may be identifiable tangible factors, or alternatively the benefits may be more psychological in nature. They can range from a specific *external* benefit (such as money from a successful insurance claim) to an *internal* benefit (such as an excuse for not reaching the expectations of others, or unconscious relief from internal stress caused by suppressed memories).

The second dimension relates to the *degree of intentionality* behind the behaviour. This can range from highly intentional, planned behaviour (such as consciously setting an internal criterion for 'not hearing', or researching hearing testing procedures so as to better subvert the test process) through to completely unintentional behaviour, where the patient is deeply identified with their assumed deafness and is not overtly seeking to deceive. From these two dimensions, three distinct categories arise (Figure 15.1).

Malingering

The first category, *malingering*, implies that the motivation driving the NOHL is an external goal, and that deliberate effort is being made to achieve that goal, for example qualifying for compensation or social security benefits; leaving the military etc. We recognise that the term 'malingering' has possible pejorative undertones, and would be

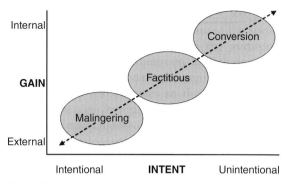

Figure 15.1 Categories on a continuum: Austen and Lynch (2004).

unhappy for audiology and ENT teams to use this term overtly in patient records: see below, 'Diagnosis of non-organic hearing loss: whose role is it?'. For the purposes of this model, however, it would be problematic to coin yet another term. It has the advantage of providing consistency with DSM-IV and will be reviewed in line with future DSM terminology updates.

Illustrative case 1: malingering

A 52-year-old motorcycle policeman became aware of colleagues receiving substantial sums for damage to their hearing through the prolonged use of powerful in-ear radio communication devices. He had been experiencing tinnitus and a dullness of hearing particularly in his left ear (the side on which he used this equipment) for several years. He instructed a solicitor and a hearing test was arranged. During the test he decided to augment the apparent 'damage' caused by the device by responding only to an intense level of loudness and above on the left side, choosing a point just beneath his threshold of discomfort. He applied considerable effort to this and thought he had managed to be consistent with his responses. When discussing the results with the ENT consultant, he was surprised, however, to find that the audiologist had stated that his hearing loss on the left was of a mild-moderate degree only. They therefore seemed aware of his plan to augment his hearing loss. He was embarrassed, became conscious of possible disciplinary action and withdrew his case, despite the fact that his unilateral hearing loss merited further diagnostic attention and that some compensation may possibly have been due (Figure 15.2).

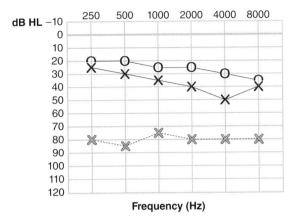

X ----- Initial audiometric thresholds for left ear

O ——— Audiometric thresholds for right ear

X ——— Revised thresholds for left ear following Stenger test

Figure 15.2 Audiogram for illustrative case 1.

Factitious

The second term *factitious* implies that the patient's motivation is internal and they are acting with less intent. A general example of the latter is the 'sick role', where persons benefit from secondary effects of their illness, such as increased attention, sympathy and support. Hearing loss may similarly be used as an excuse for perceived failure; a means of gaining attention or company; an excuse for avoiding unwanted obligations; or a 'ticket' to join the camaraderie of hearing-impaired or deaf support groups. These benefits can be so appealing to a needy individual that they may seek to ensure their supply through creating or augmenting a hearing loss.

Whereas malingering requires only a single episode or a series of occasional non-organic behaviours to achieve its (external) aim, the aim towards emotional wellbeing of factitious clients is a regular and repeated need. As behaviours are repeated to meet this need, they require less intentionality and can become part of the person's day-to-day repertoire.

A rare and extreme example of factitious behaviour in the audiological field is the Deaf Wannabee Yahoo discussion group, which pro-vides an online 'meeting place for people who have deep felt desire to wear hearing aids for pleasure, even although not deaf'. Members of the Yahoo group are unusual in their blatant intentionality and advocacy of self-harming acts. People within this group have heterogeneous motivations and include those who damage their ears or hearing in order to get attention from the medical profession; those who gain feelings of satisfaction from deceiving audiological profes-sionals; those who find noise distressing and have an unusually strong desire for silence; those who gain sexual satisfaction from deafness or hearing aids and those that believe that they have been born 'deaf in a hearing body' and wish to correct this situation.

A final factitious subgroup differentiates them-selves from the other subgroups discussed thus far by their strong desire to be and get well. This group is currently un-named, but may be provi-sionally described as 'the normal exaggerator'. This group comprises those who exaggerate symptoms in order, they believe, to get closer to a cure or solution to their difficulty: for example to get the busy clinician's full attention or to justify having taken up the clinician's time, and includes those who so desperately want a cure for their lesser degree of deafness that they exag-gerate in order to qualify for certain treatments. We postulate that media attention to interven-tions such as cochlear implants, plus perceived rationing in the United Kingdom National Health Service (NHS) may have amplified this behaviour in the UK. Certainly within cochlear implant teams we have come across people who are strug-gling so much with moderate-severe deafness that they exaggerate their loss to profound levels in the belief that the implant will solve their problems.

Illustrative case 2: factitious

A 15-year-old boy was preparing for GCSE (General Certificate of Secondary Education) examinations and was expected by his parents to do well. Due to an emotional upset at school he had fallen behind. He realised, with rising anxiety, that he did not understand some key concepts required for the maths exam. He recalled that when he was much younger he had also found school difficult for a while. Around the same time he vaguely remembered his parents visiting him after his tonsils and grommets operation, smiling and carrying presents. After a difficult day at school he found himself telling his parents that he could not hear the television clearly. His parents reacted with concern. Immediately he felt far less anxious. When he reported a few days later that he was still not hearing well, they took him for an urgent private hearing test. The audiologist seemed to take a long time with the hearing test (Figure 15.3). A different type of test was done with electrodes on his head. Following this, he and his parents were told that his hearing was normal and his parents were very relieved. The ENT consultant was concerned, however, by the young man's withdrawn behaviour and arranged a referral to clinical psychology. He later discovered that this appointment was not attended. On enquiry via the general practitioner (GP), it appeared that the boy's vision was now under investigation.

Conversion

The third category is *conversion*. It is classically defined as the conversion of intrapsychic stress

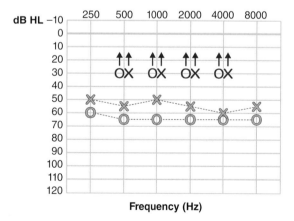

Figure 15.3 Audiogram for illustrative case 2.

into physical symptoms without the awareness of the patient, and in association with deep psychological trauma. The key difference from malingering and factitious categories is that the behaviour is wholly unintentional. There is current debate as to whether conversion disorder can be longstanding, or whether it is more likely to be characterised by a briefer conversion experience (a matter of days or weeks only), which then evolves into more intentional behaviour as a result of the perceived benefits of the deafness. The subsequent behaviour would therefore be categorised as *factitious*, e.g. the gain being the sympathy and attention, or *malingering*, e.g. financial compensation.

Illustrative case 3: conversion

A 5 year old was sexually abused and soon after was involved in a car crash in which she witnessed fatalities. She was admitted to hospital with mild head injuries and was diagnosed with severe deafness. The deafness excused her from discussing her feelings. On further testing the deafness was found to be non-organic and since she did not seem to be feigning the deafness intentionally, it appeared that this was a conversion phenomenon. As she approached adulthood, her hearing 'worsened' and, having moved to another part of the country, she was diagnosed with profound bilateral hearing loss. She was referred for a cochlear implant and provisionally accepted for surgery. Separately she was referred to a specialist deaf mental health team by her new GP to assess her longstanding health anxieties and consider whether NOHL might be present. The psychologist noticed many behaviours incompatible with profound deafness and, in discussion with the GP, was made aware of the patient's other non-organic behaviours. Objective testing showed a near-normal left ear and a mild hearing loss on the right (Figure 15.4). It seems that the conversion deafness had worn off (we don't know when) and had been replaced with a factitious presentation. The psychologist attempted a 'graceful recovery' strategy alongside broader therapy. After 6 months the client wished to be discharged. She was taking less medication for her 'medical' conditions, had improved mood and had engaged in community

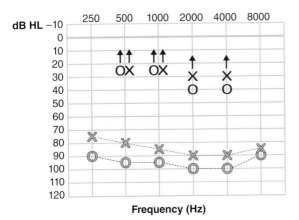

O---- Initial audiometric thresholds for right ear

X---- Initial audiometric thresholds for left ear

O   Objectively derived threshold (right) using ABR

X   Objectively derived threshold (left) using ABR

Figure 15.4 Audiogram for illustrative case 3.

activities – but was still responding at severe-profound levels when tested in clinic.

Relative prevalence of the three categories of non-organic hearing loss

In standard clinical audiological settings within the NHS, we suggest that factitious disorder is the most prevalent category. Depending on the patient population, however, the relative incidence of these three categories will vary. For example, during times of military 'call-up' or a large medico-legal campaign, malingering may increase. In cultures where emotional support is lacking or social benefits are closely linked to disability, factitious disorders are likely to increase. However, in all cases true conversion is rare.

Movement between categories

Consistent with DSM-IV it is recognised that a person may move through these categories as internal and external factors change. For example, a person may previously have experienced a genuine organic hearing loss and, having discovered some secondary benefits to the deafness, he/she becomes motivated to feign a hearing loss

so as to continue these benefits. Depending on the nature of the benefits and the degree of intent, this behaviour may fit the 'malingering' or 'factitious' category. This sequence of events was highlighted by Aplin and Rowson (1986) and is thought to be particularly common in children.

Diagnosis of non-organic hearing loss: whose role is it?

It is the role of the audiology and ENT team to be alert to the possibility of NOHL, record suspicion, proceed to identify true hearing thresholds and carry out subsequent audiological care.

Identifying the motivation (*intentionality* and *gain*) of the patient and diagnosing *malingering*, *factitious* or *conversion disorder* is the role of a trained and experienced mental health professional: usually a psychiatrist or clinical psychologist. It is never within the mandate of the audiology or ENT team to formally diagnose psychological conditions: any misapplication of psychological labels could be damaging to the patient. The Austen–Lynch model provides a useful shared framework for the audiology and ENT team to discuss possibilities and plan management options. Members of these teams, which ideally include hearing therapists and speech and language therapists, may get to know the patient well over a long period of time and obtain insight into probable intentions and gains. This is valuable information to pass to associated mental health professionals.

Portrayal of non-organic hearing loss

There have been attempts to profile psychological characteristics of persons presenting with NOHL (Trier and Levy, 1965; Aplin and Rowson, 1986). Greater degrees of emotional immaturity, social anxiety, instability and feelings of inferiority than are found in the normal population have been suggested.

Additionally we suggest that the patient's clinical presentation is linked to the category of

NOHL, for example the degree to which their deafness is 'lived out' in everyday life.

Based on anecdotal evidence, the *malingering* patient seems to limit his/her non-organic portrayal to the clinical context and has to consciously 'work' at their temporary 'act' of deafness. Thus the audiologist may therefore observe 'over-acting' or undue anxiety during testing.

The *factitious* patient is perhaps less likely to appear anxious, as they are experiencing a degree of emotional relief while portraying greater deafness, and although they have some intent, they may be less highly self-conscious about their strategy. This living-out of their deafness may have been a pattern for some time and thus has become a somewhat natural behaviour. They are likely to become anxious, however, if they feel that their deafness is not validated by others, and may insist on seeing specified clinicians with whom they feel safe.

The 'deafness' of the patient with *conversion* NOHL may also appear to be highly consistent, running through all aspects of life. Family members may be convinced by the deaf portrayal, although some may have noticed discrepancies. Persons with conversion NOHL may be less likely to give inadvertent clues during testing, as they are internally congruent with the belief in their own deafness. In conversion disorders generally, however, there is also evidence that clients are so unaware of their symptoms that they can slip in and out of them unknowingly, without overall consistency (Powsner, 2006). The rarity of this condition makes generalisation difficult.

Management of non-organic hearing loss

Successfully detecting NOHL and resolving true underlying hearing levels, although important, is not the endpoint. Although nowadays with electrophysiological testing we can detect NOHL and resolve true hearing levels very successfully, the issue of managing the subsequent interaction so that the patient's wellbeing is maximised is less well explored.

This is associated with active disagreement about the significance of NOHL. At one extreme, NOHL can be seen as simply a pattern of inconsistent responses, signifying very little. Andaz *et al.* (1995) emphasised the pragmatic value of dealing with cases of NOHL without the need for deeper analysis, particularly with children in routine settings. The problem of NOHL can be said, therefore, to disappear with the emergence of a normal audiogram. Similarly, Veniar and Salston (1983) caution against labelling. We agree that it is reasonable to hypothesise that many cases of NOHL do not indicate serious underlying psychological vulnerability. For many it may be unhelpful to have gains (such as extra attention) consolidated by referral for psychological assessment.

In contrast, some feel that NOHL (particularly when the gains are more internally derived) *does* fall within a psychological remit and therefore merits attention from healthcare services. This view fits with the body of research that associates NOHL with possible serious psychosocial dysfunction or abuse (e.g. Brooks and Geoghegan 1992; Riedner and Efros 1995). Austen and Lynch (2004) suggest that even when intention is conscious and gains are external (such as with malingering), there is occasionally scope for psychological concern, for example if the malingerer becomes suicidal at the thought of continuing in the armed services.

We suggest that the solution is to assess psychological vulnerability on a case-by-case basis. It is imperative that while the majority of cases can be dealt with pragmatically, there should also be a sensitive filter aimed at identifying the important subset of NOHL cases that may be at risk. These cases should receive prompt referral to appropriate mental health services, ideally staffed by practitioners skilled in the ramifications of both the psychology of deafness and non-organic presentation.

Management: the filter

Creating this sensitive filter is an ongoing challenge and impossible to perfect. As previously mentioned, it is *not* the job of audiology and

ENT teams to make psychological diagnoses. The crucial skill for audiological professionals is to be alert for signs of particular severity, duration and vulnerability associated with the NOHL. If in doubt as to whether an individual requires mental health input, audiology and ENT professionals should err on the side of caution.

Should an individual require referral for psychiatric or psychological treatment, a convenient way into these discussions with a patient can relate to any co-morbid anxiety or depression. Frequently these issues will be present in *factitious* cases and will also be relevant to many *malingering* cases; they can therefore act as a less emotionally loaded frame for the referral – the NOHL getting secondary mention in discussions with the patient. Indirect approaches may well be necessary as, in our experience, NOHL patients rarely wish to confront their NOHL directly and will typically default appointments if they believe disclosure is to be forced upon them.

Management: the role of the general practitioner

With the ultimate responsibility for collating information about patients, in the UK the primary care GP is the clinician who holds an overall view of an individual. Information concerning non-organic behaviour should therefore be shared with the GP in letter form. Any information that includes severe depression or suicidal intent should be communicated immediately by telephone.

Commonly, NOHL patients will have more than one type of non-organic behaviour, either at present or in the past. Such a patient, discharged after providing a normal audiogram, may find an alternative means of achieving their gain: for example, non-organic back pain, epilepsy or visual problems. In some cases it is permissible for senior staff to alert other medical establishments to non-organic treatment-seekers, although often the rules of confidentiality prevent this. By providing the GP with up-to-date information, however, he or she can detect patterns

of unhelpful behaviour and involve mental health professionals as necessary.

Guidelines for managing non-organic hearing loss

Whether or not the audiology or ENT team is planning to refer onwards for specialist opinion and management, there are some key guidelines for engaging the patient in testing and discussion, right from the moment of first suspicion. Silver (1996) suggests guidelines aimed at conversion disorder but these are able to be generalised for most non-organic presentations. To these guidelines we have added specific suggestions for each category of NOHL.

Avoid confrontation with patients regarding their non-organic hearing loss

The clinician may be tempted to 'reveal' dramatically that they know the patient has not been acting in a straightforward manner. Clearly this calls for professional restraint. The test results need to be communicated in a sensitive way with a view to maximising therapeutic outcomes.

A person in the *malingering* category is, by definition, aware of his or her intention to deceive and may feel strong anger or shame at being found out. This can result in overt hostility or acute embarrassment. Where test results have to be given in detail (in, say, a medico-legal context), the best approach is to be factual and non-judgemental, explaining what the tests have measured and how the estimation of accurate hearing levels was arrived at. Clear written copies of test results are important.

The *factitious* patient requires great sensitivity as, by definition, they have been using this behaviour to meet emotional needs. There is a possibility that if one source for soothing emotional needs is blocked by crude exposure (i.e. forcing them to lose their 'crutch'), they will attempt another route, which may possibly be more self-harming. Most patients benefit most from an opportunity to reframe and then retest with the help of a benign explanatory model (see below). It is beneficial to obtain a more accurate audiogram that is consistent with the non-behavioural test findings, as this avoids the need to draw attention to discrepancies, although it is rarely worth pursuing repeat audiograms to the point of frustration for the patient or audiologist. Indirect exploration can be made of any secondary benefits, and ideally the patient is led towards identifying for themselves a healthier route to meeting their needs. If a trained psychologist is not available, this may be best facilitated by a member of the team with recognised counselling skills.

Those with less intent (some *factitious* cases; all *conversion* cases) invariably require referral for psychiatric or psychologically based services. It is inappropriate for audiology- or ENT-based clinicians to attempt amateur psychoanalysis. In cases of *conversion*, the original precipitating trauma is likely to have been severe.

Avoid reinforcing or trivialising symptoms

Once NOHL is suspected, particularly for the *factitious* category, it is imperative that the clinicians themselves do not facilitate the gains that may be shoring up the behaviour. An appropriate, but not excessive, level of warmth and concern for the patient is required, taking care not to submit to inappropriate demands on professional time. Seeing the patient too frequently may unwittingly reinforce continuing symptoms. Equally, understanding the emotional vulnerability of factitious patients should ensure that they are not dealt with dismissively, even when it is suspected that they have positively 'enjoyed' a level of deceit.

Where possible, persuading the patient's family to change their own behaviour can be remarkably useful. A common example is asking an over-concerned parent not to mention the subject of hearing loss to their child, and to stop informal testing at home.

Benign explanatory model and expectation of recovery

Once the fact of NOHL (regardless of specific category) is clear to the clinician, he or she can create a benign explanation allowing the patient a graceful retreat from their NOHL posture. The

bigger the benefits of the NOHL (be they external or internal), the harder it will be for patients to 'give up' the behaviour, so sensitivity and tact are required. Simple options include retesting with supposedly 'better' headphones. A friendly opinion from a medical team member that the patient's hearing 'should improve' after a simple procedure such as a de-waxing can also help. Such strategies offer the patient some sense of control and dignity over the unveiling of the NOHL. Boxing a patient in a corner will result in a less elegant and therapeutic outcome and can be counterproductive.

Documentation and notation

Documenting in a clear and consistent way first the suspicion and then any subsequent fact of NOHL (including the patient's response to being told that their actual degree of hearing loss is less than their audiometric test suggested) is vital. It optimises communication within the team and creates an effective medico-legal record. We have seen cases when the audiologist was aware of possible NOHL during testing, but the obscure annotation on the audiogram was not decoded by the ENT surgeon, and potentially damaging surgery was scheduled. We suggest that every department has its own notation, perhaps using the term 'NOHL suspected' on audiograms that seem suspicious and 'NOHL probable' where electrophysiological tests have been done and all other reasonable explanations have been ruled out by the medical team.

Recent UK government legislation (Department of Health, 2003, 2007) allows patients access to their medical records and states that patients should receive copies of letters written about them. It is not acceptable to hide meaning from patients. Every audiology and ENT team should therefore be prepared to offer an explanation of the term 'NOHL' to any patient where this has been written in their records. Such teams should *not* be using the DSM-IV categories 'malingering', 'factitious' or 'conversion' formally in patient records, unless these have been validated by a qualified clinical psychologist or psychiatrist.

Emotional responses to non-organic hearing loss

Martin (2002) stresses that it is never part of the audiology team's role to make value judgements about a patient's behaviour. In the authors' opinion, this ideal is easier to achieve if the clinicians are able to manage their own feelings when faced with NOHL. It is not unusual for clinicians to feel angry at what they may interpret as an attempted personal deception and waste of valuable healthcare resources. They may also feel sympathy with the patient, or helplessness at how to assist them. It is also common for a clinician to be anxious about how to deal with the situation and what to say to the patient and their family, particularly if a vulnerable child is involved. Team awareness and discussion assists these issues and can transform negative feelings into a real interest and desire to manage these complex situations effectively.

It is also possible that a parent, spouse or other member of a patient's support network will feel strong negative emotions when the fact of NOHL is revealed. This may manifest as anger towards the patient who has 'deceived' them (of particular concern when a parent becomes excessively angry with a child, uncovering family dynamics which may necessitate the activation of child protection procedures), guilt that they have not realised their loved one's deeper needs, or frustration at the clinician who appears to have failed to acknowledge the difficulties their loved one faces.

One aim of the Austen–Lynch model is to help clinicians to conceptualise the psychological roots of NOHL. Thus, negative reactions and feelings may be replaced with interest and understanding, leading to more effective explanations for professionals, patients and patients' carers.

It vital that any prior suspicion or confirmation of NOHL does not affect the subsequent management of that person. Grady (1999) reports an anecdotal case of a woman incorrectly denied life-saving gastrointestinal treatment on the basis of her flagrant past factitious behaviour, which had blinded clinicians to the possibility of a subsequent genuine complaint.

Conclusion

This chapter opened with a quotation from Feldman *et al.* (1993). Encountering NOHL is indeed 'unlike any other consultation', and it requires that clinicians develop and blend skills from both audiological and psychological domains. We hope to have provided some structure within which audiology and ENT teams can aim for optimal outcomes for these often complex patients.

Acknowledgments

We are grateful to colleagues past and present for clinical collaboration and fruitful discussions on the subject of NOHL. We also thank Vicki Holmes BSc, MIMI, RMIP (Medical Illustrator, Royal National Throat, Nose and Ear Hospital, London) for her expertise producing the diagrams for this chapter.

References

Altschuler MW (1970) The Stenger Phenomenon. *Journal of Communicative Disorders* 3:89–105.

American Psychiatric Association (1994) *Diagnostic and Statistical Manual of Mental Disorders*. Washington DC: American Psychiatric Association.

Andaz C, Heyworth T, Rowe S (1995) Non-organic hearing loss in children: a 2-year study. *Otorhinology* 57:33–35.

Aplin D and Rowson V (1986) Personality and functional hearing loss in children. *British Journal of Clinical Psychology* 25:313–314.

Austen S, Lynch C (2004) Non-organic hearing loss redefined: understanding, categorising and managing non-organic behaviour. *International Journal of Audiology* 43:449–457.

Balko K, Fordyce D, Blankenship K, Littman T, Backous D (2003) Conversion deafness in a cochlear implant patient. *Cochlear Implants International* 4(4 suppl):19–20.

Brooks D, Geoghegan P (1992) Non-organic hearing loss in young persons: transient episode or deep-seated difficulty? *British Journal of Audiology* 36:347–350.

Coles RRA, Mason SM (1984) The results of cortical electrical response audiometry in medicolegal investigations. *British Journal of Audiology* 18:71–78.

Department of Health (2003) *Guidance for Access to Health Records Requests Under the Data Protection Act 1998.* www.dh.gov.uk/prod_consum_dh/groups/dh_digitalassets/@dh/@en/documents/digitalasset/dh_4035194.pdf (accessed 17 November 2008).

Department of Health (2007) *Copying Letters to Patients: background, issues and progress.* www.dh.gov.uk/en/Managingyourorganisation/PatientAndPublicinvolvement/Copyingletterstopatients/DH_4000431 (accessed 17 November 2008).

Feldman MD, Ford CV, Reinhold T (1993) *Patient or Pretender: inside the strange world of factitious disorders.* Boston: John Wiley and Sons Inc.

Gelfand SA (2001) Nonorganic hearing loss. In: Gelfand SA, ed. *Essentials of Audiology*, 2nd edn, pp 421–442. New York: Thieme Medical Publishers.

Glorig A (1954) Malingering. *Annals of Otology, Rhinology and Laryngology* 65:154–170.

Grady D (1999) A great pretender now faces the truth of illness. *New York Times*, 20 July 1999.

Jerger S, Jerger J (1981) Functional hearing disorders. In: Jerger S, Jerger J. *Auditory Disorders*, pp 51–58. Boston MA: College Hill Press.

Martin F (2002) Pseudohypacusis. In: Katz J, ed. *Handbook of Clinical Audiology*, 5th edn, pp 584–596. Baltimore: Williams & Wilkins.

Picton TW, John SM, Dimitrijevic A, Purcell D (2003) Human auditory steady-state responses. *International Journal of Audiology* 42: 177–219.

Powsner S (2006) *Conversion Disorder.* www.emedicine.com/EMERG/topic112.htm (accessed 17 November 2008).

Riedner E, Efros P (1995) Non-organic hearing loss and child abuse: beyond the sound-booth. *British Journal of Audiology* 42:177–219.

Silver F (1996) Management of conversion disorder. *American Journal of Physical Medicine and Rehabilitation* 75:134–140.

Sohmer H, Feinmesser M, Bauberger-Tell L, Edelstein E (1977) Cochlear, brainstem and cortical evoked responses in non-organic hearing loss. *Annals of Otology, Rhinology and Laryngology* 86:227–234.

Spraggs P, Burton M, Graham J (1994) Non-organic hearing loss in cochlear implant candidates. *American Journal of Otology* 15: 652–657.

Trier T, Levy R (1965) Social and psychological characteristics of veterans with functional hearing loss. *Journal of Audiological Research* 5:241–256.

Veniar F, Salston R (1983) An approach to the treatment of pseudohypacusis in children. *American Journal of Diseases in Childhood* 137:34–36.

Ventry IM (1976) Comment on article by Martin and Monro. *Journal of Speech and Hearing Disorders* 40:282–283.

Williamson D (1974) Functional hearing loss: a review. *Maico Audiological Library Series* 12: 334.

Tinnitus and hyperacusis

Don McFerran

16

Introduction

Tinnitus is a common but perplexing entity: there are many unanswered questions surrounding its pathogenesis, epidemiology and management. Even producing an unambiguous definition of tinnitus is difficult. Healthcare professionals regard tinnitus as a symptom rather than a disease or condition, but the general population undoubtedly regards it as a *bona fide* condition, and indeed this view receives support from the International Statistical Classification of Diseases and Related Health Problems 10th Revision (ICD-10), which lists tinnitus as a specific disorder. Tinnitus has perhaps always afflicted humankind. There are probable references to tinnitus among a series of Babylonian clay tablets dating from the 7th century BC. Definite reference to tinnitus was made in the Hippocratic Corpus, a record of the teachings of the Greek physician, Hippocrates, who lived in the 4th and 5th centuries BC. Tinnitus has afflicted many eminent people, including Ludwig van Beethoven, Charles Darwin, Jean-Jacques Rousseau, the actor William Shatner and the writer Garrison Keillor.

Definitions and tinnitus characteristics

Various definitions of tinnitus have been suggested, ranging from simplistic dictionary definitions such as 'ringing in the ears' to more sophisticated scientific definitions such as 'the perception of sound in the absence of external sounds' or 'the conscious expression of a sound that originates in an involuntary manner in the head of its owner, or may appear to him to do so'. Even the more complex definitions have shortcomings: tinnitus can appear to its owner to be outside the head; the auditory hallucinations of certain psychiatric diseases could fit these definitions but are not conventionally regarded as tinnitus. Tinnitus can be subdivided into objective and subjective types. Objective tinnitus is the awareness of a real sound within the body, generated by normal physiological or abnormal pathological processes, including blood flow or muscle activity in or around the ear. Subjective tinnitus is much more common and is a true phantom perception – the person perceives a sound in the absence of any corresponding sound in the body or environment. It is quite possible for objective and subjective tinnitus to co-exist in the same person.

Tinnitus sounds may be perceived in one or both ears, in or around the head, or even at some point distant to the person. It is not uncommon to hear someone with tinnitus describing how, at the onset of their problem, they thought that their symptom was the sound of a malfunctioning electrical appliance, distant traffic or noisy neighbours. Although most people with tinnitus describe their symptom as occurring in the same site from day to day, some people describe sounds that alter location, being sometimes in one ear, sometimes in the other, sometimes in the middle of the head.

The quality of tinnitus sounds shows enormous diversity. The popular view is that tinnitus is a ringing sound, but it can take the form of almost any auditory experience. Whistling, humming, buzzing, white noise, machinery, high-pitched tone, and hissing are a small sample of descriptors applied by people to their symptom. Some people's tinnitus is a single sound: others hear multiple sounds that may fluctuate temporally. Tinnitus can take the form of more complicated sounds, and people occasionally describe hearing musical sounds. This musical tinnitus is usually seen in elderly individuals with significant associated hearing loss. Rarely, people describe being able to hear speech, although in these cases the speech is usually distant and ill-defined. Musical and speech tinnitus are sometimes referred to as auditory imagery tinnitus and, clearly, great care must be taken to differentiate this type of tinnitus from the auditory hallucinations of schizophrenia, manic depression and other psychoses. However, just as it is important to recognise those with psychiatric illness, it is also important not to categorise someone with musical tinnitus as being insane. Differentiating auditory hallucinations from auditory imagery tinnitus can be difficult and may require assistance from an expert in mental health. One useful pointer is that sounds perceived in auditory imagery tinnitus are usually indistinct and people cannot make out clear words, in contrast to auditory hallucinations in which speech is clear and meaningful.

Epidemiology and risk factors

A study of the published literature on the prevalence and incidence of tinnitus gives confusing and sometimes apparently contradictory results, partly due to differences in the demographics of the populations being sampled, but also due to differing research methodology. The largest study into the epidemiology of tinnitus was performed by including a series of relevant questions in the UK Medical Research Council (MRC) longitudinal study of hearing. This investigation ($n = 48,313$) asked participants 'Have you ever had noises in your head or ears? Nowadays do you get noises in your head or ears?'. Other studies have used different questions such as 'Do you suffer from tinnitus?'. The MRC study made a distinction between any tinnitus experience, no matter how brief, and prolonged spontaneous tinnitus (PST), which was defined as tinnitus that arises spontaneously rather than in response to noise and lasts longer than 5 minutes at a time. Using these definitions, this study found that approximately one-third of all adults reported some tinnitus experience. About 10% of adults reported PST, and among those about 17% described it as severely annoying, with a further 28% classing it as moderately annoying. The number of people who reported tinnitus that had a severe effect on their quality of life was 0.4%.

Hearing loss increases the likelihood of a person having tinnitus, especially if that loss is at high frequencies. People who have experienced significant noise exposure also show increased risk of tinnitus, with the prevalence rising from 7.5% for those with low exposure to 20.7% for those with high exposure. Despite these observations, it is quite possible to have tinnitus with a normal audiogram, and hearing loss is not inevitably accompanied by tinnitus.

The symptom affects similar numbers of men and women, although women are more likely to describe complex tinnitus sounds.

Investigating the prevalence of PST according to age shows an increase in prevalence from about 6% of those aged 18–30 years to about

16% in those aged 61–70 years. Looking specifically at the 61–70-year age group, the number reporting a severe life quality effect was also greater than in the general population, at 0.8%. Interestingly, and perhaps counterintuitively, several studies have shown that the prevalence of PST in people over 70 years does not go on increasing but tends to fall off. This may represent the fact that the decade of life between 60 and 70 years is one of huge change, with many people taking retirement from employment at this time and suffering consequent socioeconomic upheaval.

Tinnitus is generally thought of as a disease of adulthood, and it is indeed relatively rare to see children presenting with tinnitus. There are many problems associated with trying to obtain meaningful prevalence figures in children, but the figures that have been produced suggest that awareness of tinnitus activity in the paediatric population is not dissimilar to that in adulthood. The important difference is that this awareness does not seem to translate into clinically significant tinnitus in most cases. Among those children who do complain of their tinnitus, there is a higher likelihood of associated otological or neurological pathology such as migraine, juvenile Ménière's disease, or chronic suppurative otitis media. This is therefore a group that needs especially careful investigation.

Many people with tinnitus believe – or are told – that their tinnitus has been caused or exacerbated by medication or foodstuffs. There are a small number of drugs that are definitely associated with tinnitus. Aspirin and quinine both give rise to dose-dependent reversible ototoxicity and tinnitus: the small dose of aspirin given to prevent strokes and heart attacks, or the small dose of quinine given for nocturnal cramps, is very unlikely to generate tinnitus. Certain medications including aminoglycoside antibiotics and the chemotherapeutic agent cisplatin can cause irreversible ototoxicity. This can trigger tinnitus in a proportion of individuals. However, a huge number of non-ototoxic drugs have been blamed for inducing tinnitus. There are problems associated with proving that certain agents have caused tinnitus. Firstly, coincidences can occur so it is inevitable that tinnitus and use of particular drugs will happen simultaneously purely by chance. Secondly, drugs are given for illness and illness in itself is a potent trigger for tinnitus. Finally, idiosyncratic reactions can occur so that one person may develop tinnitus when exposed to a drug, where the vast majority will not. In a similar fashion, foodstuffs including coffee, tea, alcohol, particularly red wine, chocolate, monosodium glutamate and cheese have all been blamed for producing or aggravating tinnitus. There is no good scientific basis for these accusations, and by excluding items from someone's diet, that person's life quality may be reduced thereby worsening their tinnitus. A process of exclusion followed by challenge may be required to prove that a drug or foodstuff is responsible for a person's tinnitus.

Pathogenesis

For those with objective tinnitus, the cause of the symptom would seem to be simple: there is a real sound, generated by blood flow or muscular action, which directly stimulates the auditory system. However, not every patient with a cervical or cranial bruit (a sound, usually pulsating, generated by turbulent blood flow) complains of pulsatile tinnitus: some people seem able to filter out the sound and effectively ignore it. Listening to a normal neck with a stethoscope reveals that there is a moderate amount of noise due to breathing, muscular activity and transmitted sounds from the heart. These somatosounds are generally filtered out and most people are unaware of their heart beating except in exceptional circumstances. Even when tinnitus is due to a real noise, the central auditory pathways within the brain play a significant role in determining the impact this has on that individual.

Initial theories regarding the causation of subjective tinnitus concentrated heavily on the ear, especially the cochlea, and indeed such concepts are still prevalent among both the general public and many healthcare professionals. Such suppositions, however, have distinct shortcomings.

Tinnitus can occur with a normal pure tone audiogram (PTA). Some recent research has used other more sophisticated tests of cochlear function, such as the threshold equalising noise (TEN) test, and obtained results suggesting that people with apparently normal hearing and tinnitus do in fact have subtle cochlear deficits. This remains a somewhat contentious area and it continues to be a moot point as to whether a certain degree of cochlear damage is a prerequisite to tinnitus. Whatever the rights and wrongs of this argument, tinnitus appears to be possible with either normal ears or only very minimal wear and tear. The converse argument is undoubtedly true: it is possible to have significant hearing loss without accompanying tinnitus. Looking at those people who experience tinnitus in association with hearing loss, the severity of the tinnitus correlates poorly with the degree of hearing loss. Furthermore, tinnitus can occur even after the auditory nerve has been divided, separating the central auditory system from its periphery. When people with tinnitus are questioned about the onset of their symptom, it is not infrequently associated with a stressful life event rather than a change in hearing. Functional brain imaging techniques such as positron emission tomography (PET) and functional magnetic resonance imaging (fMRI) scanning have demonstrated different patterns of cerebral activation in tinnitus patents compared to normal controls. One of the seminal observations concerning tinnitus was made by Heller and Bergman in 1953; 80 people who did not complain of tinnitus or hearing loss were put one at a time into a sound-proofed room and asked to describe what they heard. Within 5 minutes of entering the room, 94% reported being able to hear sounds such as humming, buzzing or ringing. This finding has been used to suggest that the presence of signals within the auditory system that have the potential to be interpreted as tinnitus is universal or near universal. All these factors have pointed to the importance of the central auditory system in the experience of tinnitus. Recent theories make a distinction between the point or ignition site at which a tinnitus signal is generated, which can be anywhere in the auditory system, and the subsequent physiological mechanisms that promote that signal within the central auditory pathways, thereby generating tinnitus. These central mechanisms are thought to occur through a process of neural plasticity.

Another factor that underlines the importance of the central auditory system in tinnitus is the observation that many people with tinnitus are able to modulate their symptom by an action such as clenching their jaws or touching the skin of their face. It has been postulated that this phenomenon is due to neural interaction between auditory and somatosensory centres in the brainstem.

Certain otological conditions have tinnitus as part of their symptom complex. In particular, tinnitus is common among patients with otosclerosis, Ménière's disease and vestibular schwannoma. Such forms of tinnitus are referred to as syndromic tinnitus.

Assessment

History

The key element in assessing most medical conditions is to take a detailed clinical history, and tinnitus is no different in this respect. Tinnitus-specific questions should include the nature of the tinnitus, particularly whether the percept is continuous, rhythmical or pulsatile; where the tinnitus is perceived and when it is most intrusive: people with tinnitus often complain that their sleep and powers of concentration are affected. The circumstances of the onset of the tinnitus may be revealing, and most people with tinnitus share similar fears (Box 16.1). Many people seeking help for their tinnitus have already tried other avenues of help within conventional medicine, complementary medicine or the internet. It is important to know what has been tried previously and also to find out what the person has been told – frequently they have been given negative and unhelpful advice that has exacerbated rather than helped their complaint.

Occasionally, people with tinnitus contemplate suicide. This is a rare event and research suggests that suicide is not significantly different among

> **Box 16.1** Some of the common fears expressed by patients with tinnitus.
>
> - My tinnitus will last for ever
> - My tinnitus will worsen
> - Nothing can be done about tinnitus
> - My tinnitus will drive me mad
> - My tinnitus will prevent me getting a night's sleep
> - My tinnitus will cause deafness
> - My tinnitus is caused by something potentially catastrophic

tinnitus patients in comparison to the general population. Furthermore, tinnitus is rarely the only factor in people contemplating suicide: other factors such as male gender, being unemployed, being elderly, having mental health issues and living alone are frequently relevant. There is a common feeling among healthcare professionals that it is wrong to ask about suicidal ideation as this might sow seeds in people's heads. There is no evidence that this is true. While it would be wrong to ask every tinnitus patient about suicidal thoughts, it is important to recognise the few people who are at genuine risk, and entirely appropriate to ask them straightforward questions about their intentions. Those who describe the plans that they have made for carrying out their suicide, or give a history of previous self-harm, are particularly at risk and should be referred urgently to the appropriate mental health team.

Questions about associated otological symptoms are important, particularly with reference to hearing, vertigo and hyperacusis. Because of the high degree of co-morbidity of tinnitus with anxiety and depression, it is important to check for relevant symptomatology. Some people with tinnitus have relatives with tinnitus. It is still not clear whether this represents some form of genetic predisposition, shared environmental factors or simply that being close to someone with tinnitus increases one's awareness of one's own auditory system. Questions about general health are useful, although it is unusual for other medical conditions to be directly linked to tinnitus. Symptoms that appear not infrequently in tinnitus

patients include headaches, neck pain or restriction of movements, and symptoms related to the temporomandibular joints.

Drugs are almost certainly overrated as a cause of tinnitus. Nevertheless, it is important to ask not only about prescription drugs but also about over-the-counter medication such as aspirin and the use of complementary medicine preparations. Occasionally, it is relevant to ask about the use of illicit drugs. There is no good evidence that use of the common recreational drugs causes tinnitus in the majority of people. However, some individuals who develop tinnitus worry that their symptom has been triggered by use of such agents, and they can enter a downward spiral of guilt and self-blame. While healthcare professionals cannot condone such usage, reassuring the patient that they have not caused their own problem is generally a very constructive step.

Examination

It is important to perform a thorough clinical examination, although for many patients with tinnitus this will prove normal. Basic medical observations including measurement of pulse and blood pressure should be performed. The ears should be examined using an otoscope and, if necessary, an operating microscope, which is particularly useful for detecting the tiny movements of the tympanic membrane caused by myoclonus of the middle ear muscles. Some patients are convinced that their ears are blocked with wax, infected or perforated, and it can be very helpful for this group to obtain an endoscopic picture of the ear to point out the salient anatomy and explain its normality. A rapid examination of the cranial nerves, temporomandibular joints and neck movements should be performed. If there is any suggestion that the patient may have objective tinnitus, auscultation of the head and neck should be undertaken. This may reveal the rhythmical clicking of palatal myoclonus or the bruit of a vascular anomaly. A general ear, nose and throat (ENT) examination, concentrating on the nose, mouth and pharynx should be performed, particularly if the history is suggestive of palatal myoclonus or if otoscopy has revealed findings suggestive of underlying Eustachian tube dysfunction. Fibreoptic endoscopy may be helpful in visualising Eustachian tube orifices or involuntary palatal movements. Other points to examine will be dictated by the history: on rare occasions, tinnitus may be associated with benign intracranial hypertension, and in this case fundoscopic examination of the patient is vital, if necessary calling on the expertise of an ophthalmological or neurological colleague. If the patient's clinical history includes symptoms of dizziness, a full vestibular examination should be undertaken.

Audiological investigations

When arranging tests for patients with any condition, care should be taken to request only those investigations that are going to directly influence the management of that patient. Most tinnitus patients need minimal investigation. A baseline assessment of hearing is necessary, partly to detect any underlying otological pathology or asymmetry of hearing, and partly to aid management by determining which patients will benefit from hearing rehabilitation. A PTA in the range 250 Hz to 8 kHz generally suffices. There is no good evidence that tests such as extended range audiograms or speech audiometry improve the outcome for tinnitus patients, although of course such tests may have a role in research. Tympanometry (impedence audiometry) is not an essential test for most people with tinnitus, although a sizeable minority of tinnitus patients complain that their ears feel blocked despite otoscopic evidence to the contrary. Obtaining a tympanogram can help to reassure this group of patients. Tympanometry has an undisputed role in those patients who have Eustachian tube dysfunction. Stapedial reflex estimation still has occasional value especially in the diagnosis of otosclerosis. Tinnitus-specific audiometric tests such as tinnitus pitch and loudness estimation are not necessary for the management of tinnitus. Otoacoustic emission testing similarly rarely aids the management of tinnitus. Loudness discomfort levels will be discussed in the section relating to hyperacusis.

Radiological investigations

Many patients with tinnitus do not require any additional tests, and certainly MRI scanning should not be regarded as a rite of passage for all tinnitus patients. Some, however, will need to undergo medical imaging to ensure that their tinnitus is not a manifestation of cerebellopontine angle pathology, such as a vestibular schwannoma. The indications for requesting imaging are listed in Box 16.2, although in broad terms if the patient describes asymmetry of their symptoms, or if the audiogram shows an asymmetrical sensorineural loss, further investigation is prudent. The usual imaging modality of choice is MRI scanning, and different units will use different protocols, some using gadolinium enhancement routinely, whereas others reserve gadolinium for patients whose plain scans have given equivocal results. A minority of patients will be unable to undergo MRI because of claustrophobia or the presence of metal objects in the body. Computerised tomography (CT) scanning may offer an acceptable alternative for these patients. For those who cannot be scanned, measuring the latency of wave 5 on the auditory brainstem response (ABR) may be useful. Patients with pulsatile tinnitus may require other imaging modalities which may include duplex ultrasound scanning, magnetic resonance angiography (MRA), computed tomographic angiography (CTA) or conventional angiography.

Box 16.2 Indications for requested MRI scan of internal auditory meati.

- Unilateral tinnitus
- Asymmetrical PTA: differences of 20 dB or greater in masked bone-conduction thresholds at 0.5, 1, 2 or 4 kHz
- Associated unexplained aural symptoms
- Associated neurological symptoms or signs
- Pulsatile tinnitus (may need alternative imaging mode according to clinical findings)
- Patient has morbid anxiety of intracranial pathology

Other investigations

Other tests are rarely needed unless there is clear clinical indication: someone with pulsatile tinnitus may require a full blood count to exclude anaemia causing increased cardiac output; someone with sudden or fluctuating hearing loss may need a battery of haematological investigations; someone suspected of having benign intracranial hypertension may need to be referred to a neurologist for lumbar puncture and measurement of cerebrospinal fluid pressure; someone with associated dizziness may require vestibular function tests.

Questionnaires

Because there is no simple objective test for tinnitus, various techniques have been used to try and quantify patients' distress and monitor treatment. The use of questionnaires in tinnitus clinics has helped in the assessment not only of the tinnitus itself but also in measuring associated psychological distress and allied complaints such as sleep disturbance. Table 16.1 lists some of the relevant scientifically validated questionnaires. The choice of which, if any, questionnaire to use is largely a matter of personal preference. Results from questionnaires must be seen in context and are not an alternative to a proper assessment by an appropriately qualified healthcare professional. For example, a high score in the depression questions of a HADS questionnaire (Table 16.1) does not prove a diagnosis of depression. It does, however, suggest that the patient should be assessed by a mental health expert. One recurring conundrum regarding the application of questionnaires is when to administer the instrument: before, during or after the initial consultation. Rather than agonising about which method to use, it is probably better to choose the one that fits in best with the organisation of the particular clinic, and then to be consistent.

Management

Although an outright cure for tinnitus remains elusive, there are many therapeutic options available for treating the symptom. Indeed the choice can seem bewildering, especially when resources such as the internet are consulted. This situation is further complicated by the fact that it is very difficult to produce strong scientific evidence regarding the efficacy of tinnitus treatments. Tinnitus cannot be directly quantified, so indirect

Table 16.1   A selection of some of the more commonly used tinnitus clinic questionnaires[a].

Modality	Questionnaire	Abbreviation
Tinnitus	Tinnitus Handicap Inventory	THI
Tinnitus	Tinnitus Handicap Inventory: Screening Version	THI-S
Tinnitus	Tinnitus Handicap Questionnaire	THQ
Tinnitus	Tinnitus Questionnaire	TQ
Tinnitus	Tinnitus Reaction Questionnaire	TRQ
Hyperacusis	Hyperacusis Questionnaire	HQ
Mental health	Beck Depression Inventory	BDI
Mental health	Hospital Anxiety Depression Scale	HADS
Sleep	Insomnia Severity Index	ISI
Sleep	Pittsburgh Sleep Quality Index	PSQI

[a]For further information on the questionnaires, see section at the end of the chapter.

measures have to be used. There is a strong placebo effect in tinnitus treatment, with as many as 40% of participants responding to the placebo arm of trials of treatment. Many treatments involve direct interaction between patient and therapist, making it impossible to produce double blind trials.

Explanation and reassurance

Anecdotally, a sizeable number of people with tinnitus simply want an explanation for their symptom and some reassurance that their fears are unfounded. Despite the all too frequently proffered negative advice, there are many positive statements that can be made regarding tinnitus (Box 16.3). Patients can be directed to one of the many agencies that offer practical help and advice regarding tinnitus. In the UK, charities such as the British Tinnitus Association (BTA) and the Royal National Institute for Deaf People (RNID) offer such services without charge. Self-help groups operate in many areas and details of these are listed by the BTA.

Habituation-based therapies

The most commonly available tinnitus management strategies available in the UK and most other western countries are based on the psychological or neurophysiological models of tinnitus. The psychological model was published in 1984 by Hallam, Rachman and Hinchcliffe, with the pivotal statement that tinnitus is caused by 'some neurophysiological disturbance in the auditory system at any point between periphery and cortex'. It was suggested that normally the central auditory system habituates to this disturbance. This process of habituation can, however, be disrupted, particularly if the person experiences high autonomic arousal, and if this happens, intrusive tinnitus can develop. The psychological model was used to suggest treatment strategies including the use of relaxation techniques to lessen the autonomic overactivity, and cognitive behavioural therapy (CBT) to address the emotional significance of the tinnitus.

In 1990, Jastreboff presented a treatise entitled *Phantom Auditory Perception (Tinnitus): mechanisms of generation and perception*. This work gave rise to what has subsequently been called the Neurophysiological Model of Tinnitus. This amalgamation of the available knowledge regarding tinnitus suggested that although the classical auditory system has a role in tinnitus emergence, neural pathways in the limbic system, reticular system and autonomic nervous system are also important. A management technique that was subsequently titled tinnitus retraining therapy (TRT) was extrapolated from this model. TRT uses a combination of directive counselling and sound therapy, adhering to quite a strict protocol. Many tinnitus practitioners offer therapy that uses the principles of the neurophysiological model without adhering to the strictures of TRT.

There are other management strategies that use similar principles: tinnitus activities treatment encourages patients to participate in other activities that help to distract the brain from the tinnitus; mindfulness meditation cognitive behavioural therapy utilises an ancient Buddhist technique for keeping one's thoughts focused on the present moment, thereby excluding unhelpful tinnitus-related thoughts.

Sound therapy

Most patients with tinnitus make the observation that their symptom is at its most intrusive when

---

Box 16.3   Positive statements that can be made regarding tinnitus.

- Although tinnitus is common it is very unusual for it to have a severe effect
- Most tinnitus lessens or even disappears with time
- Tinnitus is not a precursor of hearing loss
- Tinnitus is very rarely due to a serious underlying cause
- There are some very good strategies for helping tinnitus

they are in quiet surroundings, and consequently sound therapies have featured regularly among treatments for tinnitus, either as stand-alone therapy or as part of a wider tinnitus strategy. Sound can be used at a low level within the person's environment to provide some contrast and reduce the starkness of the tinnitus. This environmental sound enrichment benefits most people with tinnitus. Simple instructions to open a window and let some external sound into the house, or advice to play quiet background music can help. More sophisticated solutions include the use of electronic environmental sound generators that produce a range of quiet, repetitive, non-threatening sounds. For those who wish to use sound at night to help sleep, loudspeakers that fit under pillows or are built into pillows are available. People who have tinnitus in association with hearing loss usually derive benefit from the use of hearing aids, even if their hearing loss is not bad enough to impair communication abilities.

Sound can be used at quite high levels to drown out, or mask, tinnitus, and some patients find their tinnitus is lessened for a period even after withdrawal of the masking sound. Such residual inhibition may be complete or partial. Masking, however, usually only provides temporary respite, and various workers have criticised its usage suggesting that it may delay or prevent habituation.

Sound therapy can be used in a different fashion from masking: instead of using a sound that is loud enough to hide the tinnitus, TRT recommends using sound that is just quieter than the perceived tinnitus level. This is referred to as the mixing or blending point and proponents suggest that because the patient is still aware of their tinnitus but at a seemingly lower level, habituation should be facilitated.

Patients using sound for masking or as part of TRT may need to use a form of wearable sound generator. There are two ways of achieving this. Firstly, patients can wear a sound generator. This device, resembling a small hearing aid, produces wide-band sound: the difference between its usage as a masker or for TRT is simply the level to which its output is set. Secondly, for those patients with associated hearing loss, there are devices that combine a hearing aid with a sound generator in the same package. Although such devices have their supporters, they are complicated and difficult to set up satisfactorily.

Other forms of sound therapy include music therapy, which can help not only to provide a contrast to the tinnitus but also to promote relaxation. Neuromonics® is a form of sound therapy that is customised for each individual's hearing parameters and delivers pleasant sound interspersed by brief gaps, which allow tinnitus perception and are claimed to promote habituation.

Sound therapies are not universally favoured, and some workers, especially in the psychological field, feel that such therapies constitute a form of safety behaviour that may be unhelpful and may delay habituation. Despite the often trenchant opinions of both exponents and opponents of sound therapies, there is little hard science to support or refute their usage.

Devices and physical treatments

Masking can reduce the awareness of tinnitus, but the sound levels required interfere with hearing. Attempts have therefore been made to stimulate the cochlea by alternate routes that do not impair hearing. Both ultrasonic stimulation and vibration have been tried, but long-term results are disappointing. Sound cancellation has been suggested and devices have been produced that employ a sound that undergoes regular phase shift. Although the developers quote good results, most tinnitus experts remain sceptical; independent long-term verification is awaited.

Low-powered lasers have achieved a degree of success in the management of some forms of chronic pain, and because of similarities between pain and tinnitus this modality has been assessed for tinnitus. Conflicting results have been obtained, although the best-constructed trials showed no benefit. A functional imaging study, however, has shown evidence that laser stimulation of the ear results in activation of the cerebral cortex. Further research is clearly indicated.

Electrical stimulation of the ear with direct current does suppress tinnitus but at the not inconsiderable risk of damaging the ear. Partly because of this observation, the use of magnetic aural stimulation was tried but without success. With improved knowledge of the pathogenesis of tinnitus, focus turned from stimulation of the ear itself to stimulation of the auditory pathways within the brain. Using fMRI or PET scanning to identify abnormally activated areas of brain, electromagnetic energy in the form of repetitive transcranial magnetic stimulation (rTMS) has been used experimentally with encouraging results. This has recently been taken one step further with responders to rTMS undergoing surgical implantation of an intracranial, extradural stimulating electrode. Such techniques are very much in their infancy.

Surgery

Overall, surgery has little role in the management of tinnitus. Operations to correct conductive hearing loss in secretory otitis media and chronic suppurative otitis media probably help, although there is a surprising dearth of experimental support. Successful stapedectomy helps a majority of those patients whose tinnitus is caused by otosclerosis, with improvements in excess of 80% quoted. However, this surgery also carries a small risk of exacerbating existing tinnitus or triggering tinnitus in previously tinnitus-free patients. Surgery for Ménière's disease is generally directed at control of vertigo and there is little evidence regarding its effect on tinnitus. Surgery to remove space-occupying lesions of the cerebellopontine angle, most commonly vestibular schwannoma, does not help associated tinnitus for the majority of patients and may act as a trigger for tinnitus among those who did not have tinnitus preoperatively.

Pulsatile tinnitus may require surgery, although this is entirely dependent on the nature of the condition responsible for the symptom. For example, surgery for carotid stenosis may cure associated tinnitus, whereas a vascular lesion of the brainstem may not be amenable to surgical intervention. Small arterial loops in close association with the eighth cranial nerve are often seen on MRI scans, and there is a suggestion that

these may generate pulsatile tinnitus. Surgery in the form of microvascular decompression of the nerve is sometimes undertaken, although this is an invasive, high-risk procedure.

Surgery for subjective, non-syndromic tinnitus is generally unhelpful. Eighth nerve neurectomy or selective cochlear neurectomy has been tried, but results have been inconsistent and such surgery destroys any residual hearing.

One area of surgical success is in the management of tinnitus that is associated with profound sensorineural hearing loss. The majority of patients who undergo cochlear implantation derive benefit with regard to any concomitant tinnitus, although a small number will experience exacerbation.

Drugs

Drug treatment of tinnitus is one area where good-quality research could be expected. Unfortunately, this is frequently not the case and trials often have small sample sizes, use non-validated outcome measures, use inadequate randomisation techniques and suffer high dropout rates. Moreover, some drugs that have profound and obvious effects are tested against inert placebos, effectively unblinding supposedly blind trials.

Some of the drugs that have been evaluated have been used in the hope that they might improve cochlear function. This group, which includes vasodilators, diuretics, steroids, antioxidants, anticoagulants and hyperbaric oxygen, has been administered either systemically or intratympanically. Results have generally proved inconclusive or have shown these agents to be ineffective.

Other drugs have been studied with regard to possible action on auditory pathways in the central nervous system. Antidepressants have attracted interest partly because of the comorbidity of tinnitus with anxiety and depression, and partly because models of tinnitus and neurotic conditions show similarities. Use of antidepressants for treating concomitant psychogenic disease is certainly appropriate but the available research evidence suggests that antidepressants have little or no specific action against tinnitus.

Other psychotropic drugs have been investigated and there is some apparent support for the use of benzodiazepines. Unfortunately, these positive results derive from methodologically flawed research and in any case the tendency of benzo-diazepines to produce dependency limits their usage. Antispasmodic drugs act on similar receptors to the benzodiazepines but do not ameliorate tinnitus. Some tinnitus benefit has been described in small-scale trials of acamprosate, a drug used in the treatment of alcoholism, melatonin and botulinum toxin. Larger scale trials are required before any of these can be recommended.

A serendipitous observation established that local anaesthetic agents such as lidocaine can temporarily suppress tinnitus in approximately two-thirds of patients when administered intravenously. Unfortunately, the effect is short lived, and potential side-effects render this too dangerous to be considered as a potential treatment. Local anaesthetics are sodium channel antagonists, but orally active sodium channel antagonists such as some antiepileptic drugs have failed to show benefit for tinnitus patients.

Complementary and alternative medicine

Many forms of complementary and alternative medicine (CAM) have been administered to tinnitus patients (Box 16.4). Most of these therapies have not been rigorously tested with regard to tinnitus effect. Those that have been investigated include acupuncture, homeopathy and Ginkgo biloba, none of which have shown consistent benefit to tinnitus patients. Hypnotherapy has demonstrated benefit for some tinnitus patients, and further research with this modality would be useful. Many CAM therapies do promote non-specific feelings of wellbeing and relaxation and may have value in treating the distress of tinnitus rather than the symptom itself. Although most CAM modalities carry few risks, this is not invariable, and repeatedly trying ineffective treatments can be counterproductive, increasing feelings of despair. One form of CAM therapy, Hopi

Box 16.4 Some of the complementary medicine modalities that have been used to treat tinnitus.

- Acupuncture
- Aromatherapy
- Chiropractic
- Craniosacral
- Herbalism, particularly Ginkgo biloba
- Homeopathy
- Hopi ear candles
- Hypnosis
- Massage
- Osteopathy
- Reflexology
- Reiki
- Shiatsu

ear candles, has caused well-documented cases of aural damage, and use of these products should be avoided.

Vitamins and minerals

Many vitamins and minerals have been tried by people with tinnitus (Table 16.2), usually with

Table 16.2 Some of the dietary supplements that have been used to treat tinnitus.

Supplement	Type of supplement
Beta carotene	Vitamin precursor
Choline	Essential nutrient
Calcium	Mineral
Folic acid	Vitamin
Magnesium	Mineral
Manganese	Mineral
Omega 3 fatty acids	Essential fatty acids
Potassium	Mineral
Selenium	Mineral
Tryptophan	Essential amino acid
Vitamin A	Vitamin
Vitamin B particularly B_5, B_6 and B_{12}	Vitamin
Vitamin C	Vitamin
Vitamin E	Vitamin
Zinc	Mineral

no evidence that they are deficient in such compounds. None of these have been proven to help tinnitus, and some concerns have recently been raised that the unregulated sale of these supplements can allow people to overdose, with possibly deleterious effects.

Reduced sound tolerance (hyperacusis)

Definitions

Defining disorders of reduced sound tolerance is even more fraught than defining tinnitus. Although hyperacusis is often used as a blanket term, it does have a distinct meaning that is separate from other forms of altered sound tolerance: hyperacusis is a lowered tolerance to ordinary environmental sounds, with associated distress. Implicit in this definition is the observation that hyperacusis is a generalised sensitivity to all sounds above a certain level. This contrasts with phonophobia, literally fear of sounds, in which patients display reaction to certain sounds that have specific emotional meaning: other sounds may be tolerated in a normal fashion. A new word, misophonia, was created in 2004 to describe disorders of sound tolerance characterised by dislike of certain sounds without necessarily evoking a phobic element. With this definition, phonophobia can be regarded as a subsection of misophonia in which fear is the dominant emotion. Although there are some advantages to making this distinction, the word misophonia has yet to achieve widespread acceptance. Recruitment is a specific form of loudness tolerance disorder experienced by those who have cochlear hearing loss. These people perceive abnormally large growth in the loudness of a sound for a small increase in that sound's intensity. This results in the patient having a compressed auditory dynamic range, with consequent problems for hearing aid fitting.

Epidemiology

There are very few studies that have investigated the prevalence of hyperacusis. Prevalence figures between 8% and 15.2% have been reported, but methodological problems associated with collecting these data mean that these are almost certainly overestimates. Hyperacusis does seem to be linked to tinnitus: 40% of people with tinnitus reported hyperacusis, while 86% of those with hyperacusis reported tinnitus.

Pathogenesis

It is possible to separate hyperacusis into cases that arise in association with another medical condition and those that arise in isolation. The former group, sometimes known as syndromic hyperacusis, can be subdivided into those with a peripheral cause and those with central mechanisms. Peripheral causes are usually associated with reduced activity of the stapedius muscle, preventing the ear's normal sound protection mechanism from working. Examples include Bell's palsy, Ramsay Hunt syndrome and patients who have undergone stapedectomy. Associations with central pathology are seen in migraine, depression, post-traumatic stress disorder, multiple sclerosis, post-head injury syndrome and Williams' syndrome, which is a complex congenital syndrome caused by partial deletion of chromosome 7. Lyme disease is an interesting cause of hyperacusis: some patients develop hyperacusis due to associated facial nerve palsy, whereas others seem to have a purely central mechanism. Many of the disorders associated with central hyperacusis are postulated to be associated with dysfunction of serotonin (5-hydroxytryptamine) pathways in the central nervous system. This has been used to suggest that hyperacusis is also a manifestation of serotonin dysfunction. Other hypotheses suggest that stress generates endogenous opioids, which potentiate cochlear activity, or that defects in the medial efferent pathways of the central auditory system result in abnormal auditory gain. A cycle of fear and avoidance has been suggested, and certainly this fits in well with clinical observations. Someone exposed to a loud sound that they find unpleasant may try to protect themselves from further exposure by avoiding all types of sound. Reduced sound input causes increased central auditory gain that results in previously well-tolerated sound now seeming unpleasantly loud. This process can escalate into a downward spiral of ever-increasing central auditory sensitivity causing ever-greater sound avoidance.

Assessment

The assessment of someone with hyperacusis is essentially the same as for someone with tinnitus, except for the question of whether these patients should undergo loudness discomfort level (LDL) testing. Performing LDLs enables the problem to be quantified, allows treatment to be monitored and gives potentially valuable research information. However, measuring LDLs on a patient with hyperacusis means exposing someone to a stimulus that they find unpleasant, and possibly causing distress. In addition, measuring LDLs is notoriously difficult, with much test–retest variability. Measuring LDLs is certainly not a vital prerequisite of managing hyperacusis. Questionnaires for hyperacusis are available (Table 16.1) but have yet to be widely adopted.

Management

Any underlying condition such as Lyme disease, depression or post-traumatic stress disorder should be addressed. Patients should be carefully counselled regarding their reduced sound tolerance, and if they have instituted a programme of sound avoidance they should be advised that far from helping this may well be contributing to the problem. It should be stressed that appropriate ear defenders should be worn for truly noisy situations, such as using noisy machinery, shooting, or attending a loud music concert. Wearing ear defenders at other times should be avoided. Sound therapy has a much clearer role in the management of hyperacusis than it does for tinnitus. There are two main techniques: sound can be used to desensitise the auditory system by using ear-level sound generators and gradually increasing the volume; alternatively, sound can be used to recalibrate the auditory system by

using ear-level generators set at a constant comfortable level. Sound therapy may be instituted as a stand-alone treatment or as part of TRT. Received wisdom suggests that when tinnitus and hyperacusis co-exist, the hyperacusis should be addressed first. Psychological treatments, particularly CBT, can be used for patients with reduced sound tolerance, and anecdotally this approach seems particularly beneficial for phonophobic patients.

Conclusion

Our knowledge of the pathogenesis of tinnitus and hyperacusis has steadily improved, and the importance of central auditory pathways in the persistence of these symptoms is now well recognised. There are still unanswered questions, and a definitive cure remains elusive. Despite this, good management strategies have been developed and an optimistic approach to tinnitus patients is recommended.

References

Hallam RS, Rachman S, Hinchcliffe R (1984) Psychological aspects of tinnitus. In: Rachman S, ed. *Contributions to Medical Psychology*, vol 3, pp 31–53. Oxford: Pergammon Press.

Heller MF, Bergman M (1953) Tinnitus aurium in normally hearing persons. *Annals of Otology, Rhinology and Laryngology* 62:73–83.

Jastreboff PJ (1990) Phantom auditory perception (tinnitus): mechanisms of generation and perception. *Neuroscience Research* 8:221–224.

Further reading

Andersson G, Baguley DM, McKenna L, McFerran D (2005) *Tinnitus: a multidisciplinary approach*. London and Philadelphia: Whurr Publishers.

Baguley DM, Andersson G (2007) *Hyperacusis: mechanisms, diagnosis, and therapies*. San Diego: Plural Publishing.

Davis PB, Paki B, Hanley PJ (2007) Neuromonics tinnitus treatment: third clinical trial. *Ear & Hearing* 28:242–259.

Jastreboff PJ, Hazell JWP (1993) A neurophysiological approach to tinnitus: clinical implications. *British Journal of Audiology* 27:7–17.

Questionnaires

- **Tinnitus Handicap Inventory**: Newman CW, Jacobson GP, Spitzer JB (1996) Development of the tinnitus handicap inventory. *Archives of Otolaryngology, Head and Neck Surgery* 122:143–148.
- **Tinnitus Handicap Inventory: Screening Version**: Newman CW, Sandridge SA, Bolek L (2008) Development and psychometric adequacy of the screening version of the Tinnitus Handicap Inventory. *Otology and Neurotology* 29:276–281.
- **Tinnitus Handicap Questionnaire**: Kuk FK, Tyler RS, Russell D, Jordan H (1990) The psychometric properties of a tinnitus handicap questionnaire. *Ear and Hearing* 11:434–445.
- **Tinnitus Questionnaire**: Hallam RS (1996) *Manual of the Tinnitus Questionnaire.* London: The Psychological Corporation/Brace & Co.
- **Tinnitus Reaction Questionnaire**: Wilson PH, Henry J, Bowen M, Haralambous G (1991) Tinnitus reaction questionnaire: psychometric properties of a measure of distress associated with tinnitus. *Journal of Speech and Hearing Research* 34:197–201.
- **Hyperacusis Questionnaire**: Khalfa S, Dubal S, Veuillet E *et al.* (2002) Psychometric normalisation of a Hyperacusis Questionnaire. *ORL: Journal for Otorhino-laryngology and its Related Specialties* 64:436–442.
- **Beck Depression Inventory**: Beck AT, Ward CH, Mendelson M, Mock J, Erbaugh J (1961) An inventory for measuring depression. *Archives of General Psychiatry* 4:561–571.
- **Hospital Anxiety Depression Scale**: Zigmond AS, Snaith RP (1983) The Hospital Anxiety and Depression Scale. *Acta Psychiatrica Scandinavia* 67:361–370.
- **Insomnia Severity Index**: Bastien CH, Vallières A, Morin CM (2001) Validation of the Insomnia Severity Index as an outcome measure for insomnia research. *Sleep Medicine* 2:297–307.
- **Pittsburgh Sleep Quality Index**: Buysse DJ, Reynolds CF 3rd, Monk TH, Berman SR, Kupfer DJ (1989) The Pittsburgh Sleep Quality Index: a new instrument for psychiatric practice and research. *Psychiatry Research* 28:193–213.

Resources

The British Tinnitus Association (BTA)
- Ground Floor, Unit 5, Acorn Business Park, Woodseats Close, Sheffield S8 0TB
- Tel: 0800 018 0527 free of charge from within the UK only; 0845 4500 321 local rate from within the UK only; 0114 250 9922 national rate within the UK; +44 114 250 9922 outside the UK
- Minicom: 0114 258 5694 from within the UK; +44 114 258 5694 outside the UK
- Fax: 0114 258 2279 from within the UK; +44 114 258 2279 outside the UK
- Website: www.tinnitus.org.uk

The Royal National Institute for Deaf People (RNID)
- 19–23 Featherstone Street, London EC1Y 8SL
- Tel: 0808 808 0123 (freephone); textphone: 0808 808 9000 (freephone)
- Fax: 020 7296 8199
- Websites: www.rnid.org.uk; www.tuneout-tinnitus.org.uk/home

Psychological aspects of acquired hearing loss

17

Laurence McKenna and
Anne O'Sullivan

Introduction

We take our hearing for granted, but when we lose it, it can have a profound effect upon us. An acquired hearing loss (AHL) makes it difficult to follow speech, particularly in background noise or in group conversations, which can present many challenges in day-to-day life. Difficulty in participating in conversation can impact on personal relationships within the family, and in social and work settings. In addition to communication issues, a person with AHL may experience difficulties in hearing and appreciating non-verbal sounds such as music, traffic or doorbells.

In today's world, communication skills are of prime importance. Many more occupations are dependent on such skills rather than on the ability to carry out physical labour. A person with AHL may therefore face greater challenges, and be more disadvantaged, than a person who has physical or mobility disabilities, but good communication skills. Hearing-impaired people are three times more likely to be out of work than those with no disability, and their financial status is likely to be correspondingly poorer. Those with hearing loss and a speech problem are eight times more likely to be excluded from the workforce.

Thus AHL creates the potential for difficulties in several areas: personal, social, employment, recreation and safety. How do people respond psychologically to these difficulties? In audiology clinics, we find many examples of people with AHL reporting feelings of isolation, loneliness, loss of self-esteem, or loss of hope. In the media, people with AHL have been presented as figures of ridicule (e.g. The Deaf Guest episode of the TV series *Fawlty Towers*). In the past, people with AHL were sometimes described as suspicious and paranoid. But do all people experience and respond to AHL in a negative way, and do we have research evidence to confirm our clinical impressions? This chapter seeks to examine the current understanding of the psychological response to AHL, both negative and positive, as well as to present the psychological treatment option for which there is the strongest research backing.

Does hearing loss lead to psychological distress?

A person with AHL usually strives to maintain the identity of a normally hearing person. While hearing aids and other devices can help, it is a challenging goal, which usually has an emotional cost. Some people with AHL have likened their experience to the grief response. They grieve for their lost hearing, the things they can no longer do, and for the person they once were. This grief experience has often been cited, yet the area is not well researched, and is largely based on clinical impression. The Swiss psychiatrist Elizabeth Kubler-Ross suggested that grief reactions involve a number of stages. The relevance of these to hearing loss is described in Box 17.1. Originally, the process of grief was thought to be essentially linear, but today it is thought to be more fluid. The stages represent general emotional themes, rather than strictly defined states, through which people can move forwards and backwards, e.g.

anger one day, depression on another occasion and returning to anger before moving on again. The process of grief may make the hearing-impaired person's interactions with others, including those in the audiology service, an emotional rollercoaster. The process should, however, pass with time.

The research evidence concerning AHL and mental health problems has focused mainly on identifying enduring psychological processes such as anxiety and depression or loss of well-being. Many studies have found that the prevalence of such problems is greater among people with a hearing loss, than among the general population. In one study (Thomas, 1984), the rate of clinically significant depression or anxiety was found to be four times greater among people with AHL than among the general population. Common symptoms of anxiety and depression are listed in Box 17.2. In a study using qualitative methods, Kerr and Cowie (1997) found that 40% of people with AHL said that their hearing impairment had badly restricted their lives, and one in ten said that it had almost completely destroyed their lives.

Conflicting findings exist, however, and unfortunately many of the studies linking AHL with problems such as anxiety and depression are methodologically flawed. Some have not taken account of possible confounding variables. For example, when studies have taken account of general health as a variable, then the relationship between AHL and psychological problems is weaker than suggested above. Furthermore, many studies have focused only on people with hearing loss seen in clinical settings, rather than on the wider population of people with hearing impairment. Such shortcomings in the research do need to be addressed, but they should not lead us to reject the idea that hearing loss might lead to a poor psychological state. Some things, like judgements about general health, are not true confounding variables, but, rather, are intimately associated with hearing loss. It is likely that hearing is regarded as an important part of general health. Thus, a loss of hearing leads to a description of poor health, in which case the association between hearing loss and psychological problems remains valid. Furthermore,

---

Box 17.1   Stages of grief.

- *Denial*: the person does not believe that they have a permanent hearing loss, may feel isolated or alone with the problem and may seek a second opinion or refuse to engage in assessment and rehabilitation.
- *Anger*: the person is furious about the hearing loss. This anger may extend to those around, including the audiologist, and may lead to a refusal to engage with rehabilitation.
- *Bargaining*: the person decides that, as anger has not worked, they will do what the audiologist or physician asks them, in the hope that the problem will go away.
- *Depression*: when denial, anger and bargaining have not restored hearing to its previous level, the person experiences a sense of loss that can provoke feelings of depression, and sometimes, a sense of shame or guilt.
- *Acceptance*: after anger and depression, the person comes to an acceptance of hearing loss. This is not 'giving up', but rather working with the hearing loss rather than fighting it or ignoring it.

Box 17.2   Common symptoms of anxiety and depression.

Common symptoms of depression
- Persistent depressed mood[a]
- Loss of interest
- Loss of pleasure
- Irritability
- Restlessness/agitation
- Loss of self-confidence
- Social withdrawal
- Lack of energy/tiredness
- Trouble sleeping[b]
- Loss of libido
- Disturbed appetite – eating too much/too little
- Feeling worthless or guilty
- Difficulty making decisions
- Poor concentration
- Memory problems
- Thoughts of suicide

Common symptoms of anxiety
- Abdominal discomfort
- Diarrhoea
- Dry mouth
- Rapid heartbeat
- Muscle tension
- Tightness or pain in the chest
- Shortness of breath
- Dizziness
- Frequent urination
- Difficulty swallowing
- Sleep disturbance[c]
- On edge
- Irritability or anger
- Concentration problems
- Fear of madness/losing control
- Feeling detached (derealisation)
- Feeling unreal (depersonalisation)

[a]Often worse early in the morning or last thing at night.
[b]Especially early morning waking.
[c]Especially sleep-onset problems.

moderate associations between hearing loss and problems such as depression, anxiety and reduced wellbeing have been found in the wider population (e.g. Tambs, 2004).

Some of the latest, methodologically sound, research examining the psychological and social status of people with acquired profound hearing loss (APHL) has been conducted by Hallam *et al.* (2006, 2008). These researchers found that a substantial minority of people with APHL suffered from symptoms of post-traumatic stress disorder (PTSD). Their work, like some others', has suggested that APHL is associated with strain in relationships and greatly increased relationship breakdown. They point out that the stresses experienced by hearing-impaired people are different from the stresses experienced by those close to them with no hearing loss. This results in opportunities for misunderstandings and conflict. They found that interpersonal stress was apparent in half of the participants of their study, a similar figure to that reported by Thomas (1984). They point out that communication problems are likely to obstruct the means by which problems are usually solved, i.e. through negotiation. It also hinders spontaneous expression, and reduces the ability to 'offload' about the normal stresses of the day. Hallam and colleagues noted that a profound loss imposes a considerable burden of extra effort on partners. They point out that old habits of communication have to be changed, and many family members admitted that they were poor at making such adjustments. Domestic, social and leisure activities may have to be curtailed. Family members, including children, may have to take over responsibilities such as domestic duties or acting as go-between with the hearing world. This may alter existing power relationships as the deafened person becomes more assertive, or more dependent. An interesting and important observation that emerged from the studies by Hallam and colleagues was that close family members report levels of emotional distress that are almost as high as those evident in people with profound hearing loss.

Another aspect of mental health that merits particular mention is the connection between hearing loss and psychosis. The idea that hearing loss is associated with paranoia was widely held until relatively recently. The scientific origins of the idea stem from the work of the psychiatrist Emil Kraeplin in the early 20th century. Kraeplin, the founder of modern psychiatry, was credited with the development of the concept of dementia praecox, known later as schizophrenia.

He reported persecutory delusions in individuals with hearing impairment. Since then, several studies have investigated the association between hearing loss and paranoid illness. The evidence is again mixed. Some studies have failed to find an association (e.g. Thomas, 1984) but others have pointed to a significant link between hearing loss and psychotic experiences. The conflicting findings may arise from the use of different research methods, many of which were flawed; some studies used no more than subjective report of hearing loss, and psychological measures from which alternative conclusions could well be drawn. There is also the potential for hearing loss to complicate psychiatric diagnosis. A person who does not respond when spoken to, or who offers inappropriate answers to questions, may have a psychiatric illness or may simply not have heard. It is, of course, possible for both processes to be at work in an individual and for misperception of auditory information to exacerbate, or lead to, paranoid ideas. The idea of an association between hearing loss and psychosis has received attention again in the recent scientific literature. In a prospective general population study in the Netherlands, hearing-impaired people were found to have significantly more psychotic experiences than normally hearing people (Thewissen *et al.*, 2005). Although hearing loss was assessed only in terms of subjective report, it was found to predict psychotic experiences (hallucinations and/or delusional ideas) three years later. Later work from the same research group (Van der Werf *et al.*, 2007) assessed hearing loss in terms of subjective report and audiometry in a general population study. They again found an association between hearing loss and psychotic experiences. Interestingly, the association was significant only for self-reported hearing loss, and not for objective hearing measures. Furthermore, the association was significant only if hearing loss continued to present problems in spite of the use of a hearing aid. The evidence that supports an association between hearing loss and psychosis suggests that the hearing loss may constitute an aetiological factor in the development of psychosis. There is some evidence that this is more the case for younger age groups than for older people.

Overall, the evidence, and clinical experience, does support the idea that there is a meaningful relationship between hearing loss and psychological problems, suggesting that hearing loss is an aetiological factor in the development of psychological problems. Although less obvious, there is also the possibility that a person's psychological state may lead to the development of hearing problems. It is recognised that some people exaggerate the extent of their hearing loss, and the subject of non-organic hearing loss is dealt with elsewhere in this book (see Chapter 15). Although extremely rare, cases have been cited of people with psychological disorders and normal hearing seeking to induce an organic hearing loss through deliberate self-injury, or seeking medical and surgical assistance to induce such a disorder. Such individuals have been observed to have personality disorders (Veale, 2006) or Munchausen's syndrome (a psychological disorder that results in a person exaggerating or creating symptoms of illnesses in order to gain investigation, treatment, or other attention from medical personnel; it can result in multiple unnecessary operations).

The discussion so far has focused on negative psychological consequences of hearing loss. It should be noted, however, that people with hearing loss can also report positive effects. These effects have included an increase in mental alertness. Some artists with hearing loss, including Joshua Reynolds and David Hockney, have described an enhancement of other senses. Evelyn Glennie, an acclaimed solo percussionist, was profoundly deaf at 12 years old. She has said that she feels adjusted to herself as a deaf person and musician and that regaining her hearing would present a difficulty to her playing and her everyday life. Her deafness does present daily challenges, but she feels that it has also had a positive effect on her life, and wonders whether it has helped her to be so determined. Other positive effects that have been reported are reduced disturbance from unwanted noise, greater appreciation of successful communication, the support and sympathy of others, improved personal relationships, using hearing loss to self-advantage, and increased patience. Positive experiences have been found to account for a surprisingly high proportion of the statistical variance (10–14%) in analyses of the experience of hearing loss. Reports of positive effects of hearing loss are more likely to come from younger people and from those who have had a hearing loss for longer (Stephens and Kerr, 2003).

The relationship between hearing thresholds and measurements of psychological disturbance

It seems reasonable to expect that a greater hearing loss would lead to a greater degree of psychological distress. The research, however, presents a mixed picture. In a few studies, a strong positive relationship between scores of psychological distress and pure tone thresholds has been observed (e.g. Thomas, 1984). In a study by Sherbourne *et al.* (2002), 61% of people with acquired profound hearing loss reported symptoms indicative of clinical depression, i.e. higher than the general population and higher than that observed in groups of people with less severe hearing loss.

More common, however, is the repeated observation (including in very recent studies, e.g. Helvik *et al.*, 2006) that the level of psychological disturbance cannot reliably be predicted from the severity of hearing loss. It has also been noted that the positive effects of hearing loss referred to above are not clearly related to the degree of hearing loss. Such observations have led to the suggestion that there is not a direct relationship between psychological state and hearing loss. It has been suggested that even mild or moderate hearing loss cuts off a person from the world, and this sense of being cut off is fundamental in creating the psychological impact. The implication here is that hearing loss not only disrupts communication, but also acts at a more fundamental level of connecting the person to basic background sounds in the environment. Another suggestion has been that more severe or profound hearing losses tend to be longstanding, while milder losses reflect more dynamic processes that lead to greater changes in psychological state. As Hallam *et al.* (2008) point out,

however, the situation facing people with APHL may have similarities to that facing people with less severe losses but, in reality, the situation is likely to be more challenging for people with APHL. In particular, the options of ignoring and minimising hearing loss are not available to people with APHL in most situations.

What other possible explanations can account for the repeated observation that the levels of hearing loss and of psychological problems are poorly correlated? The observation may simply reflect the inadequacy of the research methods and assessment devices used. For example, auditory thresholds alone are unlikely to provide an adequate measure of functional hearing. It has been suggested that the relationship between extent of hearing loss and psychological (and social) problems becomes clearer when measures of speech discrimination are included; then it is apparent that a profound hearing loss is associated with greater psychosocial difficulties. It is also the case that studies have often included relatively few people with a profound hearing loss and have focused too narrowly on some measures while not taking account of others. It would certainly be surprising if greater hearing loss did not represent a greater psychological challenge for those affected and those who support them. The work of Hallam and colleagues (2006) provides some insights into the situation. They found that people with APHL fell into two groups: those who suffered from significant psychosocial problems and those who did not. This meant that bracketing these two groups together resulted in average scores on psychosocial measures being within the normal range, which therefore potentially disguised the effect of APHL.

At present, there is no way of predicting accurately how a given individual will react to a hearing loss. Overall, the evidence, including that concerning APHL, does bring us back to the conclusion that the degree of hearing loss does not fully explain the individual differences in the reactions to that loss. It has been suggested that the coping style of the individual plays some role in the process. Coping styles that involve the person assuming control for their lives, rather than seeing that control as external to them, may result in fewer psychological problems. People who respond to problems by actively trying to solve them, rather than passively ignoring them, may also fare better. Interestingly, Helvik *et al.* (2006) suggested that wellbeing after hearing impairment is associated with sense of humour. The suggestion is that sense of humour represents an aspect of coping style that allows the person to focus less on the negative aspects of an event. It has been suggested that whether or not a relationship suffers because one member has an APHL may depend on the prior state of the relationship, and the personalities involved.

The presence of other problems seems to increase the impact of AHL. In particular, people with greater hearing loss often also suffer from other neuro-otological disorders, such as distressing tinnitus or balance problems. It is clear from several studies (Stewart-Kerr, 1992; Sherbourne *et al.*, 2002; Hallam *et al.*, 2006) that such additional symptoms contribute to the overall psychosocial impact of hearing loss. The presence of other social problems, such as marital or employment difficulties, also exacerbates the impact of hearing loss. Several studies have found that the psychosocial impact of hearing loss is more closely related to employment status than to pure tone thresholds, the effect being less in people who are working (e.g. Kerr and Cowie, 1997; Ringdahl and Grimby, 2000). The evidence allows us to conclude that, as problems accumulate and interact, so the impact of hearing loss increases. The group of hearing-impaired people with significant psychosocial problems may, therefore, be distinguished from the group without, by the presence of multiple other stresses, by different attitudes and by coping styles, and by an inability of others to accommodate the communication needs of the person with hearing impairment.

A biopsychosocial model

The International Classification of Functioning, Disability and Health (ICF), developed by the World Health Organization (2001), provides a framework for coding information about health

and uses a standardised common language that permits communication about health across the world in various disciplines and sciences. It defines components of health and some health-related components of wellbeing (such as education and labour). The ICF may be used within the context of a given health-related problem, including hearing loss, to distinguish the component parts of the overall process in terms of *abnormalities*, *limitations* and *restrictions*. The relevance of this classification to audiology is discussed by Stephens and Kerr (2000). The term *abnormalities* refers to changes in bodily function and structure and, in the case of hearing loss, to changes within the auditory pathway usually measured using psycho-acoustical techniques. *Limitations* refer to reductions in activities and, in the current context, to the hearing loss or the auditory problems experienced by the person. In our context of hearing loss, *restrictions* refer to the reduction in participation, or the non-auditory problems, or disadvantages, that the person experiences. This classification is set within *contextual factors* that are social, environmental and personal variables that influence the experience of hearing loss (or other health issues). The structure and language of the ICF allows us to understand that the component parts of the overall hearing loss experience are unlikely to have a one-to-one relationship between each other. The imperfect relationship between hearing loss and psychological state is therefore accommodated by this structure. While acknowledging the idea that a hearing loss is likely to increase the chances that a person will experience psychological problems, it is clear that such problems are not an inevitable consequence of losing one's hearing. For example, a given hearing impairment will have a different impact on a concert violinist from the impact on a pavement artist. There is, therefore, an imperative that audiological assessment is not restricted to measuring hearing.

In essence, the ICF classification constructs health, and health problems such as hearing loss, within a model that recognises the contributions of biological, social and psychological factors. It has long been recognised that social barriers act as determinants of disability. For example, a person in a wheelchair is disabled because there are steps rather than a ramp. It is self-evident that hearing-impaired people face social barriers. An obvious example is that background noise will reduce a hearing-impaired person's ability to communicate. The influence of social factors also accounts for why many hearing-impaired people, particularly older people living alone, do not recognise or seek help for a hearing loss. Perhaps less obvious to those of us involved in their care, hearing-impaired people report considerable stress associated with obtaining medical and rehabilitative support, including feeling stigmatised by the professionals they encounter.

It is well recognised that psychological processes can also influence the level of *restrictions* that an individual experiences. Less well recognised is the possibility that psychological processes influence the extent of *limitations* (or disability). It has been argued that cognitive factors influence *limitations* in other health problems, and there is certainly a possibility that this is relevant to hearing loss. Clearly, processes such as anxiety and depression may make it more difficult for hearing-impaired people to obtain the help they require and therefore contribute to their disability. Clinically, it is also apparent that a highly anxious person is likely to miss elements of communication because their attention is elsewhere. A depressed person may process information more slowly, and as a consequence suffer greater *limitation* (or disability). Further research is needed to delineate the influence of psychological processes in this context.

Cognitive factors and the response to hearing loss

The ICF offers an overarching guide that allows for variation in the experience of hearing loss. A more precise model is needed in clinical practice. A cognitive behaviour therapy (CBT) therapy model provides such a model of the psychological element of the process (Beck, 1976). In recent years, CBT models have been developed to account for problems such as anxiety, pain and insomnia. These models propose that people

experience persistent distress about such difficulties because they make *overly* negative interpretations about the symptoms, or variations in them, or information regarding them. *Overly* negative appraisals of (ill-)health involve distortions in thinking such as black and white thinking, ignoring positive information and focusing on negative information, or 'mind reading', i.e. assuming another person is judging you in a certain way without evidence to support this idea. *Overly* negative or distorted thinking is somewhat similar to the way that people worry about problems in the middle of the night. The problem can seem huge and insurmountable and we feel terrible. By lunchtime the next day, the problem may not have gone away, but it may seem more manageable and we feel less terrible. We can therefore think differently about the same problem at different times, and it is the *thinking* that leads to us feeling stressed or not. We can all engage in distorted thinking at times. The problem comes about when 'middle of the night' thinking begins to take over and we end up suffering more than we need to. We know that when people are stressed, they are much more likely to think about things in an *overly* negative way, i.e. they drop into 'middle of the night' thinking most of the time. Distress persists because various processes maintain the overly negative interpretations from which anxiety or depression results. For example, changes in behaviour inspired by overly negative thoughts can maintain anxiety or depression when those changes stop the person from finding out that the thoughts are *overly* negative. These behaviours are then referred to as 'safety behaviours' because they keep the person 'safe' from the perceived threat, but they also prevent the person from finding out that the perception of the threat is worse than the threat itself.

From a clinical point of view, the CBT model also offers a useful paradigm for understanding the psychological component of the hearing-impaired patient's experience. A person who thinks that hearing loss is of little significance for their health or wellbeing is unlikely to be distressed. A person who believes that the hearing loss results in permanent and pervasive negative effects is likely to feel distressed. It is possible that such a judgement is accurate, but for many people the judgement is *overly* negative and is likely to lead to an anxious or depressed mood. Typical *overly* negative thoughts expressed by people with AHL are listed in Box 17.3.

A person who believes that others will think him stupid, or become annoyed with him, will naturally want to protect himself from such an uncomfortable situation. So he will avoid people in order to keep emotionally safe. The thought that others will think badly of him is itself distressing. In addition, avoidance of people will remove social pleasure, so increasing the distress. The increase in stress arousal associated with this thought can result in the person's attention being focused on detecting signs of annoyance in others, and so away from the communication. This increases the chances that communication will break down. The avoidance will also stop the person from discovering whether the thought is accurate, or characterised by 'middle of the night' thinking. Of course, there may be some truth in the person's beliefs. We know that people with normal hearing can be intolerant of those with a hearing loss. But to generalise this and avoid most people is likely to lead to depression.

Distortions in thinking are considered to play a central part in the development and maintenance of psychological disorders. The interrelationship between mood changes, stress arousal, behavioural changes and distortions in thinking is widely accepted. It is possible,

however, that the reduced sensory input involved in hearing loss can also contribute to the development of cognitive distortions. This might happen in a number of ways:

- in order to understand other people's behaviour we make inferences about their beliefs, thoughts and intentions (i.e. their mental state). A hearing loss might reduce the information available to help do this and so put us at risk of developing inappropriate inferences and therefore psychological disturbance
- it has been suggested that the loss of information from the environment produced by a hearing loss might interfere with a person's ability to discriminate between internally generated stimuli (especially speech) and events in the environment. This may increase the risk of psychotic experiences such as hallucinations
- alternatively, a person who does not recognise that they have a hearing loss may mistakenly interpret incomplete auditory input as other people whispering or being secretive.

These possibilities all need further investigation.

Psychological treatment

Many people will experience a hearing loss, or a change in that loss, without significant psychological distress. Others will experience a bereavement or adjustment reaction. The physician, audiologist or other therapist should understand the nature of grief reactions so that they can offer appropriate emotional support, and accommodate the changing emotional reactions of the patient. The emotional support will take the form of therapeutic listening involving empathy, warmth and a non-judgemental approach. Many patients are confused by their grief reactions. The therapist can benefit the patient by helping them understand this process, in addition to educating them about the technical aspects of the hearing loss. Most grief reactions will resolve with a little time and support for the affected person and

---

Box 17.3 Typical *overly* negative thoughts expressed concerning hearing loss.

- I will go completely deaf
- Life will never be good again
- I can't enjoy anything now
- I will never be able to enjoy life again
- I can't do normal things any more
- I must keep away from all loud sounds
- No one understands
- It is not fair that this has happened to me
- Everyone thinks I am stupid
- Everyone will become annoyed with me
- No one will accept me

Box 17.4 Distinguishing grief reactions from psychological disorder.

- The longer the time since onset the less likely it is to be grief.
- Evidence of changing emotions suggests grief.
- The degree of *overly* negative thinking – more extreme thoughts suggest a mood disorder.
- Use psychological scales, e.g. the Hospital Anxiety and Depression Scale (HADS) to assess the degree of anxiety or depression symptoms.

without the need for in-depth psychological treatment. It is therefore important to distinguish grief reactions from more enduring and pervasive anxiety or depressive disorders (Box 17.4).

When a person experiences persistent distress for more than about 3 months, it is worth offering more structured psychological therapy than the emotional support offered during a grief reaction. If the physician or audiologist has the therapy skills, then this may be done within the audiology clinic. Alternatively, a referral should be made to psychology services.

At this stage, much of the therapy effort goes into exploring the person's thoughts about their hearing loss and the changes in behaviour associated with these thoughts. The patient is helped to understand the links between thoughts, feelings and behaviour. When negative thoughts are identified, the person is helped to establish whether they are helpful (acknowledging that the person is likely to face real difficulties) or *overly* negative. This may be achieved through discussion or by changing the way the person acts in order to test the thoughts. A generic CBT model is helpful in understanding many hearing-impaired people's distress. Determining what thoughts the person has about his or her hearing problems and what they do (or don't do) as a consequence of this, is a central part of the therapeutic process. There are, however, more specific CBT models that have particular relevance in this context, e.g. CBT models of social phobia and of low self-esteem. We will use some case examples

to illustrate the CBT conceptualisation and treatment approach (see case examples 1 and 2).

Case example 1

Angela developed a hearing loss as a consequence of measles when she was 6 years old. She attended mainstream school. Although she could communicate well in a quiet environment, communication often broke down in the school playground, and the other children tended to avoid her. She had few friends and was teased. With good intentions, her parents made every effort to treat Angela the same way as her normally hearing siblings, and expected the same things of her. She, however, found it difficult to be just like them, particularly in her teenage years. During those years, her sister had a string of boyfriends, but Angela did not. She had a crush on a boy at school. Although he was kind towards her he did not become her boyfriend. She assumed that he did not want to be seen going out with the 'deaf kid'. As a young adult she had a series of jobs. Although she managed the work well, she left each job because of poor personal relationships with her colleagues. By 29 years of age, she still had not had a boyfriend, and moved jobs again, feeling very depressed. At this stage, Angela was referred to the psychology service. It emerged during the course of CBT that she had low self-esteem, believing that she was not likeable or attractive. She believed, in particular, that communication breakdowns made her unlikeable. She therefore felt anxious when communicating with colleagues and made strenuous efforts to control her listening environment. She kept her interactions to a minimum. She interpreted many other everyday events as evidence that she was not an attractive person. This was particularly true when the event had an ambiguous nature, e.g. when a man offered his seat on a crowded bus to the woman next to Angela. In order to test the accuracy of her ideas, Angela agreed to ask some of her new colleagues about how they thought she was fitting in. This 'survey' was different from her usual avoidance of conversation, particularly about something so intimate. She discovered that people thought she was generally nice and her hearing loss made her interesting, but she was hard to get to know and she was sometimes aggressive or overly controlling. It became apparent that her efforts to guard against rejection were increasing the chances of it. She then changed her behaviour by talking more to people and being less strenuous in her efforts to control the listening environment. This did lead to more communication failures, but she discovered that people did not reject her as they had in the playground. She learnt that people did not regard her as unlikeable. Having learnt that one of her ideas about herself was overly negative, she went on to test her beliefs further by placing an advert with a dating agency. After a few dates she met someone with whom she established a positive relationship. Angela certainly had some negative experiences, but her interpretation of events was *overly* negative; her belief that everyone would reject her if communication failed was an over-generalisation. Her efforts to prevent communication breakdown (while sensible at one level) represented safety behaviours. She tested her ideas by dropping her safety behaviours and discovered that she was likeable. Her distress reduced considerably and she developed a greater ease with her hearing loss.

Case example 2

Ted was a successful professional. Always anxious, he worried that others would find shortcomings in his work, and therefore in him. He was poor at delegating, and reluctant to accept help at work. He therefore worked extremely hard, double-checking everything. In his 50s he experienced sudden and progressive hearing loss. Initially he was helped by hearing aids, but within 5 years his loss was profound and hearing aids were no longer of benefit. He was now not able to cope at work, within the family, or at church were he had always spent much time. He became very anxious, as he believed his hearing loss would lead people to judge him badly. When having conversations he believed that others saw him as an object of ridicule or pity. In anticipation of conversations, and during them, he was preoccupied by this image, and this made it dif-

ficult for him to focus on the communication. He used two main coping strategies in order to deny the extent of his hearing loss to others. He controlled conversation by talking too much, and he pretended to have heard when he had not. Instead of helping, his coping strategies made matters worse. They made him appear socially inappropriate and he was aware that others reacted hesitantly towards him. Thus, by employing these unhelpful coping strategies, he brought about the thing he was trying to avoid. Because people responded unfavourably to his behaviour, this increased his anxiety levels. He went on to believe that his symptoms of anxiety were indicative of a mental breakdown that would lead to hospitalisation. His general practitioner (GP) prescribed antidepressant medication, but he was unable to tolerate the side-effects. He was referred to psychology and during a course of CBT Ted was helped to see the link between his thoughts, behaviour and feelings. He was educated about the process of anxiety and came to realise that his symptoms were not indicative of mental breakdown as he feared. He was taught relaxation and other anxiety-management techniques. He was helped to see that his efforts to keep safe stopped him from finding out the accuracy of his ideas that others regarded him as ridiculous or pitiable. Ted came to realise that his safety behaviours actually created prejudicial ideas in others. He was encouraged to tell others that he had a hearing loss and to drop his safety behaviour. Allowing others to talk more created more opportunities for his hearing loss to be evident. Having an explanation for his difficulties allowed people to react more positively towards him. His image of how others saw him therefore changed and his anxiety reduced. The use of hearing tactics is evident in this case. They were used within the context of a CB model of social anxiety.

Hearing loss and dementia

There is a strong association between hearing loss and dementia in older adults. Approximately twice as many people with dementia have a hearing loss compared with matched controls. It has proved difficult to explain the relationship between hearing loss and dementia. Some researchers have speculated that there may be a common process (other than age) linking the two things; however, the association between hearing loss and dementia is not significant when age is controlled for. Post-mortem evidence for pathology in the auditory pathway of people with Alzheimer's disease is mixed. As an alternative, it has been suggested that hearing impairment simply reduces a person's ability to attend to spoken instructions and thus their ability to perform tests of cognition. It is argued that in otherwise healthy older people, a hearing impairment increases the effort required to recognise speech. As a result, the person has fewer cognitive resources for processing and remembering that information. This argument, however, does not account for all of the observations in this context. For example, when cognitive tests are administered in written form to hearing-impaired people, they have been found to perform more poorly than hearing controls. It may be that hearing loss leads to isolation and to disorientation and that this contributes to poor functioning. Alternatively, hearing loss may lead to depression and this may reduce the efficiency of a person's cognitive processing.

Whatever the explanation for the relationship between hearing loss and dementia, it is important for those involved in the care of older hearing-impaired adults to be aware of issues relating to dementia. The growing number of older people in the population means that increasing numbers of older people with dementia will be seen in audiology clinics. The professionals in such clinics may be in a position to identify people at risk and refer them to appropriate services. A review for audiologists has been provided by Dancer and Watkins (2006). Their review includes a list of warning signs proposed by the Alzheimer's Association (www.alz.org) as helpful for early identification; these are summarised in Box 17.5.

The existing evidence does suggest that people with dementia can tolerate audiological procedures. The provision of hearing aids to people with a hearing loss and dementia has been associated with some improvements in a measure of overall wellbeing. Unfortunately, the weight of evidence suggests that the use of hearing aids does not improve cognitive functioning, activities of daily living, or psychiatric symptoms. The evidence on whether or not it reduces the burden on care-givers is mixed. Nonetheless, the benefits, although limited, suggest that the provision of hearing aids should not be restricted to people with only mild dementia. Providing hearing aids to people with more severe dementia also appears to be beneficial. As much of the burden of dementia falls on the care-giver, it is worthwhile including them, as well as the patient, in educational counselling about amplification and communication skills.

Box 17.5 Warning signs for Alzheimer's disease.
• Memory loss
• Misplacing things
• Disorientation in time and place
• Difficulty performing familiar tasks
• Problems with language
• Loss of initiative
• Poor judgement
• Problems with abstract thinking
• Changes in mood and behaviour

Conclusions and future directions

A clear conclusion from the literature is that there are non-auditory dimensions to the experience of hearing loss. Indeed, the non-auditory aspects of the experience may outweigh the auditory ones. It has been suggested that AHL can result in both good and bad consequences. The audiology professional should be careful not to make assumptions about the patient's experiences, particularly on the basis of audiometry alone. The bad consequences are more relevant from a clinical point of view. AHL has been associated with psychological problems such as grief, anxiety, depression, PTSD symptoms and psychotic-like experiences. There is evidence that

AHL affects relationships and places a significant strain on close family members. There is also a strong relationship between AHL and dementia. When the associations are examined carefully, it seems that psychological problems arise from an interaction between hearing loss and factors such as individual differences in attitudes and coping styles, social problems and health problems. A model that includes psychological, social and biological factors is needed to account for the observations surrounding AHL. Whatever the exact mechanisms, the reality is that professionals may be confronted by the package of problems that the patient brings to the audiology clinic. Therefore, care needs to be taken when devising assessment and rehabilitation programmes to ensure that psychological aspects of AHL are addressed. Interventions should focus on helping the whole family adjust to the loss.

Clearly, clinical psychologists have a role in the care of hearing-impaired people. Existing CBT models offer a structured and validated approach to resolving many of the problems that people with AHL face. CBT is becoming more available as an internet-based psychology service and this may be particularly useful for people with AHL. The new wave of cognitive therapies, involving mindfulness and acceptance approaches, is highly applicable to the issues surrounding hearing loss. These approaches will extend the help available to hearing-impaired people. Another future role for psychologists may be to provide expertise in solving the difficult problem of how to change attitudes and behaviour towards harmful noise exposure.

Ideally, clinical psychologists should be integrated into audiology clinics, but this is still relatively rare. Professionals working with hearing-impaired people should therefore seek to establish close links with their local psychology services. Unfortunately, there are currently too few clinical psychologists to meet the demands upon their services. This means that some of the burden of dealing with psychological problems will fall on audiologists and their close colleagues. The result will be a considerable expansion of audiologists' responsibilities. This expansion is in keeping with the current vision for psychological health services. This vision anticipates that professionals such as audiologists, supervised by more experienced mental health workers, will provide basic psychological care. Clearly, this development will require an extension of audiology training.

References

Beck A (1976) *Cognitive Therapy and the Emotional Disorders*. Madison, CT: International University Pess.

Dancer J, Watkins P (2006) *Remember Me? A guide to Alzheimer's Disease and hearing loss.* http://www.audiologyonline.com/articles/article_detail.asp?article_id=1503 (accessed 1 December 2008).

Hallam R, Ashton P, Sherbourne K, Gailey L (2006) Acquired profound hearing loss: mental health and other characteristics of a large sample. *International Journal of Audiology* 45:715–723.

Hallam R, Ashton P, Sherbourne K, Gailey L (2008) Persons with acquired profound hearing loss (APHL): how do they and their families adapt to the challenge? *Health* 12:369–388.

Helvik A-S, Jacobsen G, Hallberg L (2006) Psychological well being of adults with acquired hearing impairment. *Disability and Rehabilitation* 28:535–545.

Kerr P, Cowie R (1997) Acquired deafness: a multidimensional experience. *British Journal of Audiology* 31:177–188.

Ringdahl A, Grimby A (2000) Severe profound hearing impairment and health related quality of life amongst post lingual deafened Swedish adults. *Scandinavian Audiology* 29:266–275.

Sherbourne K, White L, Fortnum H (2002) Intensive rehabilitation for deafened men and women – an evaluation study. *International Journal of Audiology* 41:195–201.

Stephens SDG, Kerr P (2000) Auditory displacements: an update. *Audiology* 39:322–332.

Stephens D, Kerr P (2003) The role of positive experiences in living with hearing loss. *International Journal of Audiology* 42: S118–S127.

Stewart-Kerr P (1992) *The Experience of Acquired Deafness: a psychological perspec-*

tive. PhD thesis, Queens University of Belfast.

Tambs T (2004) Moderate effects of hearing loss on mental health and subjective well being: results from the Nord-Trondelag hearing loss study. *Psychosomatic Medicine* 66:776–782.

Thewissen V, Myin-Germeys I, Bentall R *et al.* (2005) Hearing impairment and psychosis revisited. *Schizophrenia Research* 76:99–103.

Thomas A (1984) *Acquired Hearing Loss: psychological and social implications*. Orlando, FL: Academic Press.

Van der Werf M, van Boxtel M, Verhey F *et al.* (2007) Mild hearing impairment and psychotic experiences in a normal aging population. *Schizophrenia Research* 94:180–186.

Veale D (2006) A compelling desire for deafness. *Journal of Deaf Studies and Deaf Education* May:1–4.

World Health Organization (2001) *The International Classification of Functioning, Disability and Health – ICF*. Geneva: World Health Organization.

Mental health and pre-lingual deafness

Sally Austen

18

Introduction

This chapter will consider mental health in the context of congenital and pre-lingual deafness (deafness acquired before language has developed). It will also focus on the severe to profound range of deafness which limits speech perception. It will argue that deafness itself does not directly cause mental health problems but that some of the causes and consequences of deafness may well be associated with increased risk of mental health problems.

Causes of mental health problems in children

Factors associated with the cause of deafness

Congenital or perinatally acquired deafness is not itself responsible for mental health problems. However, the factors that caused the deafness may also be responsible for brain damage, learning difficulties and, in some cases, more subtle cognitive deficits, in the absence of obvious dis-

ability (Van Reekum et al., 2000; Deb et al., 2001). About one-third of congenitally deaf people have additional difficulties (cognitive, visual, motor, linguistic or physical) (Crocker and Edwards, 2004). These factors include the consequences of prematurity and low birth weight, meningitis, congenital cytomegalovirus (CMV) infection and some syndromic causes of congenital deafness. Increased survival rates for infants with these problems during the next 20 years are likely to result in a 20% increase in deafness (Davis, 2001) and also to increase the proportion of deaf people who have additional difficulties.

Parental attitudes and behaviours

Social factors take higher precedence in the early childhood years, when parenting and language acquisition are important. During these years the deaf individual's perception of their situation is less influential than that of their parents.

Diagnosis of deafness usually comes as a great shock to parents, particularly to hearing parents. Regardless of when the diagnosis occurs it may be viewed by the parents as a tragedy and a sign that their child is irreparably damaged. In contrast, some parents may come to view deafness as an unexpected difference, complete with its own set of challenges that they will expect to get over. Some parents (usually those who are themselves congenitally deaf) are genuinely pleased to discover that their child is deaf.

The reaction of the parents is the first in a long line of social factors that influence the mental health of that deaf individual. The way that a diagnosis is explained to parents and the information and support they are offered can have a huge effect on the wellbeing of the parents and subsequently the child (Hindley and Kitson, 2001). The beliefs of the parents are seen as a crucial place to start psychological interventions (Woolfson, 2004).

Deaf children of hearing parents are three times more likely to have behaviour problems than hearing children and this is, in part, put down to parental beliefs (Meadow, 1981; Hindley, 2000). Hearing parents, who are more likely to view deafness as an insurmountable disability, are significantly more likely to indulge and overprotect their child. In contrast, those that perceive a positive identity of deafness are more likely to parent the deaf child as hearing parents would a hearing child and insist upon socially acceptable behaviour. Style of parenting not only affects the child's current behaviour but, over time, affects the older child's beliefs about their responsibility for their own behaviour. The negative effects of this may endure into adulthood (Kentish, 2007).

Deaf children of deaf parents do not have the same degree of emotional or behavioural problems as deaf children of hearing parents (Meadow, 1980; Bailly *et al.*, 2003). This may be for a number of reasons. The deaf parent is likely to see the child's deafness more positively and set boundaries for unacceptable behaviours without feeling a need to compensate the child for his deafness (Kentish, 2007). Due to the relatively higher proportion of hereditary causes of deafness, deaf children of deaf parents are also less likely to be at neurological risk, compared with deaf children of hearing parents. The latter include a higher proportion deafened by factors such as perinatal hypoxia or meningitis, causes of deafness that place them at neurological risk. Finally, the deaf child of deaf parents has social and linguistic role models from an early age, just as hearing children with hearing parents do, and are less likely to suffer from isolation or language deprivation.

Pollard and Rendon (1999), however, caution that deaf/hearing issues are rarely the sole link to family dysfunction, but that normal family relations depend on the family's general mental health. Examples of 'at risk deaf parents' (Charlson, 2004) alert us that deaf people who have suffered additional linguistic, social, mental health or parental deprivations will not automatically find parenting a deaf child easy.

Language deprivation

The human brain has a window of opportunity for full language ability that closes around the time a child goes to primary school (5–7 years). Without a rich language environment in these early years, language deprivation (permanently stunted language) is possible. Unfortunately this is all too common among pre-lingually deaf children. In a study of deaf children and their families, Gregory *et al.* (1995) found that 20% of their sample was unable to be interviewed either in speech or in sign because of poor language skills and despite normal non-verbal IQs (intelligence quotients).

Late diagnosis of deafness deprives the child of early enough exposure to aided oral language or to sign language. Some profoundly deaf children may have been prevented from signing in the belief that this will improve their oral abilities. This hypothesis has never, however, been backed up, and in hearing children who are being taught to sign there is evidence that this helps their language development (Meier and Newport, 1990).

Language deprivation can have huge effects on daily functioning (communicating with one's friends and family) and emotional stability (preventing tantrums and inappropriate behaviours through explanation, reasoning and education). Language is also one of the ways in which longer-term cognitive and social ability is either developed or stunted, for example via the acquisition of 'theory of mind'.

Theory of Mind

'Theory of Mind' (ToM) describes the ability to understand that others might think or feel differently to ourselves, or that they might have access to different information from us. For example, my shy friend and I are planning a night out. I require ToM to appreciate that my friend is nervous in social situations and therefore needs my support. A more sophisticated level of ToM is required for my friend to appreciate that, although I do usually provide this extra social support, this evening, since I have a bad cold, I might not be able to provide the support to such a great extent.

The absence of theory of mind seriously affects interpersonal relationships and behaviour as it is crucial to cognitive planning, reasoning skills, empathy and the understanding that behaviours have consequences. Delay in acquiring ToM is linked to poor language acquisition (Woolfe *et al.*, 2002). Without language it is difficult to achieve the degree of social interaction to learn about the mental states of other people and how their behaviour may relate to these. While deaf children of deaf parents develop ToM at the same time as hearing children of hearing parents (around 3–5 years), deaf children of hearing parents often have significant delays in ToM. Peterson (2002) found that 40% of deaf children with hearing parents did not succeed in measures of ToM in the 13–16-year group. The social and cognitive purpose of ToM is to allow the person to deal with new learning and social situations such as interacting effectively with peer groups, authority relationships and romantic relationships. Delayed acquisition of ToM results in many missed learning opportunities.

Lack of, or poorly developed, ToM is also a feature of autistic spectrum disorder (ASD). Differential diagnosis between poor ToM as a result of language deprivation and poor ToM as a result of ASD can be challenging.

Identity

Although *adjustment* is often discussed in association with *acquired* disability, those *born* deaf or deafened pre-lingually will also need to assimilate their deafness into their identity and make sense of their position as a deaf person in a predominantly hearing world. Poor adjustment can lead to depression, anger and, ultimately, to personality difficulties.

The tasks of childhood and adolescence are clustered around social communication. This enables children to share vast amounts of interpersonal detail with each other, to calculate norms and differences, and to find their place among their peers. This place defines us for years to come. Thus, the role of school is not only to provide academic education but also to provide an environment that facilitates social growth.

Identifying oneself as part of a deaf or hearing world was clearer cut for the older generation. Deaf people went to deaf schools and one way or another learnt to sign; hearing people went to hearing schools where speech was the norm. Primitive technology and lack of interpreters did not allow for much mixing. Now advances in hearing aid and cochlear implant technology have increased the proportion of severely and profoundly deaf people who have some useful access to speech, and have resulted in a more 'patchwork' deaf–hearing society. However, identity may be harder to glean. For example, child A functions as although severely deaf when he has his cochlear implant in during a noisy class, profoundly deaf while swimming, and only moderately deaf when communicating one-to-one with his mother. He is identified by his lack of hearing during class but also by his sporting prowess during football. 'Mainstreaming' deaf children into hearing schools has increased the number of groups to which a deaf child has the opportunity to belong – the football crowd, the science crowd, the bus travel crowd – but might still fail to provide a 'deaf crowd'. Finding one's place in this complicated social network can be difficult. Furthermore, if the deaf child still fails to find a place, his sense of isolation will be increased and the risk of mental health difficulties will also increase as adolescence ensues.

Some children may utilise difficult behaviour in order to combat their sense of invisibility and get attention from their peers or adults. However, the negative feedback that the child then receives for his behaviour can negatively affect self-esteem; this either results in further externalised displays of unhappiness, such as more challenging behaviour, or internalised displays such as anxiety, low mood and withdrawal (Edwards and Crocker, 2008).

Isolation

Isolation is an issue for most deaf people that follows them from cradle to grave. Ninety per cent of deaf children are born into hearing families: this can make them isolated in their experience, their identity and often their language. Being deaf in a hearing world can be a lonely experience. For deaf children born into deaf families this is less likely, since they have immediate social and linguistic role models in their family; this can be reflected in their higher self-esteem (Woolfe, 2001).

There are now significantly fewer deaf specialist schools, and more deaf children are being integrated into mainstream generic (hearing) schools. Those in favour say that mainstreaming helps integrate deaf children into a predominantly hearing world; those against say that mainstreaming is an excuse for cutting resources for deaf children to save money. While it does potentially maximise the exposure of deaf children to their hearing peers, mainstreaming can result in a lone deaf child in a school of hearing children. Not only does this isolate the child, affect their chances of good peer relationships and emphasise their 'difference', but economies of scale mean that specialist resources are stretched, and that facilities for training teachers and preparing hearing pupils how best to work with the deaf individual may be reduced.

Psychologically, each individual has the capacity to react differently to the same situation, including their deafness (Austen, 2004a). Individual differences in cognition determine how isolation or bullying is received, and determine the resulting emotions. For those that perceive these experiences negatively – 'I am not good enough', 'No one will ever like me' – the result can be fear, helplessness and depression. Others may reframe the experience – 'They are ignorant, I am doing fine' – and survive this isolation with their mental health intact. Cole and Edelmann (1991) found that deaf teenagers often perceived their social problems as being directly caused by their deafness rather than being a factor of their developmental stage. For example, many believed that they had problems with their parents or getting girlfriends because they were deaf, whereas in fact most teenagers are likely to have these difficulties.

Children of any age or audiological status who have no one to share their experience will have no access to the social supports that are generally thought to protect us from mental health problems (Gray and du Feu, 2004). For deaf adolescents who have limited shared language with either their parents or their peers, this is often a precursor to mental health problems.

An isolated child (or adult) is vulnerable to bullying and abuse of all kinds. Deaf children who cannot communicate effectively are obvious, easy targets. Compared to hearing people, deaf children, male and female, are more likely to be victims of sexual abuse, particularly those who went to boarding school (Sullivan *et al.*, 2000). Previous abuse is linked to behavioural and emotional problems, particularly if the individual receives no therapy (Sullivan *et al.*, 2000).

Education and opportunity for learning

Much of a hearing person's learning is incidental, picked up informally from peers, elders or the media. For deaf people who cannot 'overhear' conversations, learning becomes more of a directed experience. Extremely bright deaf people may still have gaps in their learning that are indicative of lack of opportunity, not of lack of ability. Even directed learning experiences such as school, evening classes, TV and the workplace are relatively inaccessible to deaf people if they do not have access to communication equipment such as loop and FM systems, sign language interpreters, or when their instructors lack specialist knowledge of deafness. Underachievement in terms of qualification is commonplace. Literacy is known to be a particular problem, with the reading age of pre-lingually deaf adults averaging less than 9 years (Mayberry, 2002). This has implications for the use of forms, handouts, questionnaires etc. Writing is therefore *not* a reliable means of assessing or treating profoundly pre-lingually deaf patients.

Prevalence of mental health problems in deaf children

Determining the prevalence of psychological and behavioural difficulties in deaf children is difficult. The presence of additional disabilities, lack of valid assessment tools, and a scarcity of mental health professionals with sufficient communication skills or experience of deafness are but some of the factors responsible for this difficulty (Hindley, 1997). Although deaf children appear to experience the same range of mental health problems as hearing children (Bailly *et al.*, 2003), the prevalence of these mental health problems is between two and five times greater than it is in hearing children (Hindley, 2000). Hindley and Kitson (2001) report that language limitation in deaf children, and the tendency for many non-specialist mental health professionals to mis-attribute all problems to the child's deafness, result in frequent under-diagnosis of mental health problems in deaf children.

A number of studies have suggested greater impulsiveness in deaf children. However, the incidence of attention deficit hyperactivity disorder (ADHD) does not appear to be higher than for the general child population, with the exception of children with acquired hearing loss, and/or additional disabilities (Hindley and Kroll, 1998; Bailly *et al.*, 2003).

Overall, deaf children of deaf parents are reported to attain better emotional and cognitive outcomes than do deaf children of hearing parents (Bailly *et al.*, 2003). They are also reported to have better self-image and less difficulty with impulse control (Meadow-Orlans, 1990).

Protective factors against childhood mental health problems in deaf children may include the early provision of sign language to all severely to profoundly deaf infants from as soon after diagnosis as possible (Hindley and Kitson, 2001). In Scandinavian countries, where native sign languages have been introduced to all deaf children and their parents, the rate of mental health problems among deaf children is no higher than in hearing children (Sinkkonen, 1994). Remedial interventions to promote social and emotional development for deaf children in secondary school levels include the Promoting Alternative Thinking Strategies (PATHS) programme (Greenburg and Kusche, 1993), which can be used in signed or oral environments. The programme promotes emotional understanding, self-control, social problem solving and reflective thinking skills. It has been shown to prevent a range of behavioural, emotional and personality difficulties (Hindley and Kitson, 2001)

Adulthood

Prevalence of mental health problems in pre-lingually deaf adults

In adulthood, mental health or behaviour problems that started to appear in childhood either diminish or become more persistent. Demographic studies are still quite scarce but the increased prevalence of mental health problems in deaf children is unlikely to have lessened as this cohort reaches adulthood. Two factors contribute to the ongoing vulnerability of deaf adults to mental health problems. The first is the continued experience of discrimination. Deaf people still overall have higher rates of unemployment and lower rates of pay than hearing people. Isolation and bullying continues from childhood through to adulthood, with significant discrimination, for example, in the workplace where deaf people are often passed over for promotions or training (Hogan, 2001). Eighty-six per cent of deaf people report suffering prejudice and ill-treatment from people they have just met (Royal National Institute for Deaf People (RNID), 1998), with 20% saying they had been the victims of abusive language or gestures (McCrone, 1994).

The second factor is difficulty accessing mental health services.

Access to mental health services

One of the greatest problems in assessing the prevalence, treatment and prevention of mental health problems is that mental health services are often relatively inaccessible. In order to know that an experience or symptom requires help, the patient must have had access to information about normal and abnormal mental health. Without incidental learning (overhearing others discussing mental health issues, accessing a discussion programme on TV or reading a leaflet in a general practitioner (GP) waiting room), the deaf person will not understand when they should ask for help or where to go for help.

Once a deaf person decides to seek help, the physical process of attending for an appointment may carry its own difficulties. Some clinic buildings may have a voice phone and an intercom rather than a minicom or video phone. Once in the building it is possible that staff have limited ability to work knowledgeably with a deaf patient or to understand the need to book an interpreter who has appropriate physical or mental health knowledge. Should a mental health problem be suspected, staff may not know how and where to refer the patient (Gray and du Feu, 2004; Kitson and Austen, 2004).

The paradox that deaf people both have difficulty accessing services and are over-represented in psychiatric hospitals (Timmermans, 1989; Denmark, 1966) reflects the fact that a deaf person is more likely to be taken seriously by members of the care professions if he or she is very ill. One purpose of primary care is to prevent the escalation of problems and the need for hospitalisation. However, many deaf people have difficulty gaining access even to the simplest of GP services (RNID, 2004; Department of Health, 2005). Extremely few protective environments such as youth clubs, drop in centres, telephone help lines, substance misuse services, doctors' surgeries, hospitals or mental health services, are accessible to deaf people. This not only prevents useful preventative or rehabilitative work, but can increase the sense of isolation and reinforces the difference between deaf and hearing worlds. Developments in mental health care such as early intervention teams, assertive outreach teams, and preventative programmes are unlikely to reach deaf people (Gray and du Feu, 2004). Where mental health services are available, the deaf person's problem may be picked up very late and/or be dealt with inadequately.

The average length of stay of a deaf person in psychiatric hospital is twice that of a hearing person (Patterson and Baines, 2005). This is the result of a number of factors: the mental health problem of a deaf patient is likely to have remained untreated for a much longer time, additional disabilities may make treatment more difficult and the markedly reduced options for community support or supported living can delay discharge dramatically.

There are three specialist deaf mental health services for adults in Britain, based in London, Birmingham and Manchester, and three for children, based in London, Dudley and York. There are also a small number of deaf adult forensic services, including a deaf-specific ward in Rampton high-security psychiatric hospital. Two charities, RNID and SignHealth provide the bulk of specialist housing for deaf people with mental health problems. Specialist services with signing- and communication-skilled staff reduce the likelihood of misdiagnosis, which is common in deaf people. Historically, perfectly well deaf people were diagnosed as 'mad' and languished in psychiatric hospitals. Even today, failing to diagnose severe mental illness in deaf people, leaving them untreated, is also relatively common (Austen *et al.*, 2007).

The disadvantage of specialist services is that some patients may have long distances to travel or cannot access the services at all. To this end, the *Mental Health and Deafness: towards equity and access* document (Department of Health, 2005) recommends that deaf specialist services, local generic (hearing) mental health teams and primary care teams find ways of working together to ensure that patients do not fall through the net.

Types of mental health problems

Deaf adults are likely to experience the same range of mental health problems as hearing people, with some having a higher prevalence. Substance misuse, anxiety and depression appear to have a similar prevalence in deaf people, with their impact being more severe due to lack of preventative measures or accessible treatment facilities (Evans and Elliot, 1987; Austen and Checinski, 2000; Connolly *et al.*, 2006).

It is probable that personality disorder and schizophrenia have either an equal or higher prevalence in deaf people. Some of the factors that increase the risk of personality disorder, such as a history of abuse, neurological risk, behaviour problems and an unstable family life, are more common in deaf children, so may increase the prevalence of personality disorder in deaf adults. Schizophrenia is known to have a strong genetic component, not associated with deafness. However, the other social and biological predisposing factors such as neurological risk and disadvantaged backgrounds (social isolation, poor job prospects, poverty, victimisation, separation from family of origin and lack of social role) are common to deaf people (Gray and du Feu, 2004).

There is no evidence to show that the three times higher prevalence of challenging behaviour in deaf children is likely to fall when they become adults. Causes remain similar to those among children, with a greater emphasis on the increasing years of less-effective learning and boundary setting. Neurological vulnerability can be a cause of temper control difficulties and poor 'executive functioning' (the part of our brain that double checks our behaviour, morals, manners and complex reasoning). The frustration from being isolated is likely to continue from childhood but now the adult has less contact with their family, school peers or teachers. The impact of poor learning becomes more noticeable in adulthood. For example, in a child with poor theory of mind who fails to consider the feelings of others, this behaviour can go unnoticed. However, adults' behaviours in the workplace, while driving and in intimate behaviour will have a much greater impact and can no longer be passed off as 'a phase' the child is going through. An adult with a poor understanding of boundaries now becomes more problematic than the equivalent small child, and the potential for harm to self or others increases. Unfortunately, those with the potential to educate adults about boundaries (e.g. bus conductors, police, judges) often regard the deaf person as unfortunate and not in control of their own behaviour, so are reluctant to do so.

Deafness and Challenging Behaviour: the 360° degree perspective (Austen and Jeffery, 2007) maintains that 'communication is the key to large parts of the cause, prevention, and resolution of challenging behaviour'. Isolation, learning inequalities and boundary setting are social factors that may have been preventable earlier in life but become more deeply entrenched if left into adulthood.

Deaf older adults

Whether deafened pre-lingually or by acquired presbyacusis (age-related progressive hearing loss), the greatest issue for deaf older adults is isolation, which can lead to a myriad of mental health problems ranging from anxiety and depression to psychosis and cognitive decline. As a group they are often 'invisible'. This is reflected in the fact that little has been published about their plight. The high prevalence of progressive deafness in older age tends to obscure the needs and existence of the severely to profoundly pre-lingually deaf people who have also got older. The needs of these two client groups are very different.

Our deaf older adults were born in a generation where immunisation and antibiotics were yet to be invented. Deafness resulting from measles, mumps, meningitis and rubella were relatively common. However, survival rates from such illness were lower, and survival was usually restricted to those without multiple disabilities. Thus, the older deaf population are less likely to have additional disabilities than their younger counterparts.

Service provision for deaf older adults is severely limited, with many ending their days in a generic old people's service with no specialist communication provision or knowledge of deafness and mental health. This often leads to misdiagnosis of communication frustration or misunderstanding as mental illness (Feldman and Eck, 2007). Signs of cognitive decline, such as decreasing language proficiency in stroke patients, may be passed off as idiosyncrasies associated with the patient's deafness. Specialist, deaf geriatric professionals are extremely scarce, internationally. None of the UK's three national deaf mental health services or the three deaf forensic services provides services routinely to people over 65 years. These services would be able to advise on mental health problems, such as depression, anxiety or schizophrenia, originally diagnosed while the patients were of working age, that have persisted into old age. However, they may be limited in the help they can give in relation to age-related ailments such as dementia.

Follow-on services, such as specialist housing, are equally sparse. Group homes for deaf older adults are only a partial solution to this problem as, although they would provide the right geriatric care in the right communication environment, their relatively small numbers mean that most of the occupants would be a long way from their families.

As well as the lack of specialist clinicians and services, there is also a dearth of validated psychometric tests and measures. This is common throughout the deaf lifespan but is particularly problematic in older age mental health services. Comparison of premorbid *versus* current functioning is regularly used to identify decline and to diagnose conditions such as dementia. However, premorbid functioning tests are mostly inappropriate for use with a pre-lingually deaf population. Premorbid measures, such as the National Adult Reading Test (NART) tend to rely on reading ability (some aspects of which are thought to remain intact during brain injury). This is not appropriate for pre-lingually deaf people, due to the reduced average literacy rate and the fact that this test measures aural memory of the word rather than phonetic construction. In hearing people, premorbid functioning may be estimated by subjective measures of lifestyle such as job, income, hobbies. However, in deaf people, whose access to education and work is so restricted, this is not a reliable measure of their true ability.

For those older deaf people who suffered from early language deprivation or additional disabilities such as brain damage, the effects of these problems will continue into old age. It is likely that with the cognitive decline that normally occurs with ageing, and the social stresses of isolation, the risk of challenging behaviour will increase (Austen and Paijmans, 2006). Protective factors for the mental health of older people include the presence of an intimate confidant, social skills such as assertiveness and communication skills, accessibility of day centres, and counselling related to life events such as bereavement. The linguistic and social isolation of deaf elderly people means that when these protective factors are not available to them, the likelihood of mental health problems will increase (Austen, 2004b).

Conclusion

Although biological damage associated with cause of deafness is partially to blame, most of the causes of mental health difficulty in deaf children, adults and older adults are socially created and are therefore preventable. To reverse this situation, discriminatory attitudes of hearing people towards deaf people will need to change, language acquisition and social competence training need to be a priority for pre-school and school-age children, and specialist deaf mental health provision for all ages needs improving such that mental health problems can be prevented from starting or from escalating.

References

Austen S (2004a) Cognitive behavioural models in deafness and audiology. In: Austen S, Crocker S, eds. *Deafness in Mind. Working psychologically with deaf people across the lifespan*, pp 101–104. London: Whurr Publishers Ltd.

Austen S (2004b) Older adults who use sign language. In: Austen S, Crocker S, eds. *Deafness in Mind. Working psychologically with deaf people across the lifespan*, pp 329–341. London: Whurr Publishers Ltd.

Austen S, Checinski K (2000) Addictive behaviour and deafness. In: Hindley P, Kitson N, eds. *Mental Health and Deafness*, pp 232–252. London: Whurr Publishers Ltd.

Austen S, Gray A, Carney S (2007) Diagnosis and challenging behaviour of deaf people. In: Austen S, Jeffery D, eds. *Deafness and Challenging Behaviour: the 360° perspective*, pp 52–72. Chicester: John Wiley and Sons Ltd.

Austen S, Jeffery D, eds (2007) *Deafness and Challenging Behaviour: the 360° perspective*. Chicester: John Wiley and Sons Ltd.

Austen S, Paijmans R (2006) *Challenging Behaviour in Deaf Seniors*. Presentation to Spring Conference (Deaf Elderly Special Interest Group of the European Society of Mental Health and Deafness), Ede, Holland, April 2006.

Bailly D, Dechoulydelenclave MB, Lauwerier L (2003) Hearing impairment and psychopathological disorders in children and adolescents: review of the literature. *Encephale* 29(4 pt 1):329–337.

Charlson E (2004) At-risk deaf parents and their children. In: Austen S, Crocker S, eds. *Deafness in Mind. Working psychologically with deaf people across the lifespan*, pp 222–234. London: Whurrs Publishers Ltd.

Cole SH, Edelmann RJ (1991) Identity patterns and self- and teacher-perceptions of problems for deaf adolescents: a research note. *Journal of Child Psychology and Psychiatry* 32: 1159–1165.

Connolly C, Rose J, Austen S (2006) Identifying and assessing depression in prelingually deaf people: a literature review. *American Annals of the Deaf* 151:49–60.

Crocker S, Edwards L (2004) Deafness and additional difficulties. In: Austen S, Crocker S, eds. *Deafness in Mind. Working psychologically with deaf people across the lifespan*, pp 252–270. London: Whurr Publishers Ltd.

Davis A (2001) The prevalence of hearing impairment. In: Graham J, Martin M, eds. *Ballantyne's Deafness*, 6th edn, pp 10–25. London: Whurr Publishers Ltd.

Deb S, Thomas M, Bright C (2001) Mental disorder in adults with intellectual disability. 1: Prevalence of functional psychiatric illness among a community-based population aged between 16 and 64 years. *Journal of Intellectual Disability Research* 45:495–505.

Denmark J (1966) Mental illness and early profound deafness. *British Journal of Medical Psychology* 39:117–124.

Department of Health (2005) *Mental Health and Deafness: towards equity and access*. London: Department of Health Publications.

Edwards L, Crocker S (2008) *Psychological Processes in Deaf Children with Complex Needs. An evidence-based practical guide*. London: Jessica Kingsley Publications.

Evans J, Elliot H (1987) The mental status examination. In: Elliot H, Glass L, Evans J, eds. *Mental Health Assessment of Deaf Clients: a practice manual*, pp 83–92. Boston: Little, Brown and Company.

Feldman D, Eck K (2007) Challenging behaviours and the deaf older adults. In: Austen S, Jeffery D, eds. *Deafness and Challenging Behaviour: the 360° perspective*, pp 144–155. Chicester: John Wiley and Sons Ltd.

Gray A, du Feu M (2004) The causes of schizophrenia and the implications for Deaf people. In: Austen S, Crocker S, eds. *Deafness in Mind. Working psychologically with deaf people across the lifespan*, pp 206–219. London: Whurr Publishers Ltd.

Greenberg MT, Kusche C (1993) *Promoting Social and Emotional Development in Deaf Children: the PATHS curriculum*. Seattle, WA: Washington University Press.

Gregory S, Bishop J, Sheldon L (1995) *Deaf People and Their Families: developing understanding*. Cambridge: Cambridge University Press.

Hindley PA (1997) Psychiatric aspects of hearing impairments. *Journal of Child Psychology and Psychiatry* 38:101–117.

Hindley P (2000) Child and adolescent psychiatry. In: Hindley P, Kitson N, eds. *Mental Health and Deafness*, pp 42–74. London: Whurr Publishers Ltd.

Hindley P, Kitson N (2001) Deafness and mental health. In: Graham J, Martin M, eds. *Ballantyne's Deafness*, 6th edn, pp 272–287. London: Whurr Publishers Ltd.

Hindley P, Kroll L (1998) Theoretical and epidemiological aspects of attention deficit and overactivity in deaf children. *Journal of Deaf Studies and Education* 3:64–72.

Hogan A (2001) *Hearing Rehabilitation for Deafened Adults. A psychosocial approach.* London: Whurr Publishers Ltd.

Kentish R (2007) Challenging behaviour in the young deaf child. In: Austen S, Crocker S, eds. *Deafness in Mind. Working psychologically with deaf people across the lifespan*, pp 75–88. London: Whurr Publishers Ltd.

Kitson N, Austen S (2004) Mental health services for deaf people. In: Austen S, Crocker S, eds. *Deafness in Mind. Working psychologically with deaf people across the lifespan*, pp 147–160. London: Whurr Publishers Ltd.

Mayberry RI (2002) Cognitive development in deaf children: the interface of language and perception in neuropsychology. In: Segalowitz SJ, Rapin I, eds. *Handbook of Neuropsychology*, 2nd edn, vol 8, pt II, pp 71–107. Amsterdam: Elsevier.

McCrone W (1994) A two year report card on Title I of the Americans with Disabilities Act: Implications for rehabilitation counseling with deaf people. *Journal of the American Deafness and Rehabilitation Association* 28:1–20.

Meadow K (1980) *Deafness and Child Development.* London: Edward Arnold.

Meadow K (1981) Studies of behaviour problems in deaf children. In: Stein L, Jabeley T, eds. *Deafness and Mental Health*, pp 3–22. New York: Grune and Stratton.

Meadow-Orlans KP (1990) Research on developmental aspects of deafness. In: Moores DF, Meadow Orlans KP, eds. *Educational and Developmental Aspects of Deafness*, pp 283–298. Washington: Gallaudet University Press.

Meier RP, Newport EL (1990) Out of the hands of babes: on a possible sign advantage in language acquisition. *Language* 66:1–23.

Patterson N, Baines D (2005) *The Psycho-social Influences Affecting the Length of Hospital Stay for Deaf Mental Health Service Users.* Presentation to the British Society of Mental Health and Deafness Annual Conference, Newcastle, May 2006.

Peterson CC (2002) Drawing insight from pictures: the development of concepts of false belief in children with deafness, normal hearing, and autism. *Child Development* 73:1442–1459.

Pollard R, Rendon M (1999) Mixed deaf-hearing families: maximizing benefits and minimizing risks. *Journal of Deaf Studies and Deaf Education* 4:156–161.

Royal National Institute for Deaf People (1998) *Breaking the Sound Barrier.* London: The Royal National Institute for Deaf People.

Royal National Institute for Deaf People (2004) *A Simple Cure: a national report into deaf and hard of hearing people's experiences of the National Health Service.* London: Royal National Institute for Deaf People.

Sinkkonen J (1994) *Hearing Impairment, Communication and Personality Development.* Helsinki: Department of Child Psychiatry, University of Helsinki.

Sullivan P, Brookhouser P, Scanlan M (2000) Maltreatment of deaf and hard of hearing children. In: Hindley P, Kitson N, eds. *Mental Health and Deafness*, pp 149–184. London: Whurr Publishers Ltd.

Timmermans L (1989) *Research Project European Society for Mental Health and Deafness.* Proceedings of the European Congress on Mental Health and Deafness. Utrecht, pp 87–91.

Van Reekum R, Cohen T, Wong J (2000) Can traumatic brain injury cause psychiatric disorders? *Journal of Neuropsychiatry and Clinical Neuroscience* 12:316–327.

Woolfe T (2001) The self-esteem and cohesion to family members of deaf children in relation to the hearing status of their parents and siblings. *Deafness and Education International* 3:80–95.

Woolfe T, Want SC, Siegal M (2002) Signposts to development: theory of mind in deaf children. *Child Development* 73:768–778.

Woolfson L (2004) Family well-being and disabled children: a psychosocial model of disability-related child behaviour problems. *British Journal of Health Psychology* 9(1): 1–13.

Hearing aids

Graham Frost

19

Introduction

Once a hearing loss has been confirmed, it is the role of the audiologist to characterise the loss in terms of its severity and frequency specificity using the range of diagnostic and clinical tests available. Using this information, the audiologist will then be able to identify the cause of the loss and determine the most appropriate way in which it can be managed. In some cases a loss may be best managed through medical or surgical intervention, but for the majority the provision of a hearing aid or hearing aids will provide the best potential outcome.

It is perhaps important to differentiate between a hearing aid and an aid to hearing, as both can play a strategic part in both the alleviation of an impairment, resulting from a hearing loss, and the long-term rehabilitation and benefit of a hearing-impaired individual.

A hearing aid is a device which is, in general, worn by the user for the majority of the time to provide continual audibility of sounds within the environments in which the user may be situated. These sounds include speech, music and other inputs from their environment. An aid to hearing is generally used to provide an improvement in audibility or discrimination in a particular listening situation, for example in an educational environment or a theatre. An aid to hearing, often referred to as an assistive listening device, may be employed instead of hearing aids or used in conjunction with them (see Chapter 23).

This chapter provides a general description of the physical characteristics, main functions and features of different types of hearing aids that provide an acoustic output, where processed sound is delivered to the ear canal using an acoustic transducer known as a receiver. Specific considerations for particular users, for example special requirements for children, are not detailed. Some of the assistive listening devices, which may be used in conjunction with hearing aids, are also described (see also Chapter 23).

A hearing loss is still considered by many to be just a reduction in hearing sensitivity, which can be fully rectified by the provision of an appropriate amount of amplification. It must be emphasised, however, that the effects of a hearing loss can be very complex and subjective. It may not only result in reduced audibility but also poor discrimination of speech and a reduced ability to perform auditory processing. An example of this is localisation: our ability to determine the direction from which a particular sound travels.

Unlike the use of prescriptive optical lenses, which can provide correction for most forms of visual impairment, providing optimum benefit to a hearing-impaired individual is far more complex and requires one or two hearing aids which can provide not only appropriate frequency and input level specific amplification, to accommodate their loss in sensitivity, but also employ sophisticated signal processing strategies. There are now strategies that can not only enhance speech discrimination but also compensate for other auditory processes, such as localisation.

It must also be emphasised that it takes considerable time to gain the maximum benefit from using hearing aids. This process is known as *acclimatisation*. The user must learn to manage the aids, accept wearing a device that may initially cause some discomfort, and learn to accommodate changes in sound quality. The user will experience sounds that they may have not heard before, or for some considerable time. They must learn to use the hearing aids in order to take full advantage of them and the sound environment around them.

A hearing aid should satisfy a number of requirements:

- it should make all sounds audible to the user, making quiet sounds audible without making louder sounds uncomfortably loud. Ideally the hearing aid should be able to map the normal audible range of sound levels and frequencies to the hearing-impaired individual's residual hearing, so that they are heard at a similar perceived loudness as would be heard by a person with normal hearing in the same environment
- it should optimise the user's ability to discriminate sounds, especially speech, and in difficult listening situations. Hearing-impaired individuals often have great difficulty in discriminating speech in the presence of background noise, and a hearing aid can employ processing strategies that may improve this
- it should be comfortable when worn, provide an acceptable sound quality and be easy to manage by the user. An individual's ability to

routinely clean their hearing aid and change batteries must be considered.

Hearing aids continue to develop, taking full advantage of new technologies, and in some cases have themselves been responsible for state-of-the-art evolution. The first hearing aids were totally reliant on the passive enhancement of a purely acoustic signal. The earliest example of this is perhaps the cupped hand held behind the pinna, effectively extending the pinna and directing the acoustic signal into the ear canal. A natural development of this was the ear trumpet. With the advent of electrical devices, hearing aids were manufactured using thermionic valves (1930), followed by transistors (1953) and, more recently, integrated circuitry (1964).

Technological advances have not only led to improvements in the performance of hearing aids but also to their miniaturisation. Electronics, transducers and, just as important, batteries have all become smaller. A hearing aid, which once would have been carried in a cumbersome case over the shoulder, can now be housed in a small tailor-made plastic-like housing that can be inserted into the ear canal itself.

Perhaps the most significant change in hearing aid technology since the introduction of the first electrical device was the implementation of digital signal processing (DSP) in the mid-1990s. Although digital processing had been used in many other audio and communication engineering applications, it had not been possible to use it in a hearing aid. For this, the digital processor would be required to operate with a single cell battery of 1.3–1.4 V in order for the aid to be small enough to be acceptable to users. Hearing aids were the only audio application required to operate on a voltage this low, and the ability to achieve this eluded the hearing aid industry for some time.

DSP now provides the hearing aid manufacturer with unprecedented flexibility. For the first time, not only can hearing aids provide significantly improved filtering and amplification characterics, but DSP can provide sophisticated analysis of the sound environment around the user and adapt the processing in order to optimise their benefit.

A typical digital hearing aid (Figure 19.1) consists of a microphone system, which converts the analogue acoustic input into an analogue electrical signal, an analogue to digital converter, which converts the analogue electrical signal into a digital sequence, a digital signal processor, which can analyse the resulting digital code and provide appropriate signal processing, a digital to analogue converter, which converts the modified digital code back into an electrical signal, and a receiver (loudspeaker), which converts the electrical signal back into sound, which is then delivered to the user's ear canal.

With the introduction of DSP to hearing aids, the potential benefit to hearing aid users was no longer limited by the technology available but by the ability of manufacturers and audiologists to implement appropriate signal processing strategies and algorithms.

Types of hearing aids

The basic components of a hearing aid can be packaged in a number of ways to accommodate the type and characteristics of a specific hearing loss, the size of the user's ear canal, the ability of the user to manage the hearing aid on a day-to-day basis and the user's needs and personal preferences (Figure 19.2).

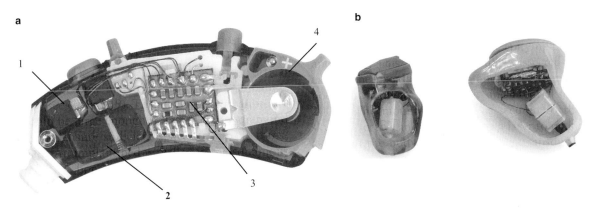

Figure 19.1   Hearing aids. **a**, The main components of a hearing aid: 1 – the microphone; 2 – the receiver; 3 – the amplifier/signal processor; and 4 – the battery. **b**, Completely-in-the-canal (CIC) (left) and in-the-ear (ITE) (right) hearing aids. (Figure courtesy of Widex A/S.)

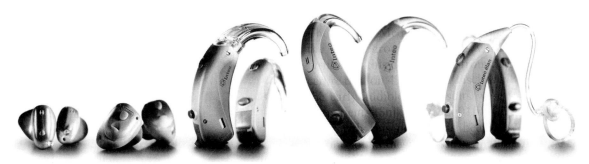

Figure 19.2   Different types of acoustic hearing aids shown as binaural pairs. From left to right, CIC, ITE, BTE, Power BTE and Open-fit. (Figure courtesy of Widex A/S.)

Behind-the-ear hearing aid

A behind-the-ear (BTE) hearing aid consists of a housing worn behind the ear which contains all the major components, including the electronics, the transducers and the battery. This housing may also carry a number of user-accessible controls. The hearing aid is supported behind the ear by means of an earhook. The sound produced by the hearing aid is carried from the earhook to the user's ear canal through a flexible tube. The other end of the tube is retained in the ear canal by means of a custom-made *earmould*.

Open-fit hearing aid

For those who have normal hearing or a mild loss in the low frequencies, but have a more severe loss in the higher frequencies, an 'open-fit' hearing aid may be used. This is similar in many respects to a conventional BTE hearing aid but, rather than using an earmould to retain the flexible tube through which the sound is carried, the thin tubing either rests freely in the ear canal or is held in place using a special open-fit ear tip. As a result there is no earmould to occlude the ear. The open-fit hearing aid is often smaller than a conventional BTE device and may use thinner tubing. This method of hearing aid fitting is becoming more popular as it allows the low frequencies to be heard directly, provides a more natural-sounding own voice and the fitting is generally more comfortable for the user.

In-the-ear hearing aid

An in-the-ear hearing aid (ITE) consists of a custom-made *shell* which contains all the hearing aid components. The shell is positioned discreetly in the entrance of the user's ear canal and delivers processed sound directly into it. The outer profile of the shell is called the faceplate and carries the microphone assembly and provides access for changing the battery. The faceplate may also carry a number of user-accessible controls. ITE hearing aids are available in a range of sizes, from those that sit in the entrance of the ear canal (in-the-canal), and those that partially fill the concha, to those that fill the entire concha bowl.

Completely-in-the-canal hearing aid

A completely-in-the-canal (CIC) hearing aid is similar in many respects to an ITE hearing aid, but the shell is positioned deeply in the ear canal and is therefore barely visible. Like an ITE hearing aid, the shell has a faceplate which carries the microphone assembly and provides access for changing the battery. However, due to its insertion depth, the faceplate does not carry any user-accessible controls. A CIC hearing aid also takes advantage of the natural acoustics of the outer ear.

Receiver-in-the-canal (receiver-in-the-ear) hearing aid

A receiver-in-the-canal (RIC) hearing aid, sometimes referred to as a receiver-in-the ear (RITE) aid, is similar to a BTE device with the exception that the receiver is not contained within the main housing but positioned in the ear canal using a special tip or a custom-made eartip. The receiver is connected via the earhook of the housing using a very fine wire which carries the electrical signal to it. Because the receiver is not contained within the housing itself, RIC hearing aids can be made to be significantly smaller than a BTE aid.

Hearing aid configurations (CROS and BiCROS)

A hearing aid fitting may be configured to provide greater benefit to those with particular types of hearing loss. Two examples of these are known as the CROS and BiCROS systems.

The CROS or contralateral routing of signal system may be used when an individual has a profound or total loss in one ear but normal or nearly normal hearing in the other. These individuals can experience problems in localising sound and discriminating speech in background noise. The CROS system comprises a BTE housing, which only contains a microphone assembly and is worn on the poorer hearing ear. The signal from this microphone is transferred to a hearing aid housing worn on the better-hearing ear, which contains all the other hearing aid components. A thin cable or a wireless link may provide this connection (Figure 19.3a). The hearing aid housing worn on the better ear is then coupled to the ear canal using thin tubing which rests freely in the ear canal or is retained using a special eartip in an *open-fit* manner. In this way the user is able to hear sounds arriving at both sides of their head.

The BiCROS or bilateral contralateral routing of signal is similar in most respects to the CROS system but may be used when there is also a mild or moderate loss in the better ear. The device worn on the better-hearing ear consists of a standard hearing aid, connected to a conventional mould placed in the ear canal, but this aid also receives input from the microphone on the contralateral (poorer-hearing) side.

Spectacle frame hearing aids

These hearing aids either form an integral part of the spectacle frame, replacing the conventional earhook on the end of the spectacle frame arm, or are attached to the frame in place of the conventional hook by means of a special adaptor (Figure 19.3b). These hearing aids are similar in construction to a BTE device and are coupled to the ear canal using a thin tube. A spectacle frame hearing aid can also be configured as a CROS or BiCROS system using the frame to carry the small cable from the microphone.

Earmoulds, custom shells and eartips

The physical characteristics of a hearing aid earmould or shell can significantly affect the acoustic performance of a hearing aid and user comfort and, therefore, the potential benefit obtained by the user.

The ear impression

Earmoulds are manufactured from an impression taken of the ear, a process which must only be carried out by someone with appropriate training. The process starts with a visual examination of the outer ear, including the pinna, ear canal and eardrum, to identify any contraindications to an impression being taken, such as wax or otitis externa. After examination, a small

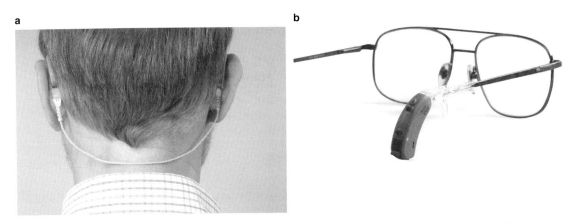

a   b

Figure 19.3   a, A hearing aid worn in a CROS configuration; **b**, a spectacle frame hearing aid using an adaptor. (Figure courtesy of Widex A/S.)

appropriately sized plug called an otostop is positioned in the canal to prevent damage to the eardrum. Impression material, which is available in a number of types, is then injected into the canal using a syringe, filling the canal and concha. This material is then left a short time to 'cure' before careful removal complete with the otostop. The ear canal is then re-examined to ensure no damage has been caused or material left behind. The resulting impression, which forms the basis for the manufacture of an earmould, shell or eartip, is checked to ensure it is a faithful replication of the ear canal and will accommodate the type of aid to be fitted. The type of hearing aid to be fitted will dictate the requirements for the impression, for example a shell for a CIC device will typically require a longer canal length than the impression for an ITE shell or earmould.

Earmould and shell manufacture

The impression of the ear is first trimmed according to the type of shell or earmould to be manufactured and, if necessary, corrected for any irregularities, for example material flow marks or shrinkage, by building up the affected area with wax from a wax bath. This process is known as rectification. A cast of the resulting rectified impression is then made in silicone or a similar material.

If an *earmould* (Figure 19.4) is to be manufactured, the earmould material is then poured into the cast and cured before being removed, finished and polished by a qualified technician. This process includes creating a bore through the earmould, which will later take the tubing which carries the sound from the hearing aid receiver to the ear canal.

If a *shell* is to be manufactured, the shell material is poured into the cast and allowed to partially cure. The cast is then inverted to allow any excess material to drain off and create a hollow cavity. The remaining cured lining within the cast then forms the hearing aid shell, which is removed from the cast, finished and polished prior to assembly as the completed device.

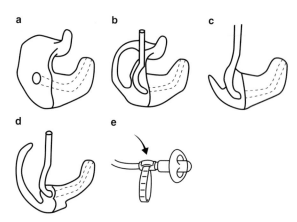

Figure 19.4 Different types of earmould. **a**, Shell mould; **b**, skeleton mould; **c**, canal lock; **d**, open mould; and **e**, standard fit eartip. (Figure courtesy of Widex A/S.)

Venting

The acoustic performance of a hearing aid can be adjusted by modifying one or more of the physical characteristics of the earmould or shell. One frequently used modification is to incorporate an additional bore through the earmould or shell, to provide an acoustic path between the outer profile of the earmould, or the faceplate of the shell, and the ear canal. This acoustic pathway is referred to as a *vent* and allows both the leakage of low frequency sound from the ear canal to the outside and sound to enter the ear canal from the outside (Figure 19.5).

A vent reduces amplification in the low frequencies, particularly at frequencies below

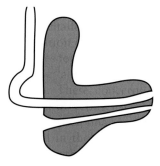

Figure 19.5 Cross-section of an earmould showing the bore, which carries the thin sound tubing, and a vent. (Figure courtesy of Widex A/S.)

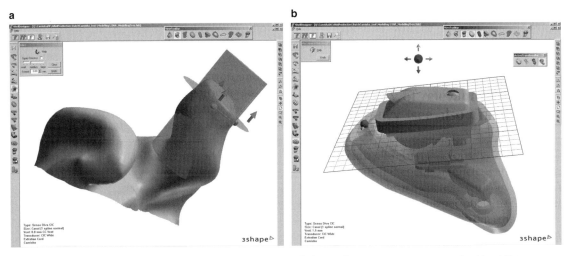

Figure 19.6 Two stages of the modelling process in computer-aided manufacture. (Figure courtesy of Widex A/S.)

500 Hz, and is useful for those with minimal or no hearing loss at these frequencies. The amount of reduction in amplification is dependent on the physical characteristics of the vent, in particular its diameter and length. In general, the greater the diameter of the vent, the greater the reduction in amplification.

A disadvantage of using a vent is that the leaking sound can re-enter the hearing aid microphone and result in acoustic feedback which may be heard as a whistle or howling. Modern hearing aids, however, provide processing strategies that can prevent acoustic feedback from occurring.

A vent can also be extremely beneficial in reducing the occlusion effect experienced by some hearing aid users. The occlusion effect is caused by the enhancement of low frequency bone-conducted sound resulting from the occlusion of the ear canal by the mould or shell, thereby giving the hearing aid wearer greater perception of their own voice and a 'blocked up' sensation.

Computer-aided shell and earmould manufacture

Computer-aided shell and earmould manufacture is a new method of producing individual hearing aid shells, earmoulds and eartips. As with traditional earmould manufacture, the first step is to take an accurate impression of the ear. The ear impression is then scanned by a laser and the resulting high-definition data are manipulated by a sophisticated computer modelling programme into a three-dimensional image (Figure 19.6). Technicians then use the image to model the final earmould, shell or eartip so that it can fit the specific ear canal precisely. The modelling process can also show the location of the components required and include any shell or earmould rectification and, when appropriate, venting.

Once the modelling has been completed, the data are transferred to a manufacturing laser printer unit, where a powerful laser is used to cure a light cure material, building the shell or earmould layer by layer with great precision. In the case of a shell, the resulting structure is a hollow cavity which will later accommodate the components of the hearing aid. For an earmould, the structure is solid, with the exception of the bore which will carry the sound tubing and, if to be used, a bore for a vent.

Hearing aid performance

Hearing aids are designed to provide a range of electroacoustical characteristics, signal processing strategies and other features, in order to match the user's hearing loss and meet their specific needs.

Hearing aid electroacoustical characteristics are specified in accordance with a series of international standards. This series of standards, IEC 60118 'Electroacoustics – Hearing aids', is published by the International Electrotechnical Commission. The standards are also published as harmonised standards by the British Standards Institution as BS EN 60118. Characteristics are derived using strictly defined methods of measurement and, where the output characteristics

of a hearing aid are specified, measured in a reference device known as an ear simulator or acoustic coupler. These devices are used to simulate the acoustic performance of a 'normal' adult ear.

Electroacoustical characteristics may be specified as numerical values or may take the form of a graphical representation drawn as a function of frequency (Figure 19.7). Specifications include the acoustic gain (amplification) of the hearing aid, the difference between the output sound pressure level (SPL) measured in an acoustic coupler and the input SPL at the microphone at

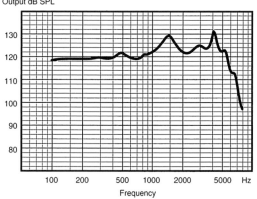

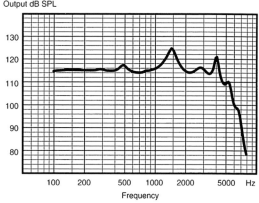

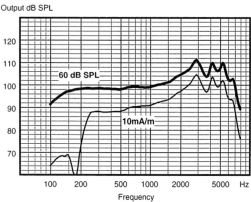

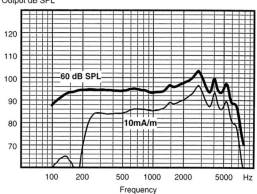

Figure 19.7   A typical hearing aid specification sheet showing the output and frequency response characteristics in graphical form. (Figure courtesy of Widex A/S.)

a particular frequency, the maximum output and nominal frequency response. The input–output characteristics of the aid at certain frequencies may also be specified. Manufacturers may, in addition, show the range of hearing loss for which that particular hearing aid may be suitable.

Digital signal processing strategies

All DSP strategies and algorithms are designed to provide the user with optimum benefit when listening to a range of different sounds in a variety of listening environments. To provide optimum benefit, a digital hearing aid may accommodate more than one listening programme, with each programme designed for a specific listening environment. In some devices, a particular programme may be selected automatically by the hearing aid itself; in others the user may manually select the programme.

The principal function of a hearing aid is to make sounds audible that would otherwise be inaudible to a hearing-impaired individual. Emphasis is normally placed on providing appropriate amplification of speech, but it is important that hearing aid users can also hear other sounds, for example music or sounds from their environment.

Adaptive signal processing

Signal processing strategies can either be fixed, where the processing acts continually, or adaptive, where the processing is automatically modified in response to a change or changes in one or more defined parameters. Examples of this are compression, which may adapt to changes in input, and noise-management algorithms that may adapt to changes in background noise characteristics.

Compression

The signal processing priority is to amplify the spectrum and dynamic range of speech so that after amplification it becomes comfortably audible to the hearing aid user. To achieve this, the amplified dynamic range of speech should ideally be placed above the individual's threshold yet below their discomfort level. Soft sounds need to be amplified more than louder sounds, and greater amplification has to be provided for the frequency bands where the loss may be more severe. In order to achieve this, the amplification characteristics of a hearing aid need to be not only frequency specific, but also dependent on the level of input. There is also a need to limit the output of the hearing aid to prevent discomfort.

This non-linear amplification is referred to as compression and is used to restore normal loudness to the wearer. When applied to the majority or all of the dynamic range of a hearing aid input, it is known as wide dynamic range compression (WDRC), and the digital signal processor is ideally suited to this application. By processing the input signal in different frequency bands and applying sophisticated WDRC strategies, the digital hearing aid can provide very effective 'mapping' of the amplified input signal to the user's residual hearing, helping to make all sounds audible yet comfortable. It is generally agreed that the more sophisticated the compression algorithm and the greater the number of frequency bands used, then the more accurate the mapping.

Compression systems take a short time to respond to changes in input. The time taken to respond to an increase in input level is known as the attack time, and the time to return to its original characteristics, or a reduction in input level, the release time. These times may be fixed or adaptive and can be selected to provide the wearer with optimum sound quality in different listening environments. Compression characteristics are generally described by the compression ratio, the ratio of the change in output level to a change in input level, together with the attack and release times.

Other signal processing strategies

Many hearing aids also incorporate processing strategies and algorithms which are designed to provide the user with enhanced signal quality, in order that they may achieve improved speech discrimination, communicate better in noisy environments and be more comfortable in a diverse range of listening situations.

Directional microphones

In early generations of hearing aids, the microphones used were usually *omni-directional*, which made them equally sensitive to sounds from all directions. This meant that a hearing aid user could have great difficulty in understanding a conversation in a noisy situation, even when facing the speaker and with the competing noise source to their side or even behind them.

Directional microphone systems, which consist of one or more microphones, were later introduced enabling the hearing aid to be more sensitive to sounds arriving from the front compared to those arriving from other directions. This meant that a hearing aid user had a greater chance of understanding a conversation and communicating in noise. Microphone systems at this time were, however, either of a fixed omni-directional type or a fixed directional type. Both provided benefits in some listening situations but had disadvantages in others.

The use of *adaptive digital signal processing strategies* in conjunction with microphone systems now enables the microphone characteristics to be optimised for the user's listening environment. By analysing the incoming signal to the microphone, the directional sensitivity of the hearing aid can be adjusted to provide optimum listening in any environment. If the characteristics of the environment should change, the directional characteristics can be automatically adapted if required.

Noise reduction

The majority of those with a sensorineural hearing loss will, to a greater or lesser extent, experience problems in understanding speech in the presence of background noise. An example of this would be trying to hold a one-to-one conversation when there may be others holding conversations in the same room or when music is being played.

This difficulty in discriminating speech is predominantly caused by the masking of speech by the low-frequency components of the noise, often referred to as the upward spread of masking. Someone with normal hearing is more able to cope in these difficult listening environments as they have greater access to the mid and high frequencies and can process this complex signal more effectively.

The ability of an individual to discriminate speech in noise is greatly dependent upon the ratio of the level of speech to the level of noise, referred to as the *signal-to-noise ratio*. Directional microphone systems can significantly improve the signal-to-noise ratio in difficult situations but other digital signal processing strategies can also help.

A general approach to managing noise within the processing of a hearing aid is to reduce the amplification in the lower frequencies, where the majority of the conflicting noise occurs. This process can prove very effective. With digital signal processing, the effect can be further enhanced to make the process more selective. The spectral and temporal characteristics of speech and noise are very different and, by performing a statistical analysis of the incoming signal within a particular frequency band, the hearing aid can determine whether the information in that band is predominantly speech or noise. If it is predominantly speech, the hearing aid can provide appropriate amplification for the user. If predominantly noise it can reduce the amplification and also the potential for masking. This processing strategy continually monitors the incoming signal and modifies the amplification accordingly; it has the added advantage that not only can it improve speech discrimination but it can also make noisy environments more acceptable.

Feedback management

Acoustic feedback takes the form of a loud high frequency whistle or howling, which may not always be heard by the hearing aid user. Hearing aids have always been susceptible to acoustic feedback, where some of the amplified sound from the hearing aid finds a pathway back into the hearing aid microphone. It is then further amplified and this process continues until instability and whistling or howling occurs. Feedback is more likely to occur from hearing aids worn by those with a more severe loss, or those with a predominantly high frequency loss. Feedback may also result from a poor-fitting mould or shell, or the use of venting. However, blocking a vent to eliminate feedback may affect the hearing aid response or user comfort and should be considered carefully.

Lowering the level of amplification in the frequency range where the feedback occurs can reduce the risk of feedback. This can, however, have an adverse effect on the user as it may deprive them of the level of amplification required for their loss.

An alternative strategy, often employed in digital hearing aids, is known as feedback suppression or feedback cancellation. This is an active process where the signal causing the feedback sound is monitored, reproduced in the opposite phase (inverted) and then added to the original feedback signal thereby cancelling it out. Feedback cancellation has the advantage that it does not reduce the amplification available to the user, so the whistle is prevented and the user still has the amplification necessary to accommodate their loss.

Frequency transposition

With a very profound hearing loss, where there is very little residual hearing, the provision of acoustic amplification can be relatively ineffective. In order to make sounds audible, high levels of non-linear amplification are required and the significantly reduced dynamic range of the residual hearing results in extremely poor discrimination.

These types of losses are often best managed using alternative methods of aiding. However, if the profound loss is limited to the higher frequencies, and there is better residual hearing in the lower frequencies, a signal processing strategy known as frequency transposition may be used.

In principle this strategy, which has only been implemented in a very small number of hearing aid models, moves higher frequencies, where there is little or no residual hearing, down into a frequency range where the residual hearing can benefit from amplification. This is particularly

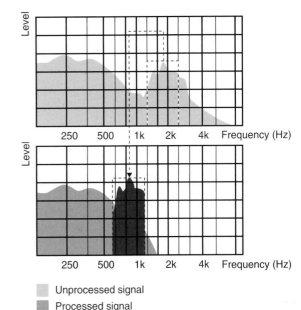

Unprocessed signal

Processed signal

Transposed high frequency signal

Figure 19.8 The principle of frequency transposition. The figure illustrates how a band of high frequencies is transposed to the lower frequency region. (Figure courtesy of Widex A/S.)

useful when there are 'dead regions' in the high frequency part of the cochlea, and the ability to detect pitch in these regions is lost.

The resulting sound at first appears strange to the listener, as for example the sound of a bird or a voice is heard at a lower pitch, but it gives the user access to sounds they would not otherwise hear.

A number of methods of frequency transposition have been used, including linear, where, as the name suggests, a band of high frequencies is shifted down in the spectrum in a linear manner, and non-linear (Figure 19.8), where the frequency spectrum is compressed downwards. These methods are sometimes referred to as non-proportional and proportional frequency transposition respectively.

Hearing aid connectivity

With current technology it is possible to channel other sources of sound input into the hearing aid, either using a direct electrical connection via a suitable plug and cable or using various forms of wireless connection.

Direct audio input

Many hearing aids have traditionally provided a direct audio input (DAI) facility through which an assistive device can be connected. This facility has mainly been used for FM radio receivers in an educational environment. These radio systems are now used more extensively in a number of applications. Some infra-red audio receivers can also be connected in this manner, for example for use in theatres. A DAI input can also accept devices such as personal music players.

Inductive telecoil ('T' setting)

Contained within the housing of many hearing aids is a small inductive coil which is often referred to as the telecoil. This coil is designed to provide a wireless inductive coupling with a telephone handset so the hearing aid user can receive a better quality signal direct from the telephone, without having to worry where the hearing aid microphone is positioned in relation to the handset. In some hearing aids the microphone can be disabled when using the telecoil, to reduce masking from environmental noise.

The telecoil can also be used in conjunction with an inductive loop system in locations such as school classrooms, banks, theatres and churches. A notice is usually displayed indicating that a loop system is available (Figure 19.9).

Remote control

The majority of hearing aids, with the exception of completely-in-the-ear hearing aids, are provided with user-accessible controls so that the programmes can be changed or the volume adjusted. Some hearing aids can alternatively or additionally be adjusted using a small hand-held remote control (Figure 19.10). This not only makes adjustment much easier, but the remote

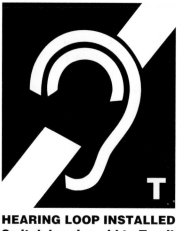

HEARING LOOP INSTALLED
Switch hearing aid to T-coil

Figure 19.9   Notice showing availability of inductive loop system.

control can often be used when in a pocket or handbag, so the user can make changes without bringing attention to their hearing aids.

Bilateral communication

The benefits of bilateral listening are well known; however, when a person wears a pair of hearing

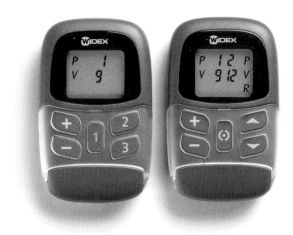

Figure 19.10   Hearing aid remote controls. (Figure courtesy of Widex A/S.)

aids, and the two aids function independently of each other, these benefits may be reduced. To address this problem, some hearing aids are now capable of communicating with each other when used in a bilateral fitting. This sharing of data enables the devices to complement each other through their adaptive processing, to provide optimum binaural benefit.

Audio streaming

In order to provide greater connectivity with hearing aids, audio streamers are available. These consist of a small body-worn device which is able to accept a range of inputs, both hard-wired, for example the output of a personal music player, and wireless, for example a Bluetooth connection with a mobile phone. The audio streamer then connects *wirelessly* with the hearing aid, providing the user with direct access to an input of their choice. This greatly improves signal quality in many listening situations.

Hearing aid selection, fitting, and performance verification and validation

The potential benefit that may be gained from the use of hearing aids is dependent upon the type of loss, i.e. whether the loss is conductive, sensorineural or mixed, its severity, and the overall shape of the audiogram.

Those with a conductive loss do not, in general, have a significant reduction in dynamic range or loudness perception and can benefit greatly from the use of hearing aids. Auditory processing functions are often unimpaired, and appropriate amplification alone will normally compensate for much of the loss without the need for other more sophisticated signal processing strategies.

Those with a sensorineural loss, however, usually have a significant reduction in dynamic range and loudness perception, which results in poor speech discrimination, particularly in difficult listening situations such as background noise. Hearing aids can, in general, make sounds audible to someone with a sensorineural loss, but do not necessarily provide good speech discrimination. This type of loss generally requires additional signal processing to improve the signal quality, in order to provide the user with some improvement in speech understanding.

Even with the same type and severity of hearing loss, there may be significant variation in the benefit that two different hearing aid users may obtain. The audiometric data will therefore only determine some of the considerations made when selecting appropriate hearing aids. The audiologist will also need to consider what other functions and signal processing may be beneficial.

Selection and fitting

Based on the characteristics of an individual's hearing loss and particular needs, the audiologist will select an appropriate hearing aid or aids. The selection process will look at the user's lifestyle, their ability to manage the hearing aid and their potential needs for connectivity to other assistive devices.

From the information available the audiologist will help the user select the type of aid to be fitted, together with appropriate functions and features. They will also take impressions so that earmoulds or shells can be manufactured.

The fitting of a hearing aid involves setting the available parameters, including the amplification characteristics, to meet the specific needs of the individual user. In a digital hearing aid these parameters are set using special fitting software provided by the manufacture. This will use fitting strategies designed to provide the user with the most appropriate amplification characteristics for their specific hearing loss. These strategies programme the hearing aid to optimise audibility, sound quality, speech discrimination and listening comfort.

Manufacturers may use their own amplification strategies that have been developed in conjunction with their hearing aids and that have demonstrated quantifiable user benefit in clinical trials. Other manufacturers may use strategies that are based on established fitting rules developed over many years and that have been subsequently optimised for the current generation of signal processing strategies.

The two most commonly used amplification strategies have both been revised to accommodate multichannel non-linear hearing aids. The NAL fitting method, developed by the National Acoustic Laboratory in Australia, is based on the principle of amplifying conversational speech so that it is heard by the hearing aid user at their most comfortable listening level. This rationale attempts to optimise potential speech intelligibility by amplifying all speech components so that they are heard by the user at the same perceived loudness. This amplification strategy is often referred to as loudness equalisation.

The DSL or desired sensation level fitting method has been developed by the University of Ontario in Canada and is based on the principle of making all speech components, at conversational speech level, audible by the hearing aid user at a comfortable level.

Hearing aid performance verification

Once fitted, the performance of a hearing aid should be verified to confirm that it is performing according to the programmed parameter settings. The amplification rationales employed in hearing aid programming use targets that are normally derived from the residual hearing characteristics of the hearing aid user. Hearing aid manufacturers' fitting software will often display these targets graphically together with the predicted performance of the hearing aid at the programmed settings. The audiologist is then able to see from the graphics if these targets have been met, thereby verifying the programming.

Fitting software may include a facility to show how, by using the proposed programming settings, speech may be mapped to the user's residual hearing. This facility is often referred to as *speech mapping* (Figure 19.11). Some software is also capable of showing this mapping process with the hearing aid active and worn by the user, while live speech or other source is presented to the hearing aid microphone.

The performance of a hearing aid in actual use may differ from the performance predicted by the fitting software because of the acoustic properties of the ear to which it is fitted. These differences can be a consequence of a number of variables including ear canal dimensions, the effect of any venting used, leakage around the earmould or shell and other parameters unique to that particular fitting.

Real-ear measurement

In order to take into account these acoustic variables, performance measurements may be made

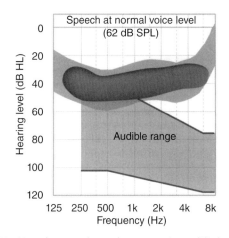 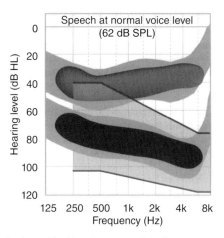

Figure 19.11   How the normal speech spectrum is amplified to lie in the residual hearing range of the hearing-impaired hearing aid user. The graph on the left shows the unaided speech spectrum lying outside the audible range. The graph on the right shows the aided speech spectrum lying within the audible range. (Figure courtesy of Widex A/S.)

with the hearing aid *in situ*, using a method known as *real-ear measurement*. These measurements are made by recording the actual output of the hearing aid as measured close to the eardrum. This uses a small acoustic probe tube connected to a measuring microphone. The output of the hearing aid is measured using specific inputs under strictly defined conditions. The real-ear measurement instrumentation will normally include facilities to compare a measured response with the target response derived from the fitting strategy chosen. This method of measurement may also be used to make minor adjustments to the hearing aid.

Some real-ear measurement systems also provide a method of presenting live or recorded speech to the hearing aid, while it is being worn, and displaying graphically how the amplified speech is being mapped to the user's residual hearing. This graphical representation includes the true effects of the real-ear acoustics.

Hearing aid performance validation

Benefit gained from a hearing aid can only really be validated through subjective measures that require a response from the hearing aid user. The simplest validation test is to perform sound-field audiometry. Audiometry is performed in a sound field without the hearing aid worn, and then repeated with the hearing aid fitted. Normally there should be an improvement in the threshold values obtained. This improvement, known as functional gain, is, however, limited in its use as it only demonstrates the audibility of low-intensity sounds and not how the wearer may benefit at conversational speech levels.

In order to validate hearing aid performance with speech, aided speech audiometry may be performed. This will not only give an indication of how the wearer's ability to hear speech may have improved, but also provide a measure of improvement in speech discrimination. There is a range of speech material and test protocols available which are designed to assess different aspects of detection and recognition (see Chapter 6).

The validation process may also include questionnaires. One commonly used example of this is the Glasgow Hearing Aid Benefit Profile (GHABP) protocol (Gatehouse, 1999). Developed by the Medical Research Council's Institute of Hearing Research, this protocol has established itself as a leading tool for hearing aid user management. It takes the form of a patient-centred structured interview that establishes the wearer's initial disability and handicap prior to fitting and their residual disability and satisfaction at a follow-up appointment, normally 8–12 weeks following the fitting.

Future developments

The application of digital signal processing to hearing aid technology provides the potential for ever-increasing flexibility, versatility and sophistication in the processing employed in hearing aids.

Manufacturers, working closely with audiologists and other hearing healthcare professionals, continue to develop new solutions to meet the requirements of hearing aid wearers and to address the problems they experience. Each new generation of hearing aid provides an improvement in sound quality, better discrimination or greater user comfort. With digital signal processing, only the ability to continue to develop effective processing strategies limits the potential of the hearing aid.

Reference

Gatehouse S (1999) The Glasgow Hearing Aid Benefit Profile: derivation and validation of a client centred outcome measure for hearing aid services. *Journal of the American Academy of Audiology* 10:80–103.

Standards

BS EN 60118-0 Hearing Aids – Part 0: Methods for measurement of electroacoustical characteristics.

BS EN 60118-7 Electroacoustics – Hearing Aids – Part 7: Measurement of the performance characteristics of hearing aids for quality inspection and delivery purposes.

BS EN 60118-4 Electroacoustics – Hearing Aids – Part 4: Induction loop systems for hearing aid purposes – Magnetic field strength

ISO 12124 Acoustics – Procedures for the measurement of real-ear acoustical characteristics of hearing aids.

Cochlear implants

Huw Cooper

20

Introduction

In recent years, cochlear implants have continued to develop, mature and become accepted as a safe, effective and hugely beneficial treatment for severe or profound deafness. Looking back, it is apparent that the fundamentals of how cochlear implants function have not changed significantly, but there have been ongoing developments that have emerged on the cochlear implant scene, some of which are discussed in detail here. These include:

- typical speech discrimination performance obtained using cochlear implants has steadily improved, such that good open-set speech recognition (without lip-reading) is now commonplace immediately following first activation of the implant following surgery
- selection criteria (expressed in terms of the level of speech recognition that can be achieved with optimally fitted hearing aids) have steadily relaxed, so that adults or children with moderate amounts of usable residual hearing can now be considered for implantation, sometimes in conjunction with

continued use of a hearing aid in the opposite ear to achieve bimodal hearing
- bilateral implantation has become increasingly accepted, and evidence of the benefits of bilateral implant use has steadily accumulated
- subgroups of deaf people who previously would not have been considered for implantation (and who would have been unlikely to request it) now often receive implants with measurable benefit – for example, adults deaf from birth or from a very young age
- although perception of music frequently remains poor for many implant users, there has been a growing interest in musical appreciation by implant listeners and this a fast-developing area for research.

General principles and speech processing

All modern implant systems share common features, although minor design features vary between manufacturers (Figure 20.1). Sounds are picked up by microphones situated either behind the ear (on the top of a behind-the-ear speech

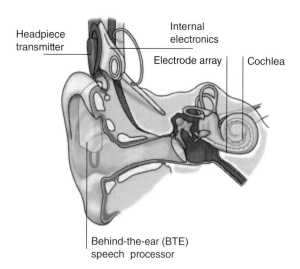

Headpiece transmitter

Internal electronics

Electrode array   Cochlea

Behind-the-ear (BTE) speech processor

Figure 20.1   Schematic representation of a typical cochlear implant shown *in situ* in cross-section of the ear.

processor) or in the ear canal (at the tip of an ear hook over the pinna, as in the case of the 'T-mic' used in the Advanced Bionics 'Harmony' speech processor). The speech processor applies analogue-to-digital conversion and a speech-processing strategy which determines how the input signal is represented in the pattern of stimulation applied to the array of electrodes in the cochlea. Crucially, the speech processor also applies compression and output limiting so that all electrical stimulation applied to each electrode is within the comfortable listening range for the implant user and does not exceed a maximum comfortable level. The output of the speech processor is transmitted via a radio-frequency carrier transcutaneously to the implanted receiver-stimulator package under the skin on the side of the head. The received signal is decoded and converted to pulsatile electrical stimulation applied to an array of electrodes inserted into the cochlea. This stimulation then reaches the auditory nerve fibres within the modiolus of the cochlea and results in auditory sensations.

Design of the intracochlear electrode array varies somewhat between manufacturers; for

example, the Cochlear Corporation Nucleus CI24 system employs 22 electrodes in a 'modiolus hugging' array that attempts to place the electrodes close to the spiral ganglion that it is intended to stimulate.

A variety of approaches to speech-processing strategies have been applied, and performance with cochlear implant listening has improved steadily over the years since their invention. In all cases, the input signal is divided by band-pass filtering into channels that are allocated to individual electrodes. All represent the spectral content of sounds by place of stimulation in the cochlea; in other words, sounds of different pitches are delivered at approximately their appropriate positions, following the tonotopic organisation found in the normal cochlea. The number of channels used varies with device; the largest number of actual electrodes in clinical use is 22, in the Nucleus CI24 system. Recently, there have been attempts to create up to 120 'virtual channels' using current steering in the Advanced Bionics device (more details below). In most cases, the stimulus delivered to the electrodes is pulsatile, and charge-balanced biphasic pulses are used (this ensures that there is no net transfer of charge to the surrounding tissue). The perception of loudness can be varied through changes in pulse amplitude or pulse width, or a combination of both. In one commonly used strategy, 'ACE' (advanced combination encoders) or 'n of m', n channels are selected from a total possible m channels for stimulation in each 'sweep' across the electrode array (Wilson, 2006). Those channels with the highest energy are picked out and stimulus pulses only delivered to a subset of the m channels available. In the Nucleus CI24 device, m is equal to 22 as there are 22 electrodes available for stimulation. The value of n in clinical use is variable between 6 and 16. Thus, spectral peaks in the stimulus waveform are represented in the pattern of stimulation across the electrode array, and this pattern is updated very rapidly with each sweep of stimulation from one end of the array to the other.

Another frequently used strategy is CIS (continuous interleaved sampling). This strategy uses relatively high rates of stimulation to represent rapid temporal variations within channels, and not all electrodes in the implanted array are stimulated, typically around eight or more. No particular features of speech are extracted or deliberately represented in the CIS strategy. Instead, envelope variations in each of multiple bands are presented to the electrodes through modulated trains of interleaved pulses (see Wilson, 2006 for a more detailed explanation of CIS and other strategies). Stimulation of individual electrodes is temporally interleaved to avoid the problem of channel interaction. An implementation of CIS in the Advanced Bionics implant system is 'HiRes' (abbreviation of hi-resolution). This uses stimulation of all implanted electrodes (up to 16) at very high pulse rates (up to over 2000 pulses/s (pps)) and is the default strategy for that implant system.

Speech recognition in quiet and noise with cochlear implants

It is now well established that present-day cochlear implants can provide remarkably good speech recognition ability to many recipients in quiet environments. For example, Wilson and Dorman (2007) recently reported results on a set of nine tests of speech recognition from a Clarion CII implant user, compared with the results on the same tests carried out by a group of normally hearing listeners; they found that scores for this particular implant user were no different from the scores for the normally hearing subjects for seven of the nine subtests. Differences were only apparent on two tests that involved sentences in a background of multi-talker babble, when the performance of the implant listener was impaired somewhat compared to the control group. However, in practice a wide variability in performance for implant listeners on tests of speech discrimination is common. Figure 20.2 shows the results on a standard measure of 'open-set' (sound alone, without lip-reading) speech discrimination in quiet at 9 months post-implant surgery for a series of 125 adult users of the Nucleus CI24 implanted at the University Hospital Birmingham NHS Trust (Birmingham, UK). The median score in this series is 69% correct,

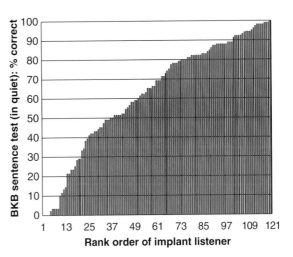

Figure 20.2 Open-set (sound alone) speech recognition scores for a series of 125 adult cochlear implant users with the Nucleus CI24 device, 9 months after surgery. Speech materials were BKB (Bamford–Kowal–Bench) sentences, presented in the sound field at 70 dB(A). Implant users were able to adjust the sensitivity or volume settings on their speech processors as desired. The *y* axis shows the percentage correct word score for a list of 30 sentences. Implant users are placed in rank order of their performance along the *x* axis.

but as can be seen the performance ranges from zero to 100% correct.

It is also well established that speech recognition performance with cochlear implants is often badly impaired by interfering noise. For example, Nelson and Jin (2002) showed that competing speech can impair performance in implant listeners, even at a signal-to-noise ratio of +16 dB (more favourable than many real-life listening situations). Nascimento and Bevilacqua (2005) reported speech recognition performance in a series of 40 users of five different types of cochlear implant; their median sentence recognition scores fell from 90% in quiet to 50% correct in the +10 dB signal-to-noise condition (i.e. a speech level 10 dB higher than the noise), and only 20% correct in the +5 dB condition. They found no statistically valid difference in the performance with the different types of implant tested, suggesting that this problem is largely independent of the implant designs that are currently commercially available.

Many modern cochlear implant systems endeavour to improve the potential for speech understanding in noisy listening conditions by the use of directional microphones, multi-microphone strategies or pre-processing of input sounds in the speech processor. For example, the Nucleus Freedom system gives the option of various strategies aimed at enhanced performance in noisy conditions. One option available is the directional 'Beam' strategy, which can provide some benefit in noisy conditions when listening to a single talker in front of the implant user. Spriet *et al.* (2007) reported improvements of up to 16 dB in the speech reception threshold (i.e. the signal-to-noise ratio at which a speech recognition score for words in sentences of 50% correct is obtained) for five Nucleus implant users when employing the 'Beam' strategy compared with the standard microphone.

Similarly, continuing research on development of speech-processing strategies is aimed at improving speech recognition performance in general, and particularly in noise. David *et al.* (2003) reviewed the performance of 139 cochlear implant users and concluded that improvements in performance could be attributed to evolving speech coding strategies and speech processors rather than to changes in patient selection criteria.

One factor that is probably a major contributor to the impaired performance of cochlear implants in noise is the limited quality of the spectral information that implants are able to convey. Spectral resolution in implant listeners may be limited by:

- the number of functioning implanted electrodes (this varies between 12 in the MedEl system and 22 in the Nucleus Freedom system)
- quality and quantity of available neural tissue in the vicinity of the electrode array
- current spread and spread of excitation between stimulating electrodes.

Also, as noted earlier, the speech-processing strategies used by modern cochlear implants use input filters for individual channels that are typically too broad for individual harmonics to be

resolved or 'heard out', and the spread of current across the cochlea would further increase the 'mixing' of harmonics (Moore and Carlyon, 2005).

Fu and Nogaki (2004) proposed that the difficulties that implant listeners experience in noise may be attributed to their reduced spectral resolution and the resulting spectral 'smearing' associated with channel interaction. They found that the performance of cochlear implant listeners in discriminating speech, in either steady-state or gated noise, was comparable to that of normally hearing listeners listening to an acoustic noiseband vocoder implant simulation, when spectral cues were 'smeared' by applying shallow filter slopes (thus reducing the frequency resolution of the vocoder channels).

Shannon *et al.* (2004) pointed out that the number of channels required for speech recognition depends on the difficulty of the situation; several studies have shown that for normally hearing listeners, only around four to six spectral channels are necessary for 100% correct recognition of simple sentences in quiet. The number of channels needed for speech recognition increases for more difficult speech materials, or for listening in noise; Shannon *et al.* (2004) suggested that up to 30 channels or more may be required for complex materials. Shannon (2005) also pointed out that speech and music have different requirements for spectral resolution; music requires at least 16 spectral channels even for identification of simple melodies. Dorman *et al.* (1998) reported the performance of a group of 21 normally hearing listeners on a speech recognition task in which they were presented with sentences processed through a simulation of a cochlear implant speech processor. In quiet conditions, they achieved 100% correct recognition with only six channels. When listening to sentences in noise at a signal-to-noise ratio of −2 dB (not uncommon in everyday situations), their performance fell well below 100% correct recognition even with 20 channels available.

The actual number of independent channels available to cochlear implant listeners may be quite limited; Friesen *et al.* (2001) reported, based on their study of 19 implant users with either the Nucleus 22 or Clarion devices, that even those implant listeners with the best speech recognition performance appeared to be unable to make use of more than seven to ten channels of spectral information, regardless of how many spectral channels were presented to them. They hypothesised that this may result partly from channel interactions. Baskent (2006) reported that speech recognition in the best cochlear implant listeners saturated around eight channels, and is not improved by the activation of more electrodes – presumably due to the reduced frequency selectivity resulting from channel interactions. Similarly, Wilson and Dorman (2007) suggest that the spread of stimulation in the cochlea produced in a multi-electrode implant array probably limits the number of perceptually separate channels to four to eight, even if more than eight electrodes are stimulated. It is therefore not surprising that cochlear implant listeners' ability to discriminate speech is so impaired in noisy conditions.

Despite this, efforts continue to increase the number of available spectral channels in implant devices; for example, Koch *et al.* (2007) reported results from 57 implanted ears for a new approach to current 'steering' recently developed by the Advanced Bionics corporation. Through simultaneous delivery of current to pairs of adjacent electrodes, it is hypothesised that the effective locus of stimulation can be 'steered' to sites between the real electrodes by varying the proportion of current delivered to each electrode of the pair. This can then provide an increased number of pitch percepts along the electrode array, theoretically much higher than that available from stimulation of the actual electrodes in the normal way. These are referred to as 'virtual channels'. Koch *et al.* found that the number of intermediate pitch percepts ranged from zero to 52, with an average number of between-electrode pitch percepts of 8.7. Overall, this meant a range in the total number of pitches from 8 to 466. Koch *et al.* (2007) suggest that 'the average cochlear implant user may have significantly more place-pitch capability than is exploited presently by cochlear implant systems'. However, evidence that an increased number of spectral 'channels' can effectively transmit more spectral information, and that implant listeners

can make use of that information to obtain improved performance for speech (or music) recognition, is not yet available. In particular, it should be noted that increasing the number of discriminable pitches does not necessarily improve the spectral information available for more complex stimuli at all.

In summary:

- speech recognition performance with cochlear implants has improved significantly with advances in speech-coding strategies
- despite this, speech recognition in implant listeners is generally badly impaired by background noise
- evidence suggests that the number of perceptually distinct spectral channels available to implant listeners is probably limited to around eight, which is not sufficient for reliable speech recognition in noise (depending on the signal-to-noise ratio)
- spread of excitation in the cochlea leads to channel interactions and spectral 'smearing', which severely impair the ability to discriminate speech in noise
- cochlear implant listeners are unable to make use of differences in fundamental frequency as a means of segregating concurrent speech.

Pitch and music perception with cochlear implants

Pitch

Multi-electrode cochlear implants rely mainly on stimulation of discrete groups of auditory neurons and the tonotopic arrangement of the cochlea to convey a sense of pitch. However, the quality of pitch percepts that can be obtained by most implant users is variable and limited. The perception of pitch by cochlear implant users was explored extensively by Moore and Carlyon (2005). As they point out, perception of pitch in normal (acoustic) hearing involves both timing (phase locking) and place cues. In cochlear implant listening, use of temporal coding is limited to low frequencies; most implant users are unable to detect changes in pulse rate above about 300 pps. Also, most commonly used speech-processing strategies use the same pulse rate on all electrodes; pitch information based on phase locking and temporal cues is not normally transmitted, and so implant listeners are dependent solely on place cues derived from peaks in the excitation pattern across the electrode array. Thus, the quality of percepts conveyed by place of electrical stimulation via a cochlear implant may only be loosely defined as pitch; although they can be described on a scale from 'low to high' or 'dull to sharp', it is not clear that they meet a strict definition of musical pitch (Moore and Carlyon, 2005).

Another limitation imposed by the most commonly used speech-processing strategies is the fact that the frequency allocations to each channel are generally too wide to enable implant listeners to resolve individual harmonics; if two harmonics have frequencies that fall within the filter bandwidth allocated to a particular channel, they will be summed and produce identical stimulation on the electrode assigned to that channel. Also, spread of excitation in the cochlea around the stimulated electrode will lead to mixing of harmonics. One consequence of this is the poor transmission of F0 (fundamental frequency or voice pitch) by cochlear implants. Some early speech-processing strategies (so called feature-extraction strategies) attempted to convey F0 via pulse rate; this approach has largely been abandoned in current approaches to speech processing, in which pulse rate is normally constant across electrodes. Research efforts to improve the transmission of F0 for implant listeners are ongoing (e.g. Stickney *et al.*, 2007). The inability of implant listeners to exploit F0 differences between competing voices is a major difficulty in multi-talker 'cocktail party' situations. Unlike normally hearing listeners, there is some evidence that they cannot benefit from a gender difference when attempting to segregate speech sounds (e.g. Stickney *et al.*, 2004).

In summary, perception of pitch by implant listeners is at best limited, and this severely restricts their ability to utilise important cues for sound segregation that are available in normal hearing. A great deal of research effort is concentrated on improving speech-processing strategies so that F0 is conveyed better, but cochlear implants are not able to reproduce faithfully the pattern of auditory nerve activation that is elicited by sound in a normal ear; this represents a substantial limitation in the cochlear implant listener's ability to interpret complex sounds, and in particular to segregate competing sounds.

Music

Cochlear implant listeners are traditionally thought to obtain poor perception of music; indeed, the main thrust of implant development has focused on improved speech recognition, with appreciation of music as an almost accidental side-effect when it occurs, although recently more research effort has gone into improving the experience of music for implant users. Reports of poor music perception in implant listeners are several, and were reviewed by McDermott (2004). He summarised the findings of previous research in these terms:

- on average, cochlear implant users perceive rhythm about as well as listeners with normal hearing
- even with sophisticated multiple-channel sound processors, recognition of melodies is poor, especially without rhythmic cues, with performance at little better than chance levels for many implant users
- perception of timbre, as used to identify musical instruments, is unsatisfactory
- implant users tend to rate the quality of musical sounds as less pleasant than do normally hearing listeners
- auditory training programmes aimed at listening to music may help to improve enjoyment of music
- perception of pitch may be improved by enhancements to speech-processing strategies
- combined electrical and acoustic hearing may help to improve music perception.

This disappointing aspect of cochlear implant performance is attributed to the inability of current implant speech processors and electrode arrays to provide listeners with sufficient spectral detail for music appreciation, combined with inadequate transmission of pitch, as already discussed. However, many implant users enjoy listening to music to varying degrees, although often their musical experience is restricted to genres that emphasise rhythm over complex harmonic structure. Also, as more research attention is directed to improving hearing for music in implant users, the importance of musical enjoyment is likely to receive greater emphasis. For example, Laneau *et al.* (2006) described a new sound-processing scheme designed to optimise pitch perception and so perhaps perception of music. In their 'F0mod' scheme, slowly varying channel envelopes are modulated sinusoidally at the F0 of the input signal, with 100% modulation depth and in phase across channels in order to maximise temporal-envelope pitch cues. The intention was to provide better F0 information to the implant listeners that should aid hearing for musical pitch. They reported that melody recognition of familiar songs, with all rhythmic cues removed, was improved by using the F0mod scheme when compared to the 'ACE' strategy, which provides no F0 information. Although this was a small study (six implant listeners), the results suggest that gains in perception of music are possible with more sophisticated sound-processing strategies, especially when they are designed to convey F0 information more explicitly.

Other potential benefits that cochlear implants can provide

Aside from the provision of access to speech recognition that has been discussed, cochlear implants can convey a range of other important (though sometimes harder to measure) benefits, including:

- *environmental sound awareness*: even in the absence of useful speech recognition, awareness and recognition of everyday sounds has enormous value to cochlear implant users
- *benefit to lip-reading/communication*: much spoken communication involves interpretation of visual cues, and many implant users can attain near-perfect recognition of speech when combining auditory and visual information (lip-reading)
- *speech and language development*: it is now well established that deaf children implanted at an appropriately early age (and with suitable auditory input) can develop remarkably successful, age-appropriate spoken language (Uziel *et al.*, 2007)
- *reduction of tinnitus*: the experience of the majority of implant users with tinnitus is that they are less aware of it following their surgery and when their implants are activated, and tinnitus is generally significantly reduced in its negative impact on their lives (Baguley and Atlas, 2007)
- *educational achievements*: there is now convincing evidence that deaf children with cochlear implants can cope with mainstream education, and that their educational achievements are significantly improved compared with children without implants but similar hearing loss (Beadle *et al.*, 2005)
- *improved employment prospects*: there is growing evidence that cochlear implantation can provide improved employment prospects, reduce unemployment, and increase job satisfaction (Fazel and Gray, 2007)
- *changes in quality of life*: long-term benefits to quality of life in deaf people with cochlear implants have been documented (Damen *et al.*, 2007)
- *psychological wellbeing*: the combination of several of the benefits listed above can significantly enhance the psychological wellbeing of deaf people (see Knutson, 2006 for a review).

Suitability and patient selection

The process of establishing which patients, adults or children, should receive cochlear implants has gained from the experience of cochlear implant teams over the years. It is generally accepted that the decision making is not purely a medical or surgical issue, and that a multidisciplinary team (MDT) including surgeons, audiologists, speech and hearing therapists, psychologists, nurses, teachers of the deaf, and radiologists is necessary. Cochlear implants are expensive technology that requires a fairly extensive surgical procedure, so careful decision making about who should receive them is vital. An example of a typical patient pathway for adults undergoing cochlear implant assessment and surgery is shown in Figure 20.3. The key components of the assessment process will include:

■ a meeting with the MDT including a detailed history and preliminary assessment

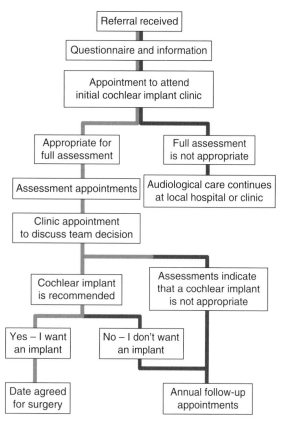

Figure 20.3 Example of a patient pathway for adults undergoing cochlear implant assessment and surgery.

■ detailed audiological and speech-discrimination testing
■ objective confirmation of hearing levels via electric response audiometry
■ optimisation of hearing aid fittings and, if necessary, repeat testing in the best-aided condition
■ detailed computed tomography (CT) and magnetic resonance imaging (MRI) scans to show the anatomy of the ears so that suitability for cochlear implant surgery may be determined
■ careful assessments of communication skills and expectations (including expectations of other family members)
■ evaluation of medical fitness for surgery
■ a meeting with an existing cochlear implant user (preferably of similar age and history)
■ team discussion followed by final meeting with the MDT to decide on agreed treatment (i.e. either a cochlear implant or an alternative treatment). If cochlear implantation is the agreed way forward, there will be further discussion on which ear should be implanted to obtain the best outcomes, and whether bilateral implants are indicated.

The key criteria that are generally used when considering adults for a cochlear implant include:

■ *age*: patients over 16 years – there is no technical reason for an upper age limit and many elderly people (i.e. aged over 70 years) can obtain great benefit from a cochlear implant, provided they are fit enough do undergo the anaesthetic and surgery. Young children under the age of 16 years should be seen by a paediatric team with the requisite skills for assessment in that age group (see 'Assessment of children')
■ *hearing loss*: patients with bilateral severe to profound sensorineural (i.e. permanent) hearing loss confirmed via behavioural and objective evaluation; patients with acquired, progressive or congenital severe to profound deafness; any aetiology of deafness, including cochlear malformation with no other radiological contraindications

- *hearing ability*: patients who get limited benefit from conventional amplification, including digital hearing aids. Current audiological criteria include patients who score up to 50% correct on open-set sentence materials presented at 70 dB(A) in quiet, in the best-aided condition
- *medical fitness*: patients should be medically fit to undergo general anaesthesia and to attend frequent appointments before and after implantation
- *communication*: patients with acquired or progressive hearing loss, whose primary communication is oral/aural; patients with congenital profound losses who show evidence of oral communication and auditory development via hearing aids, even if sign language is also used
- *motivation*: patients, or parents of children, must show the motivation to attend regular appointments over time with the MDT, patients or parents must demonstrate realistic expectations of outcome
- *psychological factors*: no psychological or psychiatric contraindications to implantation. NB: the patient may have a co-existing psychiatric illness requiring treatment, but this is not necessarily a contraindication to implantation.

The primary consideration in adults, aside from the anatomical and medical fitness to undergo surgery, is whether an individual is likely to gain worthwhile benefit from the device, over and above what they can obtain from suitably fitted hearing aids. Many patients undergoing assessment now have varying degrees of usable residual hearing, and a key assessment is of their speech recognition ability in the best-aided condition. A judgement can then be made about whether there are acceptable odds that they will achieve a better performance with an implant, based on analysis of previously obtained outcomes with a large series of implant users. The definition of acceptable odds that an implant will improve on a preoperative speech recognition score was explored by the UK Cochlear Implant Study Group (2004), and the conclusion was that cochlear implantation is an effective and cost-effective intervention, provided that implantation occurred in ears with *a priori* odds at least as favourable as 4:1 (4 chances out of 5) of improving speech recognition post-implant as compared to pre-implant. Dowell *et al.* (2004) used a 75% likelihood that postoperative performance will be better than preoperative performance as the basis to define new selection criteria. This is equivalent to accepting odds of 3:1 (3 chances out of 4). This actuarial approach to defining selection criteria has been widely applied and has led to a commonly applied criterion of a preoperative speech recognition score (in the best-aided condition) of 50% correct. This is obtained by calculating the score at the first quartile in the distribution of scores obtained by a large number of implant users ranked in order of their speech performance (see Figure 20.2). However, it may be that selection criteria will need to be further refined as performance typically obtained from cochlear implants continues to improve; in particular, measures of speech recognition in noise may provide more useful information about functional benefit both before and after implantation.

Assessment of children

In children, the assessment of when to proceed with cochlear implantation may be more complex and difficult; the well-documented importance of implantation early in a child's development must be weighed against the critical importance of making the right choice for each individual child (for a fuller review, see Osberger *et al.*, 2006). It is therefore essential that assessment of children is performed by a team with specific skills and knowledge of paediatric audiology, speech and language development, and child psychology. A large majority of children considered for cochlear implantation are born deaf, and early detection of their permanent hearing loss, rapid fitting of suitable hearing aids, and referral for assessment by a paediatric cochlear implant team are vital to their long-term success. Universal neonatal hearing screening should reduce the age of diagnosis of permanent hearing loss, and if referrals for cochlear implant assessment are made without delay, a positive outcome should be earlier implantation. The consequence should be improved results from the implant, as there is valid evidence that early implantation, particularly before the age of 2 years, is associated with better long-term outcomes (Osberger *et al.*, 2006). However, cochlear implant surgery in very small children is not without its technical challenges, and a number of anatomical obstacles may face the surgeon in such cases, for example malformed or ossified cochleas.

Bilateral implants

Historically, the overwhelming majority of adults and children who have undergone cochlear implantation have unilateral implants; these clearly can provide huge benefits, but users of single implants remain unilaterally deaf and therefore retain a level of disability. The policy of implanting one ear has been driven mainly by the factor of cost, combined with a cautious approach concerned with preservation of one ear. However, compelling evidence of the benefits of bilateral cochlear implantation has been gathering steadily in recent years and the numbers of patients receiving two implants either simultaneously of sequentially have grown substantially. The *potential* benefits of simultaneous activation of two cochlear implants were summarised by Tyler *et al.* (2006). The first and perhaps most obvious of these is sound localisation in the horizontal plane. This has clear real-life advantages in terms of (a) the ability to follow a moving sound source, (b) identifying talker location in a group conversation, (c) improved safety and spatial awareness of the acoustic environment, (d) perceptual segregation of different sound sources in the listener's surroundings and (e) locating sound sources that are out of sight. These are all aspects of the way that normally hearing listeners, processing information obtained from two ears, obtain a mental description of the acoustic environment. The second ability listed, that of identifying talker location in a group conversation, is particularly important for implant listeners, who often experience great dif-

ficulties in complex listening situations. The ability to know who is speaking in a group, then to focus attention on their speech, is key to dealing with the 'cocktail party problem' (Kidd *et al.*, 2005).

Convincing evidence that bilateral cochlear implant listeners can localise sounds in the horizontal plane (and that unilateral listeners are unable to) is now available. For example, Verschuur *et al.* (2005) reported a mean localisation error of 24° for bilateral implant users tested using an 11-loudspeaker array, compared with 67° for monaural implants (chance performance was 65°). Although impressive, they showed that the binaural performance was still worse than that obtained by normally hearing listeners and hearing aid users with the same methodology.

The second area of potential benefit from bilateral implants concerns speech perception, namely: (a) the ability to ignore one ear and to attend to the ear directed away from a competing noise source (head shadow effect), (b) improved speech discrimination when the sounds are the same in both ears and softer speech sounds are more audible (binaural summation) and (c) combining different information from each ear enabling the 'squelching' of noise (Tyler *et al.*, 2006). There is now convincing evidence available of all of these (e.g. Laszig *et al.*, 2004). The third area concerns more qualitative advantages (that are inherently harder to assess), for example:

- externalisation (sounds are perceived to originate outside the head instead of from inside)
- 'three-dimensional sound perception', i.e. location of sounds in space is perceived correctly, giving a more natural-sounding environment; this is particularly important for the process of auditory scene analysis, whereby the listener forms a 'mental image' of the world around them in which groups of sounds are allocated to their sources
- sound is more 'balanced' across the ears, richer and more natural, and listening is less effortful.

Finally, there are clear practical advantages to bilateral implantation that are often key considerations both for patients considering the surgery and for implant teams making the sometimes hard decision about whether two implants are justified. The most obvious is the fact that an implant in each ear means that if one stops working there is always a back-up; unilateral implant users find that when their single implant is out of action, they return to a world of deafness that is often distressing. Second, stimulation of both ears should prevent neural atrophy and degeneration of the auditory pathway on both sides. This is a particular consideration for the case of young children undergoing their first implant. If only one ear receives an implant, then later in life the child or parent wishes to stimulate the opposite ear, the natural concern is that performance in the second ear could be compromised by the lack of stimulation in the intervening years. Many parents of children who had a unilateral implant at a young age, but who are now older, are now pursuing implantation on the second side as they have heard about the benefits of binaural hearing.

The accumulation of evidence of the advantages of bilateral cochlear implants (compared to the well-established benefits of unilateral implants) has now led to a much stronger possibility that bilateral implants will become the norm in clinical practice. However, despite the convincing clinical evidence, the cost-effectiveness of bilateral implantation has yet to be overwhelmingly demonstrated; as a result, in any cash-limited health system this will inevitably restrict its widespread application. The incremental benefit of a second implant over and above that of a single device must be weighed up against the significant extra cost of a second implanted device, speech processor, surgery, and ongoing maintenance. Also, the potential for use of a hearing aid in the ear opposite to a unilateral cochlear implant must be considered. There is good evidence that 'bimodal hearing' provided using a combination of electrical and acoustic hearing can be highly beneficial for some patients who have sufficient usable residual hearing in the unimplanted ear (e.g. Ching *et al.*, 2004). Indeed, a recent meta-analysis (Schafer *et al.*, 2007) comparing binaural benefits between bilateral cochlear implants and bimodal stimulation found

no significant differences between the bilateral and bimodal listeners for any of the binaural phenomena studied (e.g. binaural summation, binaural squelch, and the head shadow effect). Further research is clearly needed to fully explore the longer-term benefits of both bilateral cochlear implants and bimodal hearing.

Auditory brainstem implants

The function of a cochlear implant depends on the presence of viable auditory nerve fibres that can be stimulated by intracochlear electrodes. This is the case in the majority of cases of sensorineural deafness, where deafness is a result of cochlear (hair cell) damage and the auditory nerves remain intact. However, when the auditory nerve is congenitally absent, damaged, or absent as a result of disease or surgery, conventional insertion of electrodes into the cochlea has little chance of success in delivering auditory sensations. For example, neurofibromatosis type 2 (NF2) frequently results in bilateral acoustic neuromas, the removal of which may lead to severing of the auditory nerve on both sides. The outcome for people with this condition is therefore rather bleak, as they are left without usable hearing in either ear, and no prospect that a cochlear implant could help. The auditory brainstem implant (ABI) was developed to provide some level of hearing in such cases by direct electrical stimulation of the brainstem. The ABI stimulates the auditory pathway at the level of the cochlear nucleus, and the surgery to insert an array of electrodes directly onto the brainstem is significantly more complex and difficult than that required in a 'normal' cochlear implant; as a result, the procedure is only performed by a handful of skilled surgeons with the requisite experience of skull-base surgery.

Although the numbers of ABI procedures remain relatively small as compared to the many thousands of cochlear implants around the world, there is now evidence that this approach can provide worthwhile benefit in most cases, although the outcomes are somewhat variable and unpredictable. In particular, the number of electrodes that produce auditory sensations and not other non-auditory sensations is variable and requires careful testing. Most ABI users obtain useful awareness of sound and sufficient hearing for speech to be an aid to lip-reading; however, open-set speech discrimination (without lip-reading) is very rarely achieved.

Future directions

The future of cochlear implants remains bright. Current research is directed at improvements in speech processing, the use of bilateral implants, music appreciation. Collection of long-term data on implanted children, as they grow into adults, should further establish cochlear implants as one of the great modern technological success stories.

As this book was going to press the UK National Institute for Health and Clinical Excellence (NICE) announced guidance on cochlear implants. Implants are recommended for adults who do not benefit from acoustic hearing aids, bilateral simultaneous implantation is recommended for children and deaf/blind adults. These and other guidelines are available on the NICE website: www.nice.org.uk.

References

Baguley DM, Atlas MD (2007) Cochlear implants and tinnitus. *Progress in Brain Research* 166:347–355.

Baskent DB (2006) Speech recognition in normal hearing and sensorineural hearing loss as a function of the number of spectral channels. *Journal of the Acoustical Society of America* 120:2908–2925.

Beadle EA, McKinley DJ, Nikolopoulos TP *et al.* (2005) Long-term functional outcomes and academic-occupational status in implanted children after 10 to 14 years of cochlear implant use. *Otology and Neurotology* 26:1152–1160.

Ching TY, Incerti P, Hill M (2004) Binaural benefits for adults who use hearing aids and cochlear implants in opposite ears. *Ear and Hearing* 25:9–21.

Damen GW, Beynon AJ, Krabbe PF, Mulder JJ, Mylanus EA (2007) Cochlear implantation and quality of life in postlingually deaf adults: long-term follow-up. *Otolaryngology, Head and Neck Surgery* 136:597–604.

David EE, Ostroff JM, Shipp D *et al.* (2003) Speech coding strategies and revised cochlear implant candidacy: an analysis of post-implant performance. *Otology and Neurotology* 24:228–233.

Dorman MF, Loizou PC, Fitke J, Tu Z (1998) The recognition of sentences in noise by normal-hearing listeners using simulations of cochlear-implant signal processors with 6–20 channels. *Journal of the Acoustical Society of America* 104:3583–3585.

Dowell RC, Hollow R, Winton E (2004) Outcomes for cochlear implant users with significant residual hearing: implications for selection criteria in children. *Archives of Otolaryngology, Head Neck Surgery* 130:575–581.

Fazel MZ, Gray RF (2007) Patient employment status and satisfaction following cochlear implantation. *Cochlear Implants International* 8:87–91.

Friesen LM, Shannon RV, Baskent DB, Wang X (2001) Speech recognition in noise as a function of the number of spectral channels: comparison of acoustic hearing and cochlear implants. *Journal of the Acoustical Society of America* 110:1150–1163.

Fu Q-J, Nogaki G (2004) Noise susceptibility of cochlear implant users: the role of spectral resolution and smearing. *Journal of the Association for Research in Otolaryngology* 6:19–27.

Kidd G, Arbogast TL, Mason CR, Gallun FJ (2005) The advantage of knowing where to listen. *Journal of the Acoustical Society of America* 118:3804–3815.

Knutson JF (2006) Psychological aspects of cochlear implantation. In: Cooper HR, Craddock LC, eds. *Cochlear Implants – a Practical Guide*, pp 151–178. London: Whurr.

Koch DB, Downing M, Osberger MJ, Litvak L (2007) Using current steering to increase spectral resolution in CII and HiRes 90K users. *Ear and Hearing* 28:38–41.

Laneau J, Wouters J, Moonen M (2006) Improved music perception with explicit pitch coding in cochlear implants. *Audiology and Neurotology* 11:38–52.

Laszig R, Aschendorff A, Stecker M *et al.* (2004) Benefits of bilateral electrical stimulation with the nucleus cochlear implant in adults: 6-month postoperative results. *Otology and Neurotology* 25:958–968.

McDermott HJ (2004) Music perception with cochlear implants: a review. *Trends in Amplification* 8:49–82.

Moore BCJ, Carlyon RP (2005) Perception of pitch by people with cochlear hearing loss and by cochlear implant users. In: Plack CJ, Oxenham AJ, Fay RR, Popper AN, eds. *Springer Handbook of Auditory Research, Vol 24: Pitch, neural coding and perception*, pp 234–277. New York: Springer.

Nascimento LT, Bevilacqua MC (2005) Evaluation of speech perception in noise in cochlear implanted adults. *Revista Brasileira de Otorrinolaringologia* 71:432–437.

Nelson PB, Jin S-H (2002) Understanding speech in single-talker interference: normal-hearing listeners and cochlear implant users. *Journal of the Acoustical Society of America* 111:2429.

Osberger MJ, McConkey Robbins A, Trautwein PG (2006) Assessment of children. In: Cooper HR, Craddock LC, eds. *Cochlear Implants – a Practical Guide*, pp 106–131. London: Whurr.

Schafer EC, Amlani AM, Seibold A, Shattuck PL (2007) A meta-analytic comparison of binaural benefits between bilateral cochlear implants and bimodal stimulation. *Journal of the American Academy of Audiology* 18:760–776.

Shannon RV (2005) Speech and music have different requirements for spectral resolution. *International Review of Neurobiology* 70:121–134.

Shannon RV, Fu Q-J, Galvin JJ (2004) The number of spectral channels required for speech recognition depends on the difficulty of the listening situation. *Acta Otolaryngologica* 552(suppl):1–5.

Spriet A, Van Deun L, Eftaxiadis K *et al.* (2007) Speech understanding in background noise with the two-microphone adaptive beamformer BEAM in the Nucleus Freedom Cochlear Implant System. *Ear and Hearing* 28:62–72.

Stickney GS, Assmann PF, Chang J, Zeng F-G (2007) Effects of cochlear implant processing and fundamental frequency on the intelligibility of competing sentences. *Journal of the Acoustical Society of America* 122:1069–1078.

Stickney GS, Zeng F-G, Litovsky RY, Assmann PF (2004) Cochlear implant speech recognition with speech maskers. *Journal of the Acoustical Society of America* 116:1081–1091.

Tyler RS, Noble W, Dunn C, Witt S (2006) Some benefits and limitations of binaural cochlear implants and our ability to measure them. *International Journal of Audiology* 45(suppl 1):S113–119.

UK Cochlear Implant Study Group (2004) Criteria of candidacy for unilateral cochlear implantation in postlingually deafened adults III: prospective evaluation of an actuarial approach to defining a criterion. *Ear and Hearing* 25:361–374.

Uziel AS, Sillon M, Vieu A *et al.* (2007) Ten-year follow-up of a consecutive series of children with multichannel cochlear implants. *Otology and Neurotology* 28:615–628.

Verschuur CA, Lutman ME, Ramsden R, Greenham P, O'Driscoll M (2005) Auditory localization abilities in bilateral cochlear implant recipients. *Otology and Neurotology* 26:965–971.

Wilson BS (2006) Speech processing strategies. In: Cooper HR, Craddock LC, eds. *Cochlear Implants – a Practical Guide*, pp 21–69. London: Whurr.

Wilson BS, Dorman MF (2007) The surprising performance of present-day cochlear implants. *IEEE Transactions on Bio-medical Engineering* 54(6 part 1):969–972.

Implantable devices: bone-anchored hearing aids and middle ear implants

Richard Irving

21

Introduction

Mechanical stimulation of the auditory pathway by an implantable device represents a rehabilitative alternative for patients with mild to moderate hearing loss. These devices function by exciting the otic capsule and cochlea, and unlike cochlear implants rely on some residual cochlear function. There are two main categories of device that function as mechanical stimulators of the inner ear, the bone-anchored hearing aid (BAHA) and the middle ear implant (MEI). These devices can be used in conductive, mixed and sensorineural losses. The MEI typically has been used in bilateral losses and the BAHA can benefit patients with both unilateral and bilateral hearing loss.

Bone-anchored hearing aid

The BAHA is now a well-established technology that has largely replaced traditional bone-conduction hearing aids. The main advantages of the BAHA over transcutaneous devices are the greater comfort, decreased sound attenuation

and lower levels of distortion achieved with direct bone conduction.

Physiology of bone conduction

Excitation of the cochlea by the BAHA is achieved using the phenomenon of bone conduction. We do not have a complete understanding of the physiology of bone-conduction hearing; however, the experimental work of von Bekesy has confirmed that the mode of excitation of the cochlea is identical to that achieved by air-conducted sound. According to Tonndorf (1964), the cochlea is stimulated by bone-conducted sound in three different ways: firstly by sound from the vibrating skull radiating to the external ear canal and then being transmitted via the middle ear; secondly by the inertial response of the middle ear ossicles and inner ear fluids; and thirdly by direct compression of the inner ear causing basilar membrane deflection as a result of the asymmetry of the fluid compartments.

Further work on bone-conducted sound has demonstrated that for the frequencies and vibration levels used for normal hearing, the transmission through the skull is linear and predominantly through the skull vault rather than the skull base (Håkansson *et al.*, 1996; Stenfelt *et al.*, 2000).

Osseointegration

Osseointegration describes a concept whereby the surface of an implanted material lies in direct contact with living bone without an interposing connective tissue layer. The application of this technology to the fitting of a bone-conduction hearing aid was first described by Tjellström *et al.* (1980). The BAHA fixture is made from titanium with a surface of titanium oxide that is highly biocompatible and allows for the integration of osteocytes to provide a stable interface. This integration with living bone allows long-term stability and the ability to withstand multi-directional load and stress.

History and device development

Currently there is only one device available for clinical use, the BAHA designed and developed in Gothenburg, Sweden (Figure 21.1). A second device, the Audiant, was developed in the USA, introduced in 1984 and is no longer commercially available. This was largely due to the low level of gain achieved by the device, which proved insufficient for most patients.

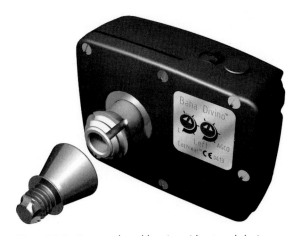

Figure 21.1 Bone-anchored hearing aid external device.

The BAHA was first developed in 1977 and has been commercially available since the mid-1980s. It is a semi-implantable percutaneous device that is secured to the skull by an osseo-integrated titanium fixture. It consists of a screw-shaped implant made of commercially pure titanium, and a sound processor attached by a snap coupling. The sound processor comprises a microphone, amplifier and vibrator. The sound processors are either ear level or body worn.

Patient selection

Otological

The BAHA was initially used exclusively in adults and children with bilateral conductive losses. Patients with absent ear canals due to congenital malformations, those with chronic ear disease, or patients unable to tolerate traditional amplification aids do especially well with this device. Some with otosclerosis have also benefited. The majority of patients at present undergo unilateral implantation; however, research on a number of bilaterally implanted patients has shown benefit (Dutt *et al.*, 2002). This suggests that the trans-cranial attenuation of bone-conducted sound is great enough to allow two different bone-conducted inputs to the two cochleae to produce binaural hearing.

More recently, the indications have been extended to include unilateral conductive loss and single-sided inner ear deafness. Unilateral inner ear deafness from a variety of causes, for example following acoutic neuroma surgery, can benefit from the BAHA. Even adult patients with longstanding congenital unilateral inner ear deafness have been successfully rehabilitated with BAHAs. In patients with unilateral losses, a trial with a BAHA attached to a headband for 2–4 weeks may be helpful in evaluating those that might derive benefit. It has also become apparent that for many children with Down's syndrome, the BAHA represents the best form of auditory rehabilitation.

Audiological

The BAHA relies on some residual cochlear function. An ear-level processor can successfully rehabilitate a patient with a residual bone-conduction level averaging 45 dB, and the body-worn device can benefit those whose average drops to 65 dB. In cases of unilateral inner ear deafness, company recommendations support the use of a BAHA only if the contralateral ear has normal (20 dB or greater) bone conduction. However, it is likely that with more experience the true level of benefit will be determined and a degree of contralateral cochlear impairment possibly down to 35 dB would not represent a contraindication.

Candidates

Children under the age of 3 years have been implanted; however, the risk of fixture loss in the very young is high and surgery is now rarely carried out in children under 5 years. For very young children, the availability of the BAHA softband, in which the vibrating part of the BAHA is held gently against the skull by an elastic headband, provides an excellent rehabilitative alternative in those with bilateral hearing losses. This device has allowed the adoption of a more conservative approach in this age group without compromising speech and language development. There is no upper age limit for the implantation of the device.

Surgical considerations

Surgery differs in adults and children in a number of respects. In adults and older children, the procedure is typically carried out as a single stage under a local anaesthetic as a day case. In children, where the bone is thinner and immature, surgery is a two-stage procedure done under a general anaesthetic. By staging the procedure, time is allowed for osseointegration; typically the second stage is done at 3 to 6 months.

The operation involves fixing the percutaneous implant behind the external ear at a site where the external device can be attached without touching the pinna and to allow spectacles to be worn. An important part of the operation is to reduce the thickness of the soft tissues around the intended fixture site and to ensure a non-hair-

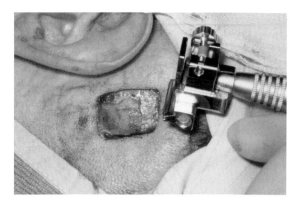

Figure 21.2 Bone-anchored hearing aid surgery showing dermatone, skin flap and soft tissue reduction.

bearing area of skin. A number of different methods of achieving this have been described. The thin skin around the fixture when healed should be immobile and directly applied to bone or periosteum (Figures 21.2 and 21.3).

Following the surgery, the patient is fitted with the external processor (Figure 21.1), typically after 8–12 weeks, allowing a short time for soft tissue healing and osseointegration before loading the fixture. Patients are then instructed on care of the abutment that normally requires cleaning on a weekly basis.

Patient outcome

Surgical complications occur in a small number of cases, the commonest being skin reactions that

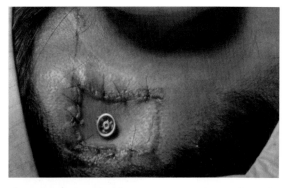

Figure 21.3 Completed surgery in a patient with single-sided deafness following acoustic neuroma removal. In these cases the device is implanted more posteriorly and superiorly to keep it at a distance from the previous incision.

are usually mild and respond to local wound care. Death of the skin flap can occur and this is again usually treated expectantly and recovery anticipated. Rarely, soft tissue overgrowth occurs and this may be overcome by the fitting of a longer abutment; if the abutment is covered by this tissue, then a small further procedure to reduce this needs to be carried out. Loss of the fixture is reported in up to 5% of cases and can be due to failure of osseointegration or to trauma.

Subjective outcome has been measured in a number of studies, and the benefit of this technology proven. Quality of life outcome studies have demonstrated an improvement with the BAHA (Browning and Gatehouse, 1994; McLarnon, 2004). In addition, patients describe a preference for the BAHA over traditional aids as it has a better aesthetic appearance, comfort and output. Additional benefits are a reduction in ear infections and ear discharge in those patients with chronic ear disease when the BAHA is compared to in-the-ear amplification aids (Bance *et al.*, 2002). Patients with hyperacusis and tinnitus are generally less satisfied with the outcome of a BAHA, although these are not considered contraindications.

Patients with inner ear unilateral deafness derive in general less benefit than those with two functioning cochleae. Many describe an ability to localise sound, but laboratory measurements do not support this. There may, however, be some ability to achieve a sense of direction in these patients due to tactile clues from vibration or the inter-aural time difference and different sound quality of the input coming from the BAHA. It appears, however, that the main value in this population group is the alleviation of the head shadow effect, since the BAHA is incapable of restoring binaural hearing when there is only one cochlea.

Middle ear implants

Middle ear implants, like the BAHA, are for patients with some residual cochlear function. They represent an alternative to amplification aids but differ in a few key aspects. In a conventional aid, the amplified signal is presented to the ear via a miniature loudspeaker situated at a distance from the middle ear. The sound signal then passes down a small-diameter conduit to the external ear canal. The loudspeaker and conduit introduce some distortion to the sound signal and represent a design limitation of conventional amplification devices. In a MEI, the transducer is directly coupled to one of the ossicles or cochlear windows. The majority of MEIs maintain an open ear canal, reducing or eliminating feedback and occlusion effects by utilising a 'hidden' external processor. By using a direct coupling and no loudspeaker or small-bore conduit, these devices aim to improve sound transmission and quality.

More recently, these devices have been employed in patients with mixed and conductive losses as an alternative to the BAHA. Their use to date has been restricted to patients with bilateral hearing loss and they are of no value in single-sided inner ear deafness. There is limited experience of these devices in children.

History and device development

Devices have been developed over the past 30 years, and much of the research has addressed the question of what is the optimal site and method of attachment of the microphone, amplifier and transducer.

The microphone can be sited post-aurally or within the ear canal. Neither site has proved to be ideal. The former is complicated by a loss of the pinna effect, and the latter has been largely unsuccessful because of problems with feedback.

Devices have predominantly used either a coil and magnet (electromagnetic) or a piezoelectric mode of transmission. The piezoelectric transducer works on the principle that when a voltage is applied to a particular ceramic (piezoceramic or piezoelectric crystal) it causes a proportional deformation and hence displacement of that ceramic. This voltage-dependent displacement can then be used to drive the inner ear. In the case of an electromagnetic transducer, the electrical signal is used to produce an electromagnetic field by means of a transduction coil. This then drives a magnet that can be attached in a variety of ways to transfer the vibrations to the inner ear.

The coupling mechanism of the device is the method by which the transducer is connected to one of the middle ear ossicles or cochlear windows. Most of the different devices so far have connected to one of the middle ear ossicles with or without need for disruption of the ossicular chain, and in some cases in conjunction with ossicular replacement prostheses. The possibility of hydroacoustic transmission, via a water-filled tube, either to the ossicles or directly to the round window membrane, has been investigated (Hüttenbrink *et al.*, 2001) and direct round window stimulation is now being increasingly employed.

A major problem with these devices has been to produce a device that is small enough to fit within the confines of the middle ear and yet powerful enough to produce the required gain. Over recent years, technological advances resulted in a number of devices that fulfilled these basic requirements. The translation from theory to a viable surgical and financial product has proved extremely difficult and many projects have ultimately ended in failure.

There are currently three devices commercially available. The Vibrant MedEl is an active semi-implantable hearing device. It consists of an internal, surgically implanted part – the vibrating ossicular prosthesis (VORP) – and an external audio processor. The VORP is made up of a receiving coil, conductor link and transducer. The transducer employs a small electromagnetic coil and enclosed magnet to produce vibrations in the floating mass transducer (FMT). The FMT can be coupled with a clip to the long process of the incus, an ossicular prosthesis, the stapes, or, with the clip removed, placed in the round window niche.

The Otologics MET ossicular stimulator is currently a fully implantable device, although the initial trials were done with a semi-implantable version, which has CE (EU certification system) approval (Kasic and Fredrickson, 2001). The device consists of a subcutaneous microphone, and an electronic receiver connected to a transducer. The transducer drives a probe coupled to the body of the incus. The tip of the probe is made of aluminium oxide and this forms a fibrous connection with a laser-made hole in the incus body. The ossicular chain is left intact. The Otologics MET ossicular stimulator is currently under FDA (Food and Drug Administration)-approved clinical trial in the United States (Backous and Duke, 2006).

The Esteem hearing implant (Envoy Medical) is a fully implantable piezoelectric device that has a CE mark and is currently under FDA trial. The device comprises a piezoelectric sensor on the incus body and a driver cemented to the stapes head. The device effectively uses the tympanic membrane as a microphone. Implantation of the device requires disarticulation of the ossicular chain, with removal of 2–3 mm of the long process of the incus (Backous and Duke, 2006).

Patient selection

Audiological

Current devices are most suitable for mild to severe sensorineural hearing losses. Recently, the Vibrant MedEl device has been proposed for use in conductive or mixed losses in combination with passive middle ear prostheses (partial ossicular prosthesis (PORP), total ossicular prosthesis (TORP) or stapes piston), or being applied directly to the round window, thereby aiming to overcome mixed losses in such cases.

For a middle ear implant, the hearing loss should ideally be stable; however, very slowly progressive losses can be considered. The worst ear is usually selected for implantation.

Otological

The classic indications for these devices required normal middle ear function. This is assessed by a combination of otologic history, otoscopic examination and the above audiological evaluation. There should be an absence of retrocochlear or central involvement in the hearing loss. Where middle ear function is abnormal, any middle ear inflammation should be controlled prior to implantation.

Candidates

The candidate for implantation at present must be an adult, although extension of this technology to children seems likely in the future. They should not have any skin conditions that may prevent attachment of any external component of the device, and should be medically fit for the surgery and anaesthesia required. In addition, the candidate should have been appropriately counselled by the surgeon and be judged to have realistic expectations.

Surgical considerations

The approach for implanting the Vibrant MedEl is similar to that for a cochlear implant, and the siting of the transducer shares similar demands to those required in stapes surgery (Figure 21.4). Different incisions are used but are mainly of one of three types: extended endaural, postaural or extended postaural (Fisch *et al.*, 2001; Fraysse *et al.*, 2001). The bone work consists of a cortical mastoidectomy and then a posterior tympanotomy (see Chapter 9). The posterior tympanotomy should be large enough to take a 3 mm diamond burr to ensure sufficient space to site the transducer. An implant bed is drilled in the squamous temporal bone to accommodate the internal receiver and conductor link. The FMT is placed in the middle ear via the posterior tympanotomy, with its attachment clip around the long process

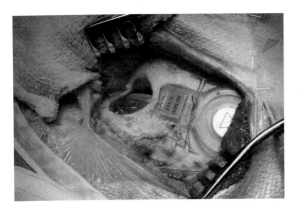

Figure 21.4 Vibrant MedEl device secured in the bony recess behind the mastoid.

of the incus. The position is checked and then the clip is crimped around the long process of the incus, using the special forming forceps provided with the implant. The main advantages of this procedure are that it utilises an approach already familiar to otologists and does not require disruption of the ossicular chain. However, bone work is required close to the facial nerve and there is also concern about crimping the clip to the long process of the incus. If the clip is crimped too tightly there is a potential for necrosis of the long process of the incus, and if it is too loose the implant may fail.

The Esteem device uses a similar approach but with more exposure of the incus. The incus long process is removed using a laser and then the sensor placed on the incus body. A sound processor and power supply is fixed in the mastoid, and the piezoelectric driver attached directly to the stapes.

Implantation of the Otologics MET device uses a more direct approach to the epitympanum and attic. This is then carefully dissected to expose the proximal antrum and then the incus body and malleus head (Kasic and Fredrickson, 2001). The mounting system is secured to the skull by screws and used to guide a laser to make a hole in the body of the incus. The transducer is then inserted into the mounting and the probe tip aligned with the laser-made hole in the incus. Fine positioning of the probe tip is made by a micrometer screw adjustment. An implant bed is again drilled in the squamous temporal bone for the receiver capsule.

Patient outcome

The Vibrant MedEl has been implanted in by far the largest group of patients worldwide. Initial results for this device came from a European 10-centre trial on 47 patients (Fisch *et al.*, 2001) and the early audiological results were presented in 63 patients (Snik *et al.*, 2001b). Clinical experience with this device has been described in a number of studies (Fraysse *et al.*, 2001; Luetje *et al.*, 2002; Sterkers *et al.*, 2003).

In the initial trials (Fisch *et al.*, 2001; Fraysse *et al.*, 2001) there were no major complications reported. One delayed-onset, temporary, partial facial weakness occurring 10 days post-surgery was reported (Fraysse *et al.*, 2001). Possible damage to the chorda tympani was reported in up to 15% but there were no reports of any lasting effects among these patients (Fisch *et al.*, 2001). No wound problems were reported in either series. One patient developed tinnitus postoperatively, who had not reported tinnitus preoperatively (Fisch *et al.*, 2001). Overall, there was no significant (defined as more than 5 dB) deterioration in the average unaided pure tone thresholds in the implanted ear pre- and post-surgery, leading both trials to conclude the safety of the device (Fisch *et al.*, 2001; Fraysse *et al.*, 2001). A further analysis of 125 patients implanted in France reported high satisfaction levels with the soundbridge device (Sterkers *et al.*, 2003).

Direct comparison with conventional aiding is difficult, as this is, by definition, a group of the population dissatisfied with conventional aids (Snik *et al.*, 2001a). Gain at threshold level was calculated by subtracting aided soundfield thresholds from unaided thresholds for 63 patients in the European trial (Snik *et al.*, 2001b). In all but one patient, a gain was demonstrated but there was a considerable range in the gain attained. Speech recognition was also measured and correlated well with the gain attained, implying that the quality of the amplification was adequate for speech recognition. Fraysse *et al.* (2001), using the Abbreviated Profile of Hearing Aid Benefit (APHAB) self-assessment questionnaire (Cox and Alexander, 1995), compared patient satisfaction with a conventional aid to the Vibrant MedEl after at least 3 months' usage. Out of 17 patients, 12 reported a significant improvement, 4 were unchanged and 1 was worse with the device. Significant patient benefit with the Vibrant MedEl has also been reported in six patients with a purely high-frequency loss (normal hearing or a mild loss at frequencies below 1000 Hz) when compared with conventional amplification (Uziel *et al.*, 2003). Overall, the results so far available for middle ear implantable devices in bilateral sensorineural loss appear encouraging and without major complications.

The application of this technology to those with conductive and mixed losses represents a new direction for this technology, and the early results with direct round window stimulation also appear encouraging (Colletti *et al.*, 2006).

The future

The use of the BAHA in single-sided deafness has shown some benefit, but further work needs to be done to decide who is likely to benefit the most from this and how can they be best assessed. The extension to children with single-sided deafness is also an area to be explored as many of these children suffer educationally as a result of their disability and are currently not being rehabilitated. Hopefully, one day, a fully implantable BAHA system will be developed.

The future of MEI technology will see increased application to patients with conductive and mixed losses, who are intolerant of conventional amplification aids and resistant to reconstructive surgery. Gain is an issue with many of these devices, and the manufacturers should look at trying to increase the potential gain of these systems. Fully implantable systems are clearly going to be more attractive for these patients, and further research will hopefully answer the issue of the best site for the microphone placement and the best method of energy transfer to the inner ear. MEI surgical development should focus on the ease of surgical placement, to simplify the process of implantation and reduce the risk of complications.

To continue to be successful, implantable devices will need to be priced in such a way as to be competitive when compared with equivalent amplification aids. This will enable them to be accessible to all patients in the developed and developing world who would potentially derive benefit from them.

References

Backous DD, Duke W (2006) Implantable middle ear hearing devices: current state of technology and market challenges. *Current Opinion in Otolaryngology and Head and Neck Surgery* 14:314–318.

Bance M, Abel SM, Papsin BC, Wade P, Vendramini JA (2002) Comparison of the audiometric performance of bone anchored hearing aids and air conduction hearing aids. *Otology and Neurotology* 23:912–919.

Browning G, Gatehouse S (1994) Estimation of the benefit of bone-anchored hearing aids. *Annals of Otology, Rhinology and Laryngology* 103:872–878.

Colletti V, Soli SD, Carner M, Colletti L (2006) Treatment of mixed hearing losses via implantation of a vibratory transducer on the round window. *International Journal of Audiology* 45:600–608.

Cox RM, Alexander GC (1995) The Abbreviated Profile of Hearing Aid Benefit. *Ear and Hearing* 16:176–186.

Dutt SN, McDermott AL, Burrell SP et al. (2002) Speech intelligibility with bilateral bone-anchored hearing aids. *Journal of Laryngology and Otology* 28 suppl:47–51.

Fisch U, Cremers CWRJ, Lenarz T et al. (2001) Clinical experience with the vibrant soundbridge implant device. *Otology and Neurotology* 22:962–972.

Fraysse B, Lavieille J-P, Schmerber S et al. (2001) A multicenter study of the vibrant soundbridge middle ear implant: early clinical results and experience. *Otology and Neurotology* 22:952–961.

Håkansson B, Carlson P, Brandt A, Stenfelt S (1996) Linearity of sound transmission through the human skull in vivo. *Journal of the Acoustical Society of America* 99:2239–2243.

Hüttenbrink K-B, Zahnert TH, Bornitz M, Hofmann G (2001) Biomechanical aspects in implantable microphones and hearing aids and development of a concept with a hydroacoustical transmission. *Acta Otolaryngologica* 121: 185–189.

Kasic JF, Fredrickson JM (2001) The Otologics MET Ossicular Stimulator. *Oto-laryngologic Clinics of North America* 34: 501–513.

Luetje CM, Brackmann D, Balkany TJ et al. (2002) Phase III clinical trial results with the Vibrant Soundbridge Implantable middle ear hearing device: a prospective controlled multicentre study. *Otolaryngology and Head and Neck Surgery* 126:97–107.

McLarnon CM, Davison T, Johnson IJM (2004) Bone-anchored hearing aid: comparison of benefit by patient subgroups. *Laryngoscope* 114:942–944.

Snik AFM, Cremers CWRJ (2001a) Vibrant semi-implantable hearing device with digital sound processing. *Archives of Otolaryngology – Head and Neck Surgery* 127:1433–1437.

Snik AFM, Mylanus EAM, Cremers CWJ et al. (2001b) Multicenter audiometric results with the vibrant soundbridge, a semi-implantable hearing device for sensorineural hearing impairment. *Otolaryngologic Clinics of North America* 34:373–388.

Stenfelt S, Håkansson BE, Tjellström A (2000) Vibration characteristics of bone conducted sound in vivo. *Journal of the Acoustical Society of America* 107:422–431.

Sterkers O, Boucarra D, Labassi S et al. (2003) A middle ear implant, the Symphonix Vibrant Soundbridge: retrospective study of the first 125 patients implanted in France. *Otology and Neurotology* 24:427–436.

Tjellström A, Håkansson B, Lindström J et al. (1980) Analysis of the mechanical impedence of bone-anchored hearing aids. *Acta Otolaryngologica* 89:85–92.

Tonndorf J (1964) Animal experiments in bone conduction: clinical conclusions. *Transactions of the American Otological Society* 52: 22–43.

Uziel A, Mondain M, Hagen P, Dejean P, Doucet G (2003) Rehabilitation for high-frequency sensorineural hearing impairment in adults with the symphonix vibrant soundbridge: a comparative study. *Otology and Neurotology* 24:775–783.

Auditory processing disorders

Doris-Eva Bamiou

22

Introduction

Over the last 20–30 years, it has become increasingly recognised that impaired structure and/or function of the brain may have little or no effect on hearing thresholds, but may cause deficits in other aspects of the hearing process. These deficits are collectively referred to as an 'auditory processing disorder' (APD). Broadly speaking, the term 'central auditory processing' refers to how the brain analyses sound to derive meaningful information. In the mid-1950s, Bocca *et al.* (1954) made the seminal observations that patients with temporal lobe tumours complained of hearing difficulties, despite the presence of normal hearing thresholds and speech recognition in quiet. Bocca and co-workers demonstrated auditory deficits by utilising a speech test in which the low frequency acoustic features of the speech signal had been removed. Around the same time, Myklebust (1954) proposed that central auditory processing ought to be considered and assessed in children with communication disorders. In the UK, the terms 'obscure auditory dysfunction' (OAD) and 'King–Kopetzky syndrome' (KKS) (Hinchcliffe, 1992) were coined in the late 1980s to describe the clinical presentation of reported difficulty understanding speech in background noise despite normal hearing thresholds. Patients with OAD/KKS are characterised by deficient performance in speech in noise tests, and personality traits such as a tendency to underestimate their hearing ability. However, OAD/KKS is not identical to APD, as it may be underlined by a variety of pathologies at both the peripheral and the central levels of the auditory pathway (e.g. mild cochlear pathology, middle ear dysfunction or medial olivocochlear efferent system dysfunction) and/or psychological problems.

APD is currently recognised as a distinct clinical entity by many practitioners in the wider field of audiology. However, accurate diagnosis remains a clinical challenge. This may be due to the lack of application of a systematic battery of diagnostic measures for APD, to current test limitations, and to the lack of universally accepted diagnostic criteria. These concerns have led to the organisation of consensus conferences, attended by a multidisciplinary audience of professionals involved in the assessment and management of APD from the wider field of audiology. The aim of these conferences is to agree on a definition of APD in order to consider the diagnostic and management approach of this entity.

In the UK, the Auditory Processing Disorder Interest Group of the British Society of Audiology (BSA) proposed that APD:

> results from impaired neural function and is characterized by poor recognition, discrimination, separation, grouping, localization, or ordering of *non-speech* sounds. It does not solely result from a deficit in general attention, language or other cognitive processes' (www.thebsa.org.uk/apd/Home.htm).

In the United States, the American Speech-Language-Hearing Association (ASHA) Working Group on Auditory Processing Disorders (2005) proposed that the term 'central' should precede the term APD, since 'most definitions of the disorder focus on the central auditory nervous system'. Thus, (C)APD is defined as 'a deficit in neural processing of auditory stimuli that is not due to higher order language, cognitive, or related factors' (ASHA, 2005). Patients with APD may show deficits, which will have both behavioural and electrophysiological correlates, in the following skills (ASHA, 1996):

- sound localisation/lateralisation
- auditory pattern recognition
- auditory discrimination
- temporal aspects of hearing (masking, ordering, integration, resolution)
- processing degraded auditory signals
- processing the auditory signal when embedded in competing acoustic signals.

APD is not as yet included in current standard classification schemes for developmental/higher-order disorders, such as the *Diagnostic and Statistical Manual of Mental Disorders* (DSM-IV), although it does fulfil several, if not all, of the criteria proposed for inclusion of a specific diagnosis in the previous edition of this manual. However, at present there is a lack of studies assessing reliability issues of this diagnosis and whether there is evidence for a syndrome. In view of the above, it would perhaps be more accurate to refer to 'disordered auditory processing' rather than 'auditory processing disorder', and although the term 'APD' will be retained for the rest of this chapter, it will be defined as 'disordered auditory processing'.

Brief overview of relevant anatomy and physiology (see also Chapter 4)

The central auditory nervous system (CANS) extends from the cochlear nucleus in the brainstem to the auditory cortex, with an increasing number of fibres from the periphery to the cortex. The CANS includes, apart from the cochlear nuclei, the superior olivary complex, lateral lemniscus, inferior colliculus in the brainstem, the medial geniculate body in the thalamus, and the subcortical internal capsule. The cortical areas include Heschl's gyrus (transverse gyrus), the planum temporale, planum polare, supramarginal gyrus, angular gyrus, inferior parietal lobe, inferior frontal lobe, and the insula (Musiek and Oxholm, 2000). Similar to the visual system, there are two parallel processing streams in the CANS, subserved by distinct pathways: the anterior or rostral 'what' stream, responsible for sound identification, and the posterior or caudal 'where' stream, responsible for sound location. In addition, the CANS is characterised by an intricate pattern of bilateral connections, ascending (from the periphery to the cortex), descending (from the cortex to the periphery) and at the same level of the CANS (e.g. from right to left cortex) (Musiek and Oxholm, 2000).

Axons from auditory and auditory-responsive cortical areas cross the midline in the forebrain commissures of the corpus callosum and the anterior commissure. Interhemispheric transfer appears to be sensory driven, context dependent, and strongly modulated by attention, and may underpin the lateralisation of functions which is characteristic of the human brain (Bamiou *et al.*, 2007). Thus, while language and speech processing is subserved by bilateral networks, some features of the speech signal are processed in one hemisphere, usually the left, while the right auditory cortex seems to be crucial for tonal processing. The interhemispheric pathway may thus contribute to the functional specialisation and increase the computational capacity of the brain (Bamiou *et al.*, 2007).

While the cochlea is fully developed at birth, maturation and myelination of the rest of the auditory system continue long after birth, from the periphery to the cortex. This is reflected in changes in auditory evoked potentials as well as improved behavioural central auditory test performance with age in normal children. The rate of myelination can vary in the normal population and is 'sound dependent', relying on afferent input from the cochlea. The brain retains an inherent capacity for plasticity throughout life, and there is ample scientific evidence of the potential of the CANS for functional and physiological change following auditory experiences such as auditory deprivation, stimulation, training and learning.

Aetiology of disordered auditory processing

In terms of aetiology, disordered auditory processing may occur (Bamiou *et al.*, 2001; Griffiths 2002) in the presence of:

- *genetic causes* – these may include:
  - □ genetic syndromes that affect the brain with structural or functional abnormalities (e.g. Bamiou *et al.*, 2007)
  - □ genetic syndromes that make the brain more susceptible to damage, e.g. in the presence of the Crigler–Najjar syndrome infants are more prone to develop bilirubin encephalopathy
  - □ the genetic basis of the auditory processing deficits that are seen in the presence of other developmental disorders also needs to be considered. However, in many such instances, it may be difficult to establish that the deficit in neural processing of auditory stimuli is not due to higher-order language, cognitive, or related factors included in the BSA and ASHA definitions
- *neurological conditions* that are known to affect the brain's structure and function, such as tumours, cerebrovascular accidents, demy-

elinating disease. These conditions may affect both children and adults, although the prevalence will differ in various age groups

- *delayed central nervous system maturation* – otitis media with effusion, i.e. glue ear, is a good example of auditory deprivation that leads to APD even after the resolution of the conductive hearing loss. In some cases, this may persist into adulthood
- *other higher-order disorders* in both adults and children, such as attention deficit hyperactivity disorder (ADHD), dyslexia, specific language impairment, etc
- *age-related changes of the central auditory system* – higher level auditory processing of sounds may be impaired in older individuals, even after peripheral hearing loss and cognitive decline have been taken into consideration
- finally, there may be an additional category of *'positive' disorders of auditory processing*, in which there is evidence of abnormal activity in the CANS, for example in tinnitus (Griffiths, 2002).

Disordered auditory processing presentation and symptoms

Disordered auditory processing may manifest itself in both children and adults with uncertainty about what the individual hears, difficulties listening in a background of competing sounds, and difficulties in following oral instructions and understanding rapid or degraded speech, despite the presence of normal peripheral hearing (ASHA, 1996; Jerger and Musiek, 2000). As a consequence of the primary auditory difficulties, children, in particular, with APD may have secondary characteristics of language, reading and spelling disorders, as well as inattention and distractibility, while both children and adults may have a higher likelihood of behavioural, emotional, social and other difficulties (ASHA, 2005). There is a paucity of studies systematically assessing auditory symptoms and clinical presentations of APD sufferers.

Smoski *et al.* (1992) developed a questionnaire, the Children's Auditory Processing Performance Scale (CHAPS), which they used to assess listening performance in 64 children with APD. The diagnosis of APD was based on findings of abnormal test results in at least two out of four validated central auditory tests. The teacher-administered questionnaire identified listening difficulties in a wide context of listening situations (in quiet, in noise, ideal listening conditions, with multiple inputs present) as well as problems with auditory memory and attention in the children with APD compared to their normal peers. However, the listening performance of children with APD, although poorer than in children without APD, varied widely (Smoski *et al.*, 1992). Meister *et al.* (2004) similarly evaluated differences between children with a 'suspected' APD (identified as clinical suspicion of APD and failure in tests unspecified by the authors) *versus* a control group, using a parent-answered questionnaire. The APD group gave significantly poorer scores on the questionnaire than the normal group. A factor analysis identified seven main components that could account for this difference, including speech understanding in demanding situations (speech in competing speech, speech in noise, degraded speech), speech/language-production abilities of the child, general behavioural issues (aggression and frustration), difficulties of the children with responses to (orally given) questions and demands, reproduction of musical cues, discrimination of speech sounds, and loudness perception.

Neijenhuis *et al.* (2003) assessed hearing disability in 24 otherwise neurologically normal adults with a suspected auditory processing disorder: patients who complained of hearing difficulties and who gave abnormal (high) scores on the Amsterdam Inventory, a validated hearing questionnaire, which assesses difficulties with the detection of sounds, distinction of sounds, intelligibility of speech in noise and in quiet and sound localisation, as part of the validation study for a central auditory test battery. Sixty-eight per cent of these adults gave abnormal results (scores below the 90th percentile of the normal control group) in the central auditory test battery. The study found that, as a group, the subjects with a suspected auditory processing disorder reported significantly more complaints regarding hearing

abilities than normal controls for all five factors assessed by the Amsterdam Inventory, with speech in noise and sound localisation as the most frequently reported difficulties. An earlier study was conducted by Blaettner *et al.* (1989) on patients with unilateral cerebrovascular lesions of the telencephalic auditory structures. These authors administered a hearing questionnaire in order to assess potential auditory perceptual problems in everyday hearing situations, as part of the validation study for a psychoacoustic pattern discrimination test. They found that about half (49%) of these patients reported auditory perceptual problems in the questionnaire, particularly in situations with simultaneous speakers, while auditory perceptual problems were reported by the vast majority (79%) of those patients who gave abnormal results in the psychoacoustic tests.

Several authors propose that the clinical profiles of patients with APD may be classified, on the basis of clinical presentation and test results, into different subcategories which may correspond to specific sites of pathology in the brain (Bellis, 2005). However, none of these clinical presentation schemes have been validated.

Diagnostic approach for disordered auditory processing

Clinical symptoms of APD are not specific for the auditory modality. In addition, the auditory processing assessment may be influenced by the presence of deficits in other higher-order disorders, which include ADHD, language impairment, reading disability, learning disability, pervasive developmental disorder, and intellectual functioning. Diagnosis of APD thus requires a test battery approach (ASHA, 2005; Auditory Processing Disorder Steering Committee of the British Society of Audiology, 2007). The test battery should include:

- baseline audiological tests, including tympanometry, acoustic reflexes, otoacoustic emissions and suppression of otoacoustic emissions with contralateral noise, and auditory brainstem electric responses. These tests are conducted in order to exclude peripheral pathology and 'auditory neuropathy/dyssynchrony'

■ behavioural central auditory tests – these include both speech and non-speech tests, that aim to assess different auditory processes

■ tests of language and cognition, and of other higher-order processes, as indicated.

In addition, electrophysiological responses such as middle-latency response, and late potentials, such as the P300 or mismatch negativity (MMN) may also be included in the test battery.

Behavioural central auditory tests

The choice of tests should be guided by several considerations, including age appropriateness, sensitivity, specificity and reliability issues, the presence of normative data, test duration, response mode and effects of higher order processes on test results, to name but a few (ASHA, 2005). Behavioural tests currently available for the evaluation of central auditory processing are broadly divided into the following main categories (ASHA, 2005; Baran and Musiek, 1999):

■ *auditory discrimination tasks*: these assess the individual's ability to discriminate between sounds that differ in frequency, intensity and temporal parameters

■ *temporal tasks*: these assess the individual's ability to analyse changes of the acoustic signal over time – temporal processing. Temporal processing can be broken down into four major subprocesses: ordering or sequencing, resolution or discrimination, integration or summation and masking

■ *monaural low-redundancy speech tests*: these assess recognition of speech material that is degraded in terms of frequency content, timing aspects or intensity

■ *dichotic tests (speech and non-speech)*, in which each of the two ears is presented with

Table 22.1 Minimal clinical test battery proposed by ASHA (Jerger and Musiek, 2000).

Behavioural measures	Electroacoustic and electrophysiological measures
Pure-tone audiometry	Immittance audiometry
Word recognition in quiet	Otoacoustic emissions
Dichotic test	Auditory brainstem electric responses
Duration pattern sequence test	
Temporal gap detection	

a different speech or non-speech sound, with these sounds aligned in time

■ *binaural interaction tests*: these assess the listener's ability to 'synthesise' intensity, time, or spectral differences of otherwise identical stimuli presented simultaneously at the two ears, in order to combine complementary input distributed between the ears.

ASHA proposed a minimal clinical test battery which incorporates a range of baseline (widely available) audiological procedures with central auditory tests that are commercially available (Jerger and Musiek, 2000) (Table 22.1).

In addition, there are a few test batteries that are either predominantly intended for research (e.g. the Newcastle Auditory Battery (NAB)) or currently in development, but not yet available for clinical practice (e.g. the Institute of Hearing Research (IHR) Multicentre Auditory Processing (IMAP) testing battery, Institute of Hearing Research).

Management of disordered auditory processing

Intervention for APD is currently based on identification and treatment of the primary deficits caused by the disease ('bottom-up') and on broader types of intervention to treat the disease-related sequelae, such as language, learning, and communication problems ('top-down'). Auditory management can be test driven: training tasks and strategies are chosen on the basis of test findings; or profile driven: the child is classified into an APD subtype, according to the test results, and intervention is decided accordingly (Bamiou *et al.*, 2006). APD management is multidisciplinary, and intervention strategies can be broadly divided into five main categories, which include environmental modifications, signal-enhancement strategies, teacher/speaker-based adaptations, formal and informal auditory training, and compensatory strategies (Bamiou *et al.*, 2006).

Environmental modifications

In a real-life acoustic environment, the presence of noise and reverberation (i.e. the reflections of sounds within a room) will distort and degrade the speech signal, due to masking of key speech elements, the smearing of temporal cues and the loss of speech energy over distance. Legislation that governs the building regulations in the UK defines the upper limit of ambient noise level as 35 dB L_{Aeq}, 30 min (i.e. the energy equivalent sound pressure level in dB(A) over 30 min) and of reverberation (<0.6 in primary and <0.8 in secondary schools). A noise survey will determine the background noise levels and the reverberation characteristics of the classroom, as well as the corrective action indicated. Simple means of acoustic treatment, such as carpets, curtains, sealing of doors, and more sophisticated methods, such as noise-absorbent partitions and acoustic panelling, may help improve background noise levels and reverberation times. Preferential sitting and use of a smaller space during direct teaching sessions will also be of benefit.

Signal-enhancement strategies

Personal or soundfield FM systems are wireless assistive listening devices that receive distant auditory input, and amplify and transmit the signal to the ear of the listener. The teacher's voice is amplified through speakers (soundfield) or a special receiver (personal system) that are wirelessly linked to a transmitter that the teacher wears around his/her neck or on his/her clothes. A microphone, worn by the speaker and connected to the transmitter, picks up the speech signal of the speaker and converts this to an electrical signal, which is transmitted via FM band waves to the receiver. These systems help counteract or minimise reverbation, masking of the speech signals by ambient noise, and the loss of critical speech energy over the distance between teacher and student.

The fitting of an FM system should be preceded by careful assessment of the child (age, motivation, setting for the use of the FM system) and evaluation and acoustic treatment, if indicated, of the classroom, while the child and the teaching environment should be educated about the use of the device, and the outcome of this intervention should be monitored.

Teacher/speaker-based adaptations

Teachers should emphasise and segment their speech in order to highlight the key points of the message; speech should also be delivered at a slightly slower pace. Repetition and rephrasing of the message, using visual or other cues, and frequent checks for understanding would also help.

Auditory training

Auditory training aims to improve the auditory system performance in the analysis of acoustic signals by capitalising on the brain's plasticity and by recruitment and facilitation of other higher-order processes. A variety of tasks may be used. Tasks should be age appropriate, presented systematically, and gradually made more difficult.

- *Informal auditory training* does not require high-tech resources and may include auditory closure activities, which teach the patient how to fill in the missing parts of the speech signal in order to perceive a meaningful whole, temporal patterning and prosody training, auditory discrimination and phonological training, or dichotic listening training (see Bamiou *et al.*, 2006 for further details).

■ *Formal auditory training* refers to tasks performed using computers or audiological equipment. Examples of computer-based commercially available auditory training programmes include Earobics (www.earobics.com/), FastForWord (www.scilearn.com/) and Phonomena (www.mindweavers.co.uk/main.asp) for children, and BrainGym for older adults (www.positscience.com). For all these programmes, auditory training tasks are presented in a computer game format with an adaptive procedure.

Compensatory strategies

Compensatory strategies may include active listening, auditory vigilance training, auditory memory enhancement, metacognitive, linguistic, metalinguistic and other strategies.

Auditory training: some outcome studies

Initial research on clinical populations indicates that auditory training may be beneficial (see Bamiou *et al.*, 2006 for a review) in groups of children with communication disorders that may overlap with APD, such as specific language impairment (SLI), dyslexia or learning disorders, as well as in normal children.

Specific language impairment

In a study by Tallal *et al.* (1996), seven children (6–9 yrs) with SLI received extensive daily training over a 4-week period. The training involved listening to audiotapes in which the speech signal was expanded in duration by 50% and the fast transitional elements of speech (3–30 Hz) were enhanced by 20 dB, in the form of computerised

games. Post-intervention, the children showed significant improvements by approximately two years in speech discrimination, language processing and grammatical comprehension. In a further study (Merzenich *et al.*, 1996), 11 children with SLI were trained with adaptive computerised games targeting temporal processing and language exercises with acoustically modified speech (group A). In addition, 11 children with SLI (group B), who were matched to group A for non-verbal intelligence and receptive language abilities, were trained with similar but non-adaptive computerised game exercises and with the same language exercises as group A, with unmodified speech. Group A showed significantly greater improvement after training than group B in temporal thresholds, speech discrimination, language processing (Token test), and grammatical comprehension.

Cohen *et al.* (2005) conducted a randomised controlled trial of FastForWord *versus* computerised educational packages targeting language development that are recommended by a national educational advisory centre *versus* no specific training, on a total of 77 children (6 to 10 years) with severe mixed receptive-expressive SLI, who were all receiving speech and language training. After training, which lasted for a mean of 24 days, each group had made significant improvements in language scores; however, there was no additional benefit for either of the computer interventions at 9 weeks or at 6 months after training.

Dyslexia

Kujala *et al.* (2001) assessed whether audiovisual training without linguistic material had a remediating effect on reading skills and central auditory processing in children with dyslexia. Forty-eight children aged 7 years, with a reading disability, were recruited and grouped into a training and a control group. After intervention, the training group showed higher reading skills and better MMN than the control group, while a significant correlation was found between the change in MMN amplitude and the change in reading skills. Using functional magnetic resonance imaging (fMRI), Temple *et al.*, (2003) showed significant improvement in word identification, passage comprehension and oral language post-training in a group of 20 dyslexic children who trained with FastForWord for 100 min/day for an average of 4 weeks. After training, the dyslexic children's scores were raised into the normal range, although there was significant variability in the extent of improvement. In addition, these children showed increased activation in a wide range of brain regions, and in some areas, activation became closer to that seen in normally reading children.

Attention deficit hyperactivity disorder and learning disorders

Hayes *et al.* (2003) recruited 27 children diagnosed with a learning disability and/or ADHD (study group), who worked with commercial auditory processing training software (Earobics) for 8 weeks, and 15 normal-learning and learning-impaired children (control group) who did not participate in any remedial programmes. After the training, the study group improved in sound blending and other measures of auditory processing, while their cortical responses were more robust than in the controls, and cortical responses in noise became more robust post-*versus* pre-training.

Russo *et al.* (2005) recently investigated whether auditory training may alter the neural brainstem encoding of speech. Nine children with a previously made diagnosis of a 'language-based learning disorder' participated in 35–40 supervised one-hour sessions of Earobics over 8 weeks, and were tested pre- and post-treatment by means of auditory brainstem and cortical evoked potentials in response to syllables, in both noise and quiet, as well as on measures of auditory processing, mental abilities and academic achievement. Ten additional children (five with learning difficulties and five without learning difficulties) underwent the same tests but did not receive any training. The group who received the training showed an increase in quiet to noise intercorrelation, reflecting greater timing preci-

sion in the frequency following response in noise after training than the control group. The trained children demonstrated significant improvement on certain tests (incomplete words, auditory processing, sentences in noise); however, the changes in brainstem responses did not correlate to these specific tests, but rather to a separate measure of auditory processing (listening comprehension). The authors concluded that auditory training improves the neural synchrony in the brainstem, thus improving the preconscious neural coding of speech sounds.

Normal children

Moore *et al.* (2005) examined the effect of phonemic contrast discrimination training on the discrimination of whole words and on phonological awareness in 8- to 10-year-old mainstream school children. Eighteen children were trained for 12 30-minute sessions over 4 weeks, using an adaptive three-interval two-alternative phonemic matching task (Phonomena). The remaining 12 children participated in regular classroom activities. Trained children showed significantly enhanced performance in the phonological assessment battery scores, while the controls showed no improvement. Enhanced performance was maintained in a delayed test 5–6 weeks following training.

Populations with disordered auditory processing

There are but a few case-control outcome studies of auditory training for management of APD. Putter-Katz *et al.* (2002) compared central auditory test results before and after intervention in 20 children with APD. Children were divided into two groups: group 1 (with problems in speech-in-noise tests) and group 2 (problems in speech-in-noise and dichotic listening tasks). The children received 13–15 weekly 45-minute training sessions, targeting the main auditory deficit, as well as environmental modification and compensatory strategies. After the training, group 1 improved on speech-in-noise scores only while group 2 improved on all tests.

Adults

The Brain Fitness Program for auditory processing (Posit Science) consists of six adaptive exercises, which aim to enhance the fidelity in auditory sensory input and language representations through 5-day weekly, hour-long training sessions for 8 weeks, and has been specifically designed for older adults. A randomised controlled study in 182 adults aged over 60 years showed that the group who performed this program significantly improved in the trained tasks and in auditory memory (*versus* no improvement of the control groups) and this improvement was maintained 3 months after training (Mahncke *et al.*, 2006).

Conclusion

Despite the lack of a uniform definition for what constitutes an 'APD', several scientific uncertainties, and absence of evidence-based guidelines for assessment and management, the field of APD is rapidly expanding. Current scientific evidence highlights the need for a multidisciplinary approach for both assessment and management of APD and indicates that appropriate intervention may be beneficial, for both children and adult APD sufferers.

References

American Speech-Language-Hearing Association (1996) Central auditory processing: current status of research and implications for clinical practice. *American Journal of Audiology* 5: 41–54.

American Speech-Language-Hearing Association (ASHA) (2005) *(Central) Auditory Processing Disorders.* www.asha.org/docs/html/TR2005–00043.html (accessed 20 November 2008).

Auditory Processing Disorder (APD) Steering Committee, British Society of Audiology (2007) *Interim Position Statement on APD – March 2007.* www.thebsa.org.uk/apd/BSA_APD_Position_statement_Final_Draft_Feb_2007.doc (accessed 20 November 2008).

Bamiou DE, Campbell N, Sirimanna TS (2006) Management of auditory processing disorders. *Audiological Medicine* 4:46–56.

Bamiou DE, Musiek FE, Luxon LM (2001) Aetiology and clinical presentations of auditory processing disorders – a review. *Archives of Disease in Childhood* 85:361–365.

Bamiou DE, Sisodiya S, Musiek FE, Luxon LM (2007) The role of the interhemispheric pathway in hearing. *Brain Research Reviews* 56:170–182.

Baran J, Musiek FE (1999) Behavioral assessment of the central auditory nervous system. In: Musiek FE, Rintelman WF, eds. *Contemporary Perspectives in Hearing Assessment*, pp 375–414. Boston: Allyn and Bacon.

Bellis TJ (2005) *Assessment and Management of Central Auditory Processing Disorders in the Educational Setting. From science to practice*, 2nd edn. New York: Delmar Learning/Singular.

Blaettner U, Scherg M, von Cramon D (1989) Diagnosis of unilateral telencephalic hearing disorders. Evaluation of a simple psychoacoustic pattern discrimination test. *Brain* 112:177–195.

Bocca E, Calero C, Cassinari V (1954) A new method for testing hearing in temporal lobe tumours. *Acta Otolayngologica* 44:219–221.

Cohen W, Hodson A, O'Hare A *et al.* (2005) Effects of computer-based intervention through acoustically modified speech (Fast ForWord) in severe mixed receptive-expressive language impairment: outcomes from a randomized controlled trial. *Journal of Speech, Language and Hearing Research* 48:715–729.

Griffiths TD (2002) Central auditory pathologies. *Brirtish Medical Bulletin* 63:107–120.

Hayes EA, Warrier CM, Nicol TG, Zecker SG, Kraus N (2003) Integration of heard and seen speech: a factor in learning disabilities in children. *Neuroscience Letters* 351:46–50.

Hinchcliffe R (1992) King–Kopetzky syndrome: an auditory stress disorder? *Journal of Audiological Medicine* 1:89–98.

Jerger J, Musiek F (2000) Report of the consensus conference on the diagnosis of auditory processing disorders in school-aged children. *Journal of the American Academy of Audiology* 11:467–474.

Kujala T, Karma K, Ceponiene R *et al.* (2001) Plastic neural changes and reading improvement caused by audiovisual training in reading-impaired children. *Proceedings of the National Academy of Sciences of the USA* 98: 10509–10514.

Mahncke HW, Connor BB, Appelman J *et al.* (2006) Memory enhancement in healthy older adults using a brain plasticity-based training program: a randomized, controlled study. *Proceedings of the National Academy of Sciences of the USA* 103:12523–12528.

Meister H, von Wedel H, Walger M (2004) Psychometric evaluation of children with suspected auditory processing disorders (APDs) using a parent-answered survey. *International Journal of Audiology* 43:431–437.

Merzenich MM, Jenkins WM, Johnston P *et al.* (1996) Temporal processing deficits of language-learning impaired children ameliorated by training. *Science* 271:77–81.

Moore DR, Rosenberg JF, Coleman JS (2005) Discrimination training of phonemic contrasts enhances phonological processing in mainstream school children. *Brain and Language* 94:72–85.

Musiek FE, Oxholm VB (2000) Anatomy and physiology of the central auditory nervous system: a clinical perspective. In: Roeser RJ, Valente M, Hosford-Dunn H, eds. *Audiology: diagnosis*, pp 45–72. New York: Thieme Medical Publishers.

Myklebust H (1954) *Auditory Disorders in Children*. New York: Grune and Stratton.

Neijenhuis K, Snik A, van den Broek P (2003) Auditory processing disorders in adults and children: evaluation of a test battery. *International Journal of Audiology* 42:391–400.

Putter-Katz H, Said LAB, Feldman I *et al.* (2002) Treatment and evaluation indices of auditory processing disorders. *Seminars in Hearing* 23:357–364.

Russo NM, Nicol TG, Zecker SG, Hayes EA, Kraus N (2005) Auditory training improves neural timing in the human brainstem. *Behavioural Brain Research* 156:95–103.

Smoski WJ, Brunt MA, Tannahill JC (1992) Listening characteristics of children with central auditory processing disorders. *Language, Speech and Hearing Services in Schools* 23:145–152.

Tallal P, Miller SL, Bedi G *et al.* (1996) Language comprehension in language-learning impaired children improved with acoustically modified speech. *Science* 271:81–84.

Temple E, Deutsch GK, Poldrack RA *et al.* (2003) Neural deficits in children with dyslexia ameliorated by behavioural remediation: Evidence from fMRI. *Proceedings of the National Academy of Sciences of the USA* 100:2860–2865.

Adult audiological rehabilitation

Lucy Handscomb

23

Introduction

Hearing loss has long been known to have far-reaching effects on quality of life. Writing in the 18th century, Dr Samuel Johnson described it as 'one of the most desperate of human calamities', and modern research suggests that, for some at least, its impact can indeed be devastating. A survey of profoundly deafened adults found rates of anxiety to be two and a half times higher amongst them than in the general population, while rates of depression were nearly five times higher (Hallam *et al.*, 2005). In a detailed investigation of the experience of both moderately and profoundly hearing-impaired people, Kerr and Cowie (1997) found evidence of significant negative effects on quality of life for both groups. They observe that these effects go beyond the immediate frustrations caused by communication breakdown to include a range of deeply felt emotions. Imperfect hearing is not merely a matter of inconvenience; it has a profound effect on one's sense of wellbeing. Given the impact that deafness can have on everyday existence, the need for aural rehabilitation should be clear.

A number of definitions of the term aural rehabilitation have been proposed: it can be taken to include many different types of intervention, from hearing aid fitting to psychotherapy. Most authors agree, however, that the fundamental purpose of aural rehabilitation is to minimise the negative effects of hearing loss on a person's quality of life. One of the more succinct summaries of its aims was proposed by Hull (1992): 'to help overcome communicative, social and psychological effects of hearing loss, to reduce barriers to communication and to facilitate adjustment'.

Hearing aids clearly have the potential to improve quality of life considerably, by offering much easier access to spoken language and environmental sounds. However, their limitations are well documented, and there are few users who experience sound quality that equates to 'normal' hearing, especially in poor acoustics or noisy conditions. Even when hearing aids are optimally fitted, they only go part way towards reducing barriers to communication. Moreover, some types of deafness cannot be helped with amplification and, of those people who can benefit from hearing aids, many choose not to use them. For all these reasons, additional intervention is frequently required.

Alternative aids to communication

The advantages of hearing aids, if they are worn, can be greatly increased by using a range of additional technology. Auditory signals may be transmitted to hearing aids via direct input – with a lead running between the hearing aid and another piece of equipment – or via a telecoil, using either an infra-red, FM radio or magnetic induction loop system. Loop systems in public places (ticket counters, theatres, churches and so on) have the great advantage of enabling the hearing aid user to tune in directly to speech (or music) being transmitted through a microphone, thus cutting out background noise and eliminating the effects of distance between speaker and listener. New hearing aid users should be made fully aware of the existence of these systems, as they are not always widely advertised. A loop system at home can enable a hearing aid user to enjoy television set at a volume that is tolerable to his or her partner – an important consideration as TV volume is one of the greatest sources of tension between hearing-impaired people and their significant others. Equally, use of a personal loop or FM system may make the difference between being able to participate in a class and failing to cope with further study. With a little creative thinking, personal listening devices may be used to help individuals in a variety of situations; a taxi driver may have a car looped in order to hear clients from behind, an audio typist may use an adapted headset which links to a hearing aid, a nurse may use an amplified stethoscope and a tourist may use a radio aid to follow a guided tour. Personal loops are also available to link to modern technology such as MP3 players (Figure 23.1).

A number of people find hearing aids inadequate for listening on the telephone, either because they do not provide sufficient amplification or because it is awkward to place the receiver close to the aid without triggering feedback. A variety of solutions are available; some amplifiers

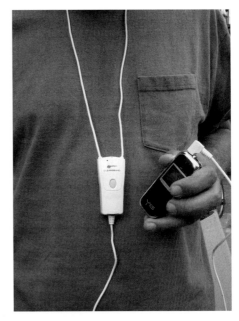

Figure 23.1 Portable loop system for MP3 player.

attach to a conventional phone (Figure 23.2), while others are integrated into a specially adapted one, meaning that incoming speech can be amplified at the touch of a button. Various devices that enable users to link hearing aids to mobile phones are also available. Patients may

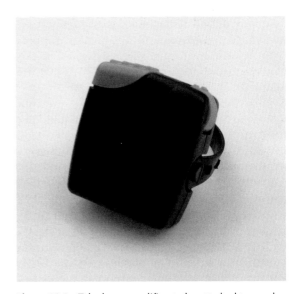

Figure 23.2 Telephone amplifier, to be attached to speaker of telephone.

well find it helpful to try out an amplified phone during a visit to audiology, and demonstration models are easy to come by. Text phones – both permanently installed and portable – may be used by those unable to hear speech even with an amplifier, and an excellent relay service is run in the UK by The Royal National Institute for Deaf People (RNID), which enables people without a text phone to talk to people with one via an operator. However, with the popularity of email, internet-based chat facilities and text messaging, the need for such technology is dwindling.

Although assistive listening devices (ALDs) such as these can make a substantial difference to quality of life, for some the introduction of new gadgets into their lives is not welcome. A questionnaire study investigating the use of ALDs amongst older people (Jerger *et al.*, 1996) found that, although subjects rated personal amplifiers with remote microphones as much clearer than hearing aids, the overwhelming majority preferred to use their hearing aids alone. ALDs were classed as too bulky, or too much bother. Younger people may have similar reactions; a qualitative study of young deaf students (Kent and Smith, 2006) identified as a common theme dislike of FM systems for being 'too much hassle'. Additionally, asking a teacher or group leader to use an ALD entails drawing attention to oneself as different, and requires a degree of assertiveness that some do not naturally possess. Support with behaviour change, discussed later in this chapter, may be needed before ALDs are adopted.

In a situation in which ALDs are not adequate, perhaps because a person does not have sufficient hearing to benefit from them, language service professionals (LSPs) are an alternative option. These people include sign language interpreters, speed typists, note takers and lip speakers (who silently voice a speaker's words in a lip-readable manner). LSPs can be booked to attend conferences, meetings or classes with a deaf person, either on a single occasion or regularly. Knowledge about these services is not particularly widespread, so audiologists can play a useful role in making people aware of them.

Inability to hear warning signals such as phones ringing, door bells, alarm clocks and smoke alarms can also be a concern, particularly for those living alone. A number of ingenious gadgets which flash brightly, activate the house lights or vibrate under the pillow at night, can help overcome some of these difficulties. Hearing dogs are an appealing alternative option for some. They are trained to respond to different sounds and alert their owners by touching them with a paw. Their benefits go beyond practical help, with many deafened owners reporting increased independence and confidence arising from the companionship the dogs offer.

Provision of ALDs, alerting devices and LSPs varies quite widely from country to country, depending on the type of disability legislation in force nationally. In general, the responsibility lies with employers and educational institutions to provide funding for any additional support needed. In some countries, a limited range of ALDs and alerting devices for domestic use is available free of charge through local social services, and audiologists can help with the application process.

Speech perception training

Regardless of their attitude towards extra technology, the majority of hearing-impaired people will be relying on hearing aids alone most of the time, and are consequently subject to all their shortcomings. The bulk of aural rehabilitation work therefore involves looking beyond technology to consider additional ways of overcoming some of the barriers imposed by hearing loss.

Those who have contact with hearing-impaired people in any capacity will be aware that most make at least some use of lip-reading in order to enhance their understanding of speech. Moreover, a number of studies (reviewed by Gagne, 1994) have indicated that normally hearing people are heavily influenced by visual speech information as well. A number of different clues can be identified on the face in addition to lip movements, and it is for this reason that many now prefer the term speech-reading to lip-reading, as a more accurate description of the skill.

Despite almost universal agreement that visual clues enhance understanding, most hearing-impaired people rate themselves as rather poor speech readers (Tye-Murray *et al.*, 1992). In reality, a wide range of speech-reading ability is revealed when formal word- and sentence-recognition tests are used (Gagne, 1994). A key question pondered by researchers is which factors account for the variation. Unfortunately, the answer remains unclear. Deaf people tend to perform better than hearing people (Bernstein *et al.*, 2001), and younger subjects better than older (Honnell *et al.*, 1991) but otherwise the correlations one might expect have not been found. Gagne (1994) summarises several studies which suggest that the degree and duration of deafness do not correlate with good speech-reading skill, nor do visual memory, intelligence or cognitive-processing style. He reports that neurophysiological differences are likely to play the largest part and these, sadly, are hard to influence.

However, this is not to say that speech-reading training is useless. In an experiment involving video training, Bernstein *et al.* (2001) reported a modest average improvement in word-identification scores, with quite large improvements for a few individuals. There is conflicting evidence from other studies, but some indication that training can result in better speech-reading ability, at least in an experimental setting.

The findings are similar for auditory training, a system that aims to enhance a hearing-impaired person's speech perception through the use of specially designed training material, which may use an analytic approach (based on phonemes and words) or a synthetic one (based on sentences and prose.) Usually, the person will be required to listen attentively to a series of exercises and repeat back what he has heard, with misheard sections being worked on in more detail. In a study involving 20 adults, Rubinstein and Boothroyd (1987) reported small but significant improvements in speech-recognition scores following eight individual auditory training sessions, and a number of other studies show similar modest improvements (Gagne, 1994). Training material in the studies varied, but whether analytic or synthetic material is used, or both, appears to make little difference (Rubinstein and Boothroyd, 1987).

Both speech-reading training and auditory training are time consuming, and an important question for clinicians is: is it worth it? What patients are actually learning from such training is rather unclear, but Gagne (1994) discusses two possibilities: they learn to extract useful information from the speech signal more effectively, or they learn to make better use of general listening strategies. Considering the latter possibility, it may be that less formal training is just as effective in teaching listening skills. In Rubinstein and Boothroyd's study (1987), all participants took part in general discussion of communication tactics as well as receiving formal auditory training, and it seems possible that this discussion was mostly responsible for the improvements noted. To investigate this idea, studies that compare formal auditory/visual training with more general communication training are needed. A further question is: what degree of improvement actually makes a difference to a person's quality of life? Does being able to speech-read a few per cent more words correctly actually enhance everyday conversation? If not, spending hours in front of a DVD machine is hardly a worthwhile exercise. Even if it does enhance conversation in ideal circumstances, is the person confident enough to ask people to speak to her in such a way as to make her new speech-reading skills usable?

Perhaps a more worthwhile approach is to look at communication from a broader point of view, and offer training in behavioural strategies that hearing-impaired people can use in real-life situations.

Behavioural strategies

Caissie and Gibson (1997) videotaped and analysed social conversations in background noise between hard-of-hearing and normally hearing people who had not previously met. They found that there were an average of 8.2 communication breakdowns per 15 minutes of conversation – an interruption to the flow every couple of minutes. Communication breakdown is a situation that is all too familiar to people with hearing loss, and inability to engage in easy, uninterrupted conversation can be regarded as one of the most frustrating aspects of deafness. Much behavioural training focuses on ways of managing or preventing communication breakdown.

Useful strategies have been categorised in a number of ways. Tye-Murray *et al.* (1992) divide them into repair (for example, asking for a repeat), corrective (changing something which is hampering conversation, such as switching off the TV) and anticipatory (preparing in advance for an upcoming situation.) Field and Haggard (1989) mention two categories: manipulating the physical environment and manipulating social interaction. However they are categorised, it is broadly agreed that a large number of possible strategies exist, but that some are used more commonly than others. Not surprisingly, Tye-Murray *et al.* (1992) found that asking for repeats is the strategy most commonly used when communication breaks down, but this is not the only strategy people are aware of. When asked to think of strategies that might be used in a variety of situations, Field and Haggard found that a group of new hearing aid users came up with an average of 5.29, which included things like sitting at the front of a hall, watching faces, and requesting clear speech, as well as asking for repeats. In the same study, however, hearing therapists were able to identify almost twice as many strategies as hearing-impaired people (including asking people not to shout and making sure there is enough light.) This suggests that the full range of strategies available is not automatically known to all people with hearing loss, and that special training can increase knowledge of these considerably.

A further purpose of training should be to increase knowledge of the most effective strategies. A study by Gagne and Wyllie (1989), in which subjects had to lip-read words on videotape, found that seeing a synonym or paraphrase of test material that had been misunderstood was more likely to result in correct identification than simply seeing it repeated. This study might be criticised for being rather artificial (when does

anyone have to lip-read single words out of context?), but the analysis of more realistic conversation by Caissie and Gibson (1997) came up with similar results. Paraphrase and confirmation of the message were the most effective strategies used. In addition, increasing the amount of semantic redundancy has been shown to enhance understanding. In other words, 'there's a variety of different choices' is more easily understood than 'there's a choice', even although not all the words in the former sentence are strictly necessary. Hearing or seeing additional words closely related in meaning to the target appears to be helpful. However, elaboration of the message (adding extra information) was found to be the least effective strategy by Caissie and Gibson, so this strategy is best avoided.

A number of different methods exist to improve people's knowledge of communication tactics, and many audiology departments hand out leaflets containing communication tips as a matter of course. It might be useful to include in this literature specific suggestions about trying less obvious strategies, such as asking people to rephrase a message. In the USA, a procedure with the acronym WATCH has been proposed by Montgomery (1994) in which audiologists advise patients to 'Watch the talker's mouth, Ask specific questions, Talk about hearing loss and Change the situation when communication is difficult' (the H stands for giving patients healthcare information). The procedure is designed to increase patients' knowledge of how to manage difficult communication situations within a short space of time. While providing information about communication tactics is important, however, it may not be adequate. Knowledge of good communication tactics does not necessarily imply use of them, because adopting them in everyday life involves changing behaviour, and this does not come easily to most of us.

Behaviour change

Much has been written about behaviour change in health psychology literature, and while most theories were developed in the context of unhealthy behaviour such as smoking, they can usefully be considered when working with hearing loss as well.

The theory of planned behaviour (Ajzen, 1985) identifies three factors that have to be in place to engender a strong intention to change: a positive attitude towards the new behaviour, a belief that the subjective norm is in favour of it (i.e. it will be approved of by others) and a high level of behavioural control (a belief that one is capable of performing it). To put this in context, knowledge about communication tactics might not be put into practice if the person believes that this misses the point: 'if only the audiologist would give me good enough hearing aids, all my problems would be solved'. Similarly, lack of support from family members or lack of confidence about making requests (such as 'please speak more slowly') reduces the likelihood of strategies being adopted. Such issues are not addressed by simply giving advice, in either written or oral form.

Even when the intention to change behaviour is strong, there remains the problem of an intention–behaviour gap. A person might go home full of determination to use better communication strategies but soon fall back into old, maladaptive ways. Gollwitzer (1993) has suggested that intentions are more likely to be carried out when specific plans are made. A plan to move to the front row at Monday's French class is more likely to be carried out than a general plan to use better positioning strategies. Much of the existing literature on audiological rehabilitation recommends using focused problem-solving strategies such as this. McKenna (1987) proposes a system of goal planning, in which the patient works towards a series of well-defined goals, graded in order of difficulty. A crucial part of goal planning is that the patient is fully involved in negotiating goals that he feels are relevant to his own life from the start, and in deciding how they might be reached.

One of the most difficult changes in behaviour for many is starting to disclose their hearing loss to other people. The instruction to 'talk about hearing loss' is given particular emphasis in the WATCH programme mentioned above, because most communication tactics cannot be used

effectively if hearing loss is not acknowledged. For some this comes naturally, but others feel awkward about admitting to hearing loss because of concerns about subjective norms; they fear that others will see them as different, talk down to them, make fun of them or give them lots of unwanted sympathy. For these reasons, it is likely that the short, one-off discussion of the advantages of disclosing hearing loss suggested within the WATCH programme will not be sufficient encouragement for a lot of people. Fear of a negative reaction will be too great a barrier.

A study by Blood and Blood (1999) demonstrated that normally hearing people actually responded more favourably to a deaf person when he acknowledged his hearing loss than when he did not. The speaker was rated as more sincere, likeable and emotionally adjusted. This suggests that, if encouraged to test out their belief that disclosure of hearing loss will result in a negative reaction, many patients will find it to be unfounded. Clinical experience backs this up. However, it is not easy for patients to take this step unsupported. Some goal planning with a clinician – considering who to disclose the hearing loss to, when would be a good time and how to word the explanation, with the opportunity for feedback afterwards – can make the behaviour change somewhat less daunting.

It can also be fruitful to challenge patients' beliefs that non-disclosure preserves an image of 'normality'. A person who frequently mishears, gives incorrect answers or ignores greetings may – if not known to have a hearing loss – be perceived as vacant, stupid or rude. Most people would prefer to be seen as deaf rather than stupid. If patients are encouraged to consider how people might be reacting to their current behaviour, a change in attitude might ensue.

Of course, it is not guaranteed that patients' fears about disclosure will prove unfounded. Many will sometimes encounter intolerant or insensitive reactions. It seems important for patients to be prepared for dealing with these, and rehearsal during an appointment of possible responses can be a useful strategy. An opportunity simply to talk about a negative encounter afterwards may also help the patient see it in perspective and move away from 'all or nothing thinking'. Just because one person reacted insensitively does not mean that the next will.

However, aural rehabilitation specialists are sometimes so keen to promote acknowledgement of hearing loss that they ignore the fact that non-disclosure can sometimes be a valid choice. In Blood and Blood's study (1999), the speaker was obviously deaf – he had a visible hearing aid – and people respected him for acknowledging this. But no comparison was made between attitudes towards him and towards somebody not seen to have a disability at all. The latter may have engendered even more favourable attitudes. Despite disability discrimination legislation, it is sadly likely that some employers have, on occasions, appointed a normally hearing person over someone equally qualified who has declared himself or herself deaf; it is all too easy to give other reasons for the choice. Hearing-impaired people have to operate in a prejudiced society, and if non-disclosure sometimes helps them to progress, it should not always be discouraged. A further consideration is that people with hearing loss do not always feel like talking about it. Perhaps our aim, then, should not be to enable people to acknowledge hearing loss in all circumstances, but to enable them to make a choice based on rational thinking rather than be guided by cognitive distortions and anxieties.

Hearing aid use

Of course, choosing to wear visible hearing aids entails acknowledging deafness (even if not verbally), and reluctance to acknowledge it can be a reason behind not wearing them. Non-use of prescribed hearing instruments is common. For example, Gianopoulos *et al.* (2002) conducted a long-term follow-up study on 116 hearing aid patients (none of whom had received post-fitting support), and found that 57% had stopped using their aids eight to sixteen years after fitting. Additionally, many adults who could benefit from hearing aids do not take steps to obtain them (Kochkin and Rogin, 2000). Embarrassment and concerns about how they might be

perceived by others are certainly amongst the reasons for non-use (Kochkin and Rogin, 2000). Other reasons include discomfort and handling difficulties (Gianopoulos *et al.*, 2002) and lack of perceived handicap (Humes *et al.*, 2003). There is a clear need for rehabilitation to pay attention to these factors.

In older people, there can be an additional barrier of lack of appropriate help from carers. In a survey of a typical American nursing home, Cohen-Mansfield and Taylor (2004) reported that 86% of residents needed help using their hearing aids, but that the majority of staff had received no training in basic hearing aid use and maintenance whatsoever, meaning that most hearing aids went unused. This regrettable situation appears to be widespread in other countries too. An important role for audiologists, which is sometimes overlooked, is to provide education for care staff who will come across actual and potential hearing aid users frequently. This might best be done via outreach visits to local residential facilities.

When dealing with psychological barriers, many rehabilitation specialists promote the use of extra patient contact in addition to basic hearing aid fitting and orientation. Discussions might address issues such as unrealistic expectations, altered self-perception and concerns about the reactions of others. Clinical experience suggests that discussion geared towards modifying attitudes towards hearing aids and feelings about wearing them in front of other people results in increased use, but there is surprisingly little research on the subject. A study by Brooks (1981) suggests that counselling does increase hearing aid use but he does not specify what type of counselling was used, and the method of measuring hours of aid use (battery consumption) is not particularly reliable. Eriksson-Mangold *et al.* (1990) report on the Swedish 'active fitting' programme, in which patients have a number of visits to the hearing centre, with structured tasks to complete at home between them, and plenty of opportunity for feedback. The aim is 'to provide a realistic picture of hearing aid use at an early stage', and participants were found to be more positive about their hearing aids, use them more often and feel more psychologically secure with them than controls. One of the principles of the programme is that, when fully supported in the adoption of new behaviour, people are more likely to maintain it. Working on similar principles, Laplante-Levesque *et al.* (2006) made daily email contact with three new hearing aid users to offer support and answers to questions. This study was qualitative and the results are not generalisable, but the response of participants was positive and the idea seems worth exploring further.

Rehabilitation groups

A difficulty with such intensive support programmes is that they are very time consuming. Rehabilitation groups are often promoted as a more time-efficient alternative, whether the goal is to encourage hearing aid use or adoption of communication tactics, or both. A number of possible group formats exist (intensive weekends or weekly meetings, large numbers or small), and a variety of activities may be included such as information sharing about hearing loss and hearing aids, practice with aid manipulation and cleaning, relaxation exercises, lip-reading instruction and communication practice. Whatever the design, most have as a common aim empowerment of the participants, and active problem solving is a central theme. In their writing on health behaviour change, Rollnick *et al.* (1999) are very clear that new behaviours are far more likely to be implemented when ideas about how to adopt them are generated by patients themselves, because there is then a sense of ownership. A number of different group rehabilitation programmes have been described, and most of these stress the importance of enabling participants to come up with their own solutions to communication problems. Scenarios are discussed or role-played and, rather than being advised by the group leader, participants suggest or act out alternative behaviours themselves. Studies comparing this type of interactive behaviour modification with straightforward advice giving in

audiology are lacking, but some investigations of interactive group rehabilitation (for example, Andersson *et al.*, 1995) do report improved use of communication tactics as key outcomes.

Of course, it is not only people with hearing loss who need to change their behaviour in order to communicate more effectively, but also their common communication partners. Simply giving information to patients to pass on to those at home does not seem to be particularly effective; Hetu *et al.* (1993) report on a study in which the majority of normally hearing partners did not think they had been given an explanation by their hearing-impaired partners following a clinic visit, even although most of the latter group stated that they had given one. A more successful approach is that suggested by Borg *et al.* (2002), who train hard-of-hearing group participants to be 'communication counsellors', and equip them with appropriate skills to express their needs to others. The big advantage here is that as many people as the participant wishes can be given their explanation. More commonly, however, significant others are invited to attend group rehabilitation themselves, enabling them to participate in the problem-solving process directly. This approach also goes some way towards addressing significant others' own difficulties. Hetu *et al.* (1993) discuss the fact that too often significant others are viewed solely as supporters, and that there can even be an 'implicit coalition' between the clinician and hearing-impaired person, who both try to persuade the partner to be more helpful. They argue that this can result in frustration within the relationship, because it does not acknowledge the partner's very real feelings of weariness at having to repeat so much, or resentment at missing out on social activities. Some programmes, such as the LINK scheme for deafened adults in the UK, run specific partners-only sessions, designed to address these emotions.

For both hearing-impaired people and their significant others, then, rehabilitation groups are not just about encouraging behaviour change, but also about dealing with emotional reactions to deafness. The reported benefits go beyond better strategy use to include reduction of perceived levels of 'handicap' and improved personal adjustment (Hawkins, 2005). In other words, it is not simply a case of managing the problem better, but of feeling better about the problem. It should be noted, however, that the evidence available so far indicates that such emotional changes tend to be rather modest. Furthermore, some work has indicated that participation in a rehabilitation group can lead to more awareness of the restrictions imposed by hearing loss. But this does not mean that groups are not providing significant emotional help. Hawkins (2005) argues that in some cases, levels of 'handicap' may not actually be reduced, but the person may learn to cope better emotionally with the reality of having a disability. The emotional benefits of being amongst others with similar problems and of fully acknowledging difficulties have not been thoroughly explored.

Individual therapy

While groups have many advantages, it should be acknowledged that they may not be the best way to address problems associated with deafness for every person. Some individuals are not 'group people', while others may feel that they do not fit in because their deafness is more severe than others', or they are older or younger, or single while everyone else is with a partner. It may also be that group members start out at different stages of change.

A 'stages of change' model was proposed by Prochaska and Di Clemente in 1982. This suggests that making a change involves five stages: precontemplation, contemplation, preparation, action and maintenance, and Di Clemente (1991) suggests adapting one's consultation style to suit whichever stage the patient is in. Although it might be assumed that patients attend audiology because they have decided things need to change, many are in fact persuaded by family members to attend (Wilson and Stephens, 2003) and may see no need to modify their communication behaviour at all; 'if only people wouldn't mumble, things would be fine'. Such people may simply not be ready to join a group that focuses on

changing behaviour. Rollnick *et al.* (1999) reject the idea of discrete stages, but do suggest asking patients to rate their readiness to change on a numerical scale. For those who do not feel themselves to be ready at all, information can be exchanged and the door left open to discuss the behaviour further later on. An option might be given to simply discuss the frustration felt when parts of conversation are missed, without any pressure to take action. If some readiness to change is expressed, the authors describe how this can be used to open further discussion of what factors might make change achievable. A skilled practitioner should be able to identify at what point a person is ready to start taking action, and consider whether a group might help them to do this.

As a further step, Rollnick *et al.* (1999) suggest asking patients to rate the importance they place on changing behaviour and their confidence in their ability to do so, the point being that importance and confidence need to be quite high in order for change to occur. If either or both are low, then the practitioner's first task is to help the patient find ways of increasing them. If a patient sees no point in learning communication tactics because he has stopped socialising anyway, a well-meaning audiologist may give guidance in them regardless, in the hope that this will make him see that there are ways of problem solving in such situations. However, this is unlikely to strengthen the patient's belief in their importance. It may be more fruitful to begin by discussing why social activities have been given up, what he misses about them, how he thinks others perceive his hearing aid, whether a few bad experiences have coloured his whole perception, and so on. This may then sow the seeds of the idea that change is possible.

Counselling

The approach described above, although designed to be used during brief consultations, has much in common with several schools of counselling. In his work on client-centred counselling, Egan (2002) describes a three-stage process which moves from exploring problems to considering possible solutions, to working out how to reach the solutions identified. In an alternative model, cognitive behavioural therapy, negative thoughts that lie behind negative emotions are identified before any behavioural modification is attempted. What all these approaches have in common is an emphasis on understanding one's perception of problems before trying to solve them. Practitioners should be wary of jumping too hastily into problem-solving mode, whether patients are seen in groups, or individually, or a combination of both. Simply allowing patients to talk through difficult feelings (for example, why is it so upsetting when people say 'oh, it doesn't matter!' when something is misheard?), before moving on to work on solutions can be enormously beneficial. Most audiologists are not trained in any particular school of counselling, it is not clear which approach is best suited to audiology, and few clinics have the capacity to offer full-scale counselling anyway. However, techniques that are common to all types of counselling, such as the establishment of a good therapeutic relationship and use of active listening skills, seem to be more predictive of a positive outcome than adherence to any particular model (Josefowitz and Myran, 2005), so a good knowledge of counselling skills will in itself be useful in helping patients explore and understand their difficulties.

Even when patients are already quite effective problem solvers, they may still experience emotional difficulties. There are emotional effects of communication breakdown; it is not just a matter of being inconvenienced but of feeling embarrassed, ashamed or undermined (Danermark, 1998). Even when a person uses several tactics for repairing breakdowns successfully, it may not stop him or her from feeling awkward about having to use them. Equally, husbands who are in the good habit of turning off the television before speaking to their hearing-impaired wives may still feel resentment at having to do so. Hallam *et al.* (2007) found that distressed profoundly deafened people knew how to use adaptive communication tactics as well as the more emotionally stable, but tended to avoid situations in which they needed to. There really is no 'technique' for accepting hearing loss, but good

counselling can help people feel more at ease with it in their own way. Although audiologists are not counsellors – and indeed need to be wary of straying beyond their boundaries – there are occasions on which listening attentively, understanding and offering support will yield more benefits to the patient than any number of technical adjustments to hearing aids.

Conclusion

The needs of hearing-impaired adults are far-reaching, and the audiologist requires more than technical expertise in order to address them adequately. Teaching, group facilitation and counselling skills are important, along with a sound knowledge of communication tactics and a basic grasp of certain psychological principles. Such things should form an integral part of every audiologist's training. It is only by considering the person behind the hearing impairment that successful rehabilitation can be achieved.

References

Ajzen I (1985). From intention to actions: a theory of planned behaviour. In: Kuhl J, Beckman J, eds. *Action-control: from cognition to behaviour*, pp 11–39. Heidelberg: Springer.

Andersson G, Melin L, Scott B, Lindberg P (1995) An evaluation of a behavioural treatment approach to hearing impairment. *Behaviour Research and Therapy* 33:283–292.

Bernstein L, Auer E, Tucker P (2001) Enhanced speech reading in deaf adults: can short-term training/practice close the gap for hearing adults? *Journal of Speech, Language and Hearing Research* 44:5–18.

Blood I, Blood G (1999) Effects of acknowledging a hearing loss on social interactions. *Journal of Communication Disorders* 32:109–120.

Borg E, Danermark B, Borg B (2002) Behavioural awareness, interaction and counselling education in audiological rehabilitation:

development of methods and application in a pilot study. *International Journal of Audiology* 41:308–320.

Brooks D (1981) Use of post-aural aids by national health service patients. *British Journal of Audiology* 15:79–86.

Caissie R, Gibson C (1997) The effectiveness of repair strategies used by people with hearing losses and their conversational partners. *The Volta Review* 99:203–218.

Cohen-Mansfield J, Taylor J (2004) Hearing aid use in nursing homes. Part 2: Barriers to effective utilization of hearing aids. *Journal of the American Medical Directors Association* 5:289–296.

Danermark B (1998) Hearing impairment, emotions and audiological rehabilitation: a sociological perspective. *Scandinavian Audiology* 27(suppl 49):125–131.

DiClemente C (1991) Motivational interviewing and the stages of change. In: Miller W, Rollnick S, eds. *Motivational Interviewing: preparing people to change addictive behaviour*, pp 191–202. London: Guildford Press.

Egan G (2002) *The Skilled Helper: a problem-management and opportunity-development approach to helping*, 7th edn. California: Brooks/ Cole

Eriksson-Mangold M, Ringdahl A, Bjorklund A-K, Wahlin B (1990) The active fitting programme of hearing aids: a psychological perspective. *British Journal of Audiology* 24:277–285.

Field D, Haggard M (1989) Knowledge of hearing tactics: (1) assessment by questionnaire and inventory. *British Journal of Audiology* 23:349–354.

Gagne J-P (1994) Visual and audiovisual speech perception training: basic and applied research needs. *Journal of the Academy of Rehabilitative Audiology* Monograph Supplement XXVII:133–159.

Gagne, J-P, Wyllie K (1989) Relative effectiveness of three repair strategies on the visual-identification of misperceived words. *Ear and Hearing* 10:368–374.

Gianopoulos I, Stephens D, Davis A (2002) Follow up of people fitted with hearing aids after adult hearing screening: the need for support after fitting. *British Medical Journal* 325:471.

Gollwitzer P (1993). Goal achievement: the role of intentions. In: Strober W, Hewstone M, eds. *European Review of Social Psychology* 4:141–185.

Hallam R, Ashton P, Sherbourne K, Gailey L, Corney R (2007) Coping, conversation tactics and marital interaction in persons with acquired profound hearing loss: correlates of distress. *Audiological Medicine* 5:103–111.

Hallam R, Sherbourne K, Ashton P *et al.* (2005) *Hidden Lives: the psychological and social impact of becoming deafened in adult life (summary report)*. Eastbourne: The Link Centre for Deafened People.

Hawkins D (2005) Effectiveness of counseling-based adult group aural rehabilitation programs: a systematic review of the evidence. *Journal of the American Academy of Audiology* 16:485–493.

Hetu R, Jones L, Getty L (1993) The impact of acquired hearing impairment on intimate relationships: implications for rehabilitation. *Audiology* 32:363–381.

Honnell S, Dancer J, Gentry B (1991) Age and speechreading performance in relation to percent correct, eyeblinks, and written responses. *The Volta Review* 93:207–231.

Hull R (1992) *Aural Rehabilitation: serving children and adults*. Australia: Singular Thomson Learning.

Humes L, Wilson D, Humes A (2003) Examination of differences between successful and unsuccessful elderly hearing aid candidates matched for age, hearing loss and gender. *International Journal of Audiology* 42:432–441.

Jerger J, Chmiel R, Florin E, Pirozzolo F, Wilson N (1996) Comparison of conventional amplification and an assistive listening device in elderly persons. *Ear and Hearing* 17:490–504.

Josefowitz N, Myran D (2005). Towards a person-centred cognitive behaviour therapy. *Counselling Psychology Quarterly* 18:329–336.

Kent B, Smith S (2006) They only see it when the sun shines in my ears: exploring perceptions of adolescent hearing aid users. *Journal of Deaf Studies and Deaf Education* 11:461–476.

Kerr P, Cowie R (1997) Acquired deafness: a multidimensional experience. *British Journal of Audiology* 31:177–188.

Kochkin S, Rogin C (2000) Quantifying the obvious: the impact of hearing instruments on the quality of life. *Hearing Review* 7:6–34.

Laplante-Levesque A, Pichora-Fuller M, Gagne J-P (2006) Providing an internet-based audiological counselling programme to new hearing aid users: a qualitative study. *International Journal of Audiology* 45:697–706.

McKenna L (1987) Goal planning in audiological rehabilitation. *British Journal of Audiology* 21:5–11.

Montgomery A (1994) WATCH: a practical approach to brief auditory rehabilitation. *The Hearing Journal* 47:52–55.

Prochaska J, DiClemente C (1982) Transtheoretical therapy: toward a more integrative model of change. *Psychotherapy: Theory, Research and Practice* 19:276–288.

Rollnick S, Mason P, Butler C (1999) *Health Behaviour Change: a guide for practitioners.* London: Churchill Livingstone.

Rubinstein A, Boothroyd A (1987) Effect of two approaches to auditory training on speech recognition by hearing-impaired adults. *Journal of Speech and Hearing Research* 30:153–160.

Tye-Murray N, Purdy S, Woodworth G (1992) Reported use of communication strategies by SHHH members: client, talker and situational variables. *Journal of Speech and Hearing Research* 35:708–717.

Wilson C, Stephens D (2003) Reasons for referral and attitudes toward hearing aids: do they affect outcome? *Clinical Otolaryngology and Allied Sciences* 28:81–84.

Disorders of balance

Peter Rea

24

Introduction

The latter half of the 20th century saw dramatic advances in our understanding and treatment of sensorineural hearing loss, as anyone who has read earlier editions of this book will recognise. The inclusion of a chapter on vestibular disorders for the first time in this seventh edition reflects the dawning of a new age in the management of patients with balance disorders. It is an exciting field to work in and one that is truly multidisciplinary.

Epidemiology

It is estimated that 30% of the UK population experience symptoms of imbalance or dizziness before the age of 65 years, and 25% of adults have 'significant' dizziness at any one time (Nazareth et al., 1999). Indeed dizziness and imbalance are the commonest reasons patients beyond the age of 75 years visit their doctor. Yet, in a London-based study only 1% of those consulting their doctor had had vestibular physio-therapy, which has been shown to be a very effective treatment for many vestibular disorders (Nazareth et al., 1999).

In contrast, vestibular vertigo was reported to have a lifetime prevalence of 7.8% in a study using the highly respected German Health Questionnaire (Neuhauser et al., 2005). In 80% of those affected, distress and disability were sufficient to interrupt daily life or lead to sick leave.

Definitions

Vertigo, dizziness and disequilibrium are terms that patients and even clinicians sometimes use interchangeably, but they have quite different meanings. Vertigo is defined as the *illusion of movement*. It may be a rotary, falling or even floating sensation. It usually arises from a peripheral vestibular disorder. Dizziness, in contrast, is a non-specific term which needs to be explored in more detail with the patient. Disequilibrium indicates a loss of balance or coordination while walking or standing, and has a multitude of causes.

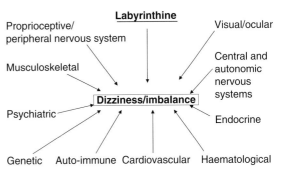

Figure 24.1 Systems that can affect balance.

Pathophysiology

Patients with dizziness can present an enormous diagnostic challenge in clinic. In patients with vestibular disorders it is common to find that one symptom (dizziness) may have several causes in the same patient – the reverse of normal medical training where one diagnosis is sought to fit several symptoms. Their symptoms are often wide ranging and non-specific (Box 24.1), and physical and psychological factors almost invariably interweave. Yet, by identifying whether their problems originate from one of three key areas in the sensorimotor control of balance (Box 24.2), over 90% of patients can be successfully diagnosed, and management pathways initiated. Non-vestibular causes also need to be considered (Figure 24.1).

The three key sensory systems that contribute to the maintenance of balance and posture are: vestibular, visual, and somatosensory.

Vestibular input derives from displacement of steriocilia bathed in the fluid-filled semicircular canals, and the utricle and the saccule of the inner ear. Displacement of fluid in the semicircular canals is caused by stimulation from *angular* movement (for example turning the head to one side), deflecting the cupula at the end of the canal and triggering neuronal impulses from the underlying hair cells (cristae ampullaris). The saccule and utricle, in contrast, recognise *linear* acceleration and *gravity* – the displacement of the otoliths (calcium crystals) triggering neural stimulation. Misplacement of these calcium crystals into the semicircular canals is a possible cause of benign positional paroxysmal vertigo (BPPV).

Visual input derives from smooth pursuit (slowly following a moving object), saccadic (refixing on a new target), and optokinetic (sensing movement in the peripheral vision such as travelling on a train looking out of the window) stimuli. Over-reliance on the visual inputs to balance causes visual (or 'supermarket') vertigo and is very common.

Somatosensory input results from pressure and joint proprioception. In peripheral neuropathies, patients struggle particularly to walk in the dark or on uneven surfaces.

Impulses from the labyrinth travel along the superior and inferior vestibular branches of the 8th cranial nerve to the vestibular nuclei, the cerebellum, midbrain and cerebral cortex, to develop conscious spatial awareness. Here information is *integrated* with inputs from the eyes and somatosensory stimuli. Anything disrupting this *central processing*, be it structural within the brain, physiological or psychological, can and will disrupt recovery from a balance disorder, and needs identifying (Figure 24.1).

Assessing visual–vestibular interaction is central to assessing the dizzy patient, as disruption of the reflexes between these two systems is the commonest cause of chronic dizziness. The *vestibulo-ocular reflex* (VOR) stabilises gaze when the head is turning and vision fixed. Head movement triggers impulses from the inner ear, which are processed centrally and result in compensatory movement of the eyes. This is the critical reflex in the dizzy patient. To appreciate the accuracy of the VOR, it is worth holding your thumb out in front of you and trying to watch it as you move it quickly from side to side. This is pure visual tracking, and gaze cannot fully be stabilised. Holding your thumb out again but this time turning your head as quickly as possible from side to side, it should be possible to maintain good visual fixation on the thumb. This is a result of the VOR.

Loss of vestibular function in one ear causes nystagmus towards the opposite ear, and veering towards the affected ear while walking. Compensation to such an injury starts with spontaneous nystagmus resolving as static suppression occurs, and is usually followed over weeks by rebalancing of central neuronal activity on head movement as the VOR adjusts. Failure of this latter mechanism is the major cause of chronic dizziness. But it can be treated!

Investigations

While many patients with vertigo or dizziness can be diagnosed without the need for investigation, specialist investigations can both aid diagnosis and better tailor treatment to an individual's needs.

Audiometry should be performed on all patients with a suspected vestibular disorder. It is particularly helpful in Ménière's disease, where a classical low-frequency sensorineural hearing

loss may be seen. It may also aid screening of those patients requiring magnetic resonance imaging (MRI) scanning to exclude acoustic neuroma.

Video nystagmography (VNG) and *electro nystagmography* (ENG) both assess eye movements in dark (with no optic fixation) and light environments. This may help distinguish between central and peripheral vestibular disorders, and the side of the lesion. While these tests are available in specialist balance centres, the use of simple infra-red goggles to observe eye movements without optic fixation should be considered a minimum requirement in any assessment of vestibular disorders beyond primary care.

A foam square for the patient to stand on will remove proprioception, and closing the eyes will remove visual inputs to balance, thus leaving the patient reliant on vestibular function. This is a very helpful screening tool, and is termed *the clinical test of sensory interaction and balance* (CTSIB). A more sophisticated way of analysing balance to help diagnosis and treatment planning is provided by *computerised dynamic posturography*. Both the floor and walls of this test booth may move with the patient (Figure 24.2). This allows detailed analysis of the interaction of the three main components of balance as well as assessments of reflex speeds, posture and centre of gravity.

Caloric testing completes the traditional test package. Irrigating the ears with warm and cold air or water, and recording the resulting nystagmus, allows a crude comparison of function between the two labyrinths. It is particularly useful prior to potentially destructive treatment of one ear (for example gentamicin instillation for Ménière's disease), as it is critical that good vestibular function is present in the non-treated ear.

Vestibular disorders

Vestibular conditions may usefully be divided into those that occur as recurrent episodes of vertigo *versus* those that cause chronic dizziness

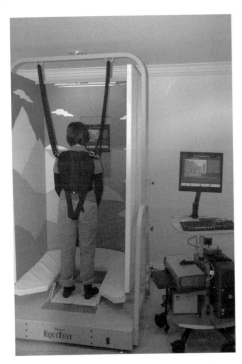

Figure 24.2 Computerised dynamic posturography.

or imbalance. The time scale of each episode and the associated neuro-otological symptoms hold the keys to diagnosis. BPPV, Ménière's disease and migraine account for the vast majority of cases of recurrent vertigo presenting to a balance clinic, while chronic vestibulopathy following vestibular neuronitis is the most common cause of chronic vestibular symptoms.

Recurrent vertigo of vestibular origin

Benign positional paroxysmal vertigo

BPPV is the most common cause of vertigo. Over 2% of people will experience it at some time in their life. It is usually a self-limiting problem lasting on average 2 weeks, but clusters may last from hours to years. Relapses are common. Intense unpleasant spinning is usually described, lasting less than a minute. While patients may claim to be 'dizzy' all day, the actual vertigo is of short duration. Spins are triggered by specific

head movement: rolling over in bed, getting up in the morning, and looking up are the classical triggers.

Aetiology

BPPV results from damage to the inner ear from a multitude of causes, so often co-exists with other inner ear disorders: common causes include head injury, vestibular neuronitis, and ageing. It seems also to occur after periods of lying flat, for example after surgical convalescence or holidays spent in deck chairs.

BPPV is most widely believed to result from *canalolithiasis*: calcium-containing particles (the otoliths) are displaced from the utricle into the semicircular canals. Here the provoking head movements lead to movement of the debris in the canals, which in turn cause movement of endolymph and so displacement of the cupula, triggering vertigo. The debris most commonly collects in the posterior semicircular canal, probably due to gravity. Debris may also less commonly stick to the cupula itself, producing *cupulolithiasis*. This produces a different Dix–Hallpike test result with no latent period observed.

Diagnosis

BPPV is diagnosed on the history and the Dix–Hallpike test (Figure 24.3). The patient is positioned seated with their head turned 30° to the right and then positioned flat on their back with the head extended 0–30° over the end of the couch – neck extension is not absolutely necessary. Posterior canal BPPV is most common, and after a latent period of 2–5 s induces torsional, upbeat, geotropic (the upper pole of the eye turns to the ground) nystagmus on dropping the head to the side of the affected ear. The patient will feel this distressing. The nystagmus fades within 30 s. Repeating the test leads to reduction of the nystagmus (fatiguing). The head is then turned through 90° to assess the opposite ear. Ageotropic (the upper pole of the eye beating away from the ground) nystagmus may be observed if the source of the BPPV is the opposite ear. A lack of distress, persistent nystagmus, lack of a latent period, absence of fatiguability, or deviation

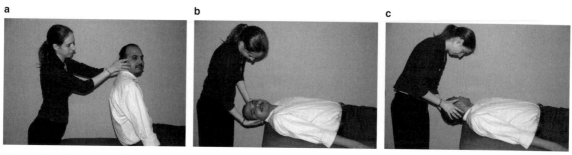

Figure 24.3 The Dix–Hallpike manoeuvre. **a**, After explaining the procedure, the patient is positioned on the examination couch facing away from the examiner, with their head turned 45° to the right. **b**, They are then smoothly dropped back, so their head is between horizontal and 30° below the horizontal when lying flat, care being taken in those with a history of neck disorders. One of the patient's eyelids is held open to observe nystagmus, and the patient reassured that any vertigo should quickly settle. Their head is firmly supported by the examiner. **c**, Their head is then turned left through 90°, and nystagmus again carefully sought. It is not usually necessary to sit the patient upright between testing the right and left ear. They are then sat back up to the sitting position.

from torsional, upbeat, geotropic nystagmus must raise the possibility of a central aetiology.

Variations may be observed. In approximately 10% of cases, posterior canal BPPV may be bilateral, and so geotropic nystagmus is seen on both left and right Dix–Hallpike's testing.

Less commonly, the debris may lie in the superior canal (figures of 0–20% are quoted), and in this case downbeat torsional nystagmus is induced. The lateral canal may also be affected in 1% of cases. To test for lateral canal BPPV, the patient is positioned lying flat on their back with the head turned 90° left and then 90° right: horizontal geotropic nystagmus is usually seen on the affected side.

All patients should have an audiogram. Atypical nystagmus on Dix–Hallpike's test, or failure to respond to treatment, may mandate MRI imaging of the internal acoustic meati.

Treatment

If an episode is self-limiting, no treatment may be required. For ongoing BPPV, a number of *particle-repositioning manoeuvres* have been described. The most widely used is the Epley manoeuvre (Epley, 1992) (Figure 24.4). First described in the early 1990s, its use has become widespread more recently. There are few medical therapies offering such rapid, safe and dramatic improvement in quality of life. This simple out-

patient procedure is well tolerated and leads to resolution of BPPV in approximately 70% of patients after one treatment session, and 90% after two. However 30% of patients will go on to experience relapses. This is most common in those whose BPPV resulted from head injury. The patient should be instructed not to lie flat for 48 h after the procedure, sleeping either in an armchair or with four pillows.

Brandt–Daroff exercises (Brandt and Daroff, 1980) (Figure 24.5) are an alternative technique that is useful in more elderly patients who cannot manage the movements of the Epley manoeuvre. They are also helpful in those whose BPPV is only partly treated by an Epley manoeuvre, and 'mop up' residual crystals. Patients are instructed to undertake the exercises three times in each position two or three times a day for two weeks. Success is achieved in 60% of treatments.

Lateral canal BPPV is treated with the glamorously named *'BBQ' manoeuvre*. The patient is log rolled in 90° steps through 360°.

For the tiny minority of patients with posterior canal BPPV who fail to respond to particle repositioning and whose BPPV remains very troublesome, *posterior semicircular canal occlusion surgery* is available. A cortical mastoidectomy is drilled and the posterior canal carefully exposed with a diamond burr before being

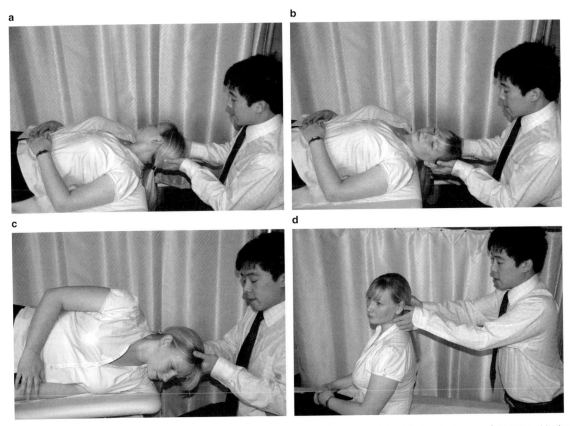

Figure 24.4 Right Epley particle-repositioning procedure. This procedure treats right-sided posterior canal BPPV. **a**, Having identified a positive right Dix–Hallpike's test, your patient will be lying horizontally with their head turned 45° to the right (the affected ear) and extended 0–30° over the end of the couch. Wait until all nystagmus and dizziness settle. **b**, Rotate the head through 90° to the left. Wait briefly and observe any nystagmus. **c**, Roll your patient onto their left shoulder, turning their head through a further 90° to the left so they will now be facing down at 45°. Intense dizziness may occur in this step. Wait for it to settle. **d**, Now sit your patient up quickly and tuck their chin just below the horizontal while supporting their back as there is often a feeling of being pushed backwards. They should not lie flat for 48 h. Repeat at one week if required.

packed with bone dust and wax. There is a small risk of imbalance and hearing loss following surgery.

Ménière's disease

In 1861, Prosper Ménière gave his name to a syndrome of paroxysmal hearing loss, tinnitus, vomiting and vertigo, which he believed arose from the inner ear. His main achievement was in linking hearing (the cochlea) to balance (the vestibular apparatus). The term *Ménière's disease* is traditionally used when no other disease process is identified, while *Ménière's syndrome* is used to describe the symptom complex when there are identifiable triggers. *Endolymphatic hydrops* is a term sometimes used synonymously, describing the fluid build-up within the scala media and endolymphatic sac, believed to be a pathological marker of the condition.

The prevalence of Ménière's disease may be approximately 0.2% of the population, although recent reports have quoted as high as 0.51% (Neuhauser, 2007). Both sexes are affected and patients typically develop symptoms between 20 and 60 years of age.

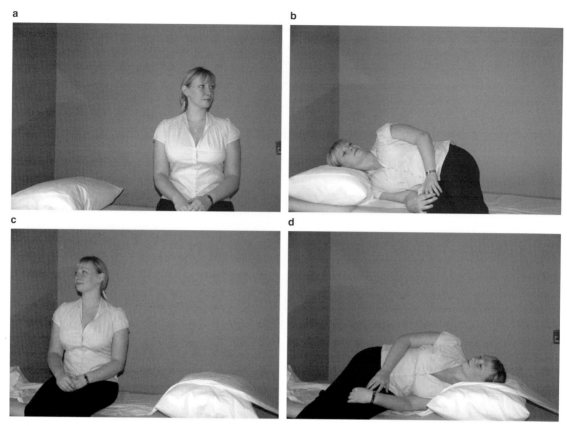

Figure 24.5 Brandt–Daroff exercises. **a**, Sit up on edge of bed with head turned 45° to the left; **b**, lie horizontally to the right with head turned up at 45°. Wait for one minute or until dizziness subsides; **c**, sit upright again before turning head 45° to the right. Wait one minute or until dizziness subsides; **d**, now lie horizontally on the left with head turned up at 45°. Wait for one minute or until dizziness subsides. Return to step **a** and repeat three times each way, 2–3 times per day, for 2 weeks.

Aetiology

The symptoms have traditionally been ascribed to an endolymph build-up in the cochlea and vestibular labyrinth. A helpful theory states that as the pressure of endolymph builds up, the membranes of the inner ear distort, causing tinnitus, hearing loss, and aural fullness in the affected ear. Then, as the pressure releases through *longitudinal flow* to the endolymphatic sac, vertigo ensues before symptoms stabilise. Alternatively, some believe that *radial flow* may occur when the pressure in the endolymph builds up and the membranes rupture between endolymph and perilymph. This dramatic event might explain Tumarkin drop attacks. However, more recent evidence suggests that this endolymphatic hydrops is itself a result of disordered fluid homeostasis within the labyrinth and it is no more than a marker for a more subtle pathological process: it may therefore not necessarily be the hydrops causing the symptoms (Merchant *et al.*, 2005). The search for the cellular abnormalities is ongoing and has already led to exciting, less invasive new treatments for Ménière's disease.

There are genetic associations (there is a family history in 10%), and attacks can certainly be triggered by stress and dietary aberrations (especially a high-salt meal). There is increasing evidence for a role for allergy, and there is a strong overlap with autoimmune inner ear disease in some patients. Infective and endocrine associations are also described.

Diagnosis

The history and the audiogram are the most helpful tools. Symptoms are unilateral in most patients initially but become bilateral eventually in 30–50%. It is a relapsing disease with attacks occurring in clusters that are sometimes interspersed by months or years without attacks. A classical attack consists of a build-up of pressure within the ear as if on a plane (aural fullness), a low-frequency roaring or humming tinnitus, fluctuating hearing loss in the low frequencies, and distressing vertigo lasting 20 min to 8 h. Attacks are associated with nausea, often vomiting, and often diarrhoea. An audiogram at the time of the attack will usually show a low-frequency sensorineural hearing loss, which improves after the attack. As the disease progresses over months or years, the hearing in the affected ear worsens, usually leaving the patient with a flat 60–70 dB hearing loss when burnt out in severe cases.

However, the onset is often much more subtle, with only one or two of the symptoms initially present. Its severity ranges from a few episodes of dizziness, which never recur, to a life-changing series of distressing attacks over many years, leaving the patient with a profound bilateral hearing loss.

In the later stages of the disease, a small number of patients report Tumarkin 'drop attacks'. Without warning, their legs give way and they fall to the floor before rapidly recovering. The good news to report to your patient is that this usually heralds the end of the disease process, at least within 12–18 months.

Investigation should include an MRI of the internal acoustic meati, syphilis serology, serial audiometry, and caloric testing if surgical intervention is considered. Auto-immune profiling is sometimes requested. *Electrocochleography* can be helpful in cases where diagnosis is difficult. This test requires an electrode to be placed on or through the tympanic membrane to measure the electrical output of the cochlea (Chapter 7).

Treatment

The 'treatment ladder' for Ménière's disease is long, and most patients can be treated conservatively. However, the increasing popularity of trans-tympanic therapies is already significantly altering the management of this condition.

Conservative treatment may merely require an explanation of the disease process in the mildest cases. Most specialists would recommend adherence to a low-salt diet, aiming for 2.5 g of sodium per day. It is the lack of fluctuation in salt intake that seems most important. Avoidance of caffeine is also often recommended.

Pharmacological intervention in the UK typically involves beta-histine, used regularly. The evidence for its benefit is sparse but many believe it helpful, and it is a safe medicine with few side-effects beyond nausea. In patients who struggle to keep their salt intake down, a diuretic such as bendroflumethiazide is often used. Anti-emetics may be required during attacks; the buccal preparation of prochlorperazine (Buccastem) is useful as it is absorbed when placed under the upper lip, so does not have to be swallowed with the risk of being vomited up. Cinnarazine is sometimes used if nausea and dizziness persist between attacks.

Surgical approaches may commence with simple grommet insertion. Why this might help is unclear, but there are definitely patients who know when their grommet blocks and symptoms return. It has the added benefit of allowing the use of a small low-pressure pump (the Meniett Device™) that is believed to reduce endolymph build-up when applied regularly to the ear. This may be most helpful in early Ménière's, especially for those patients wanting a low-risk treatment with minimal risk to their hearing.

Two intra-tympanic treatments are very popular at present. The more conservative is the trans-tympanic instillation of *dexamethasone*, usually under a local anaesthetic. This can be performed with a long, narrow spinal needle in the outpatient clinic. Alternatively, a large Silverstein grommet with a wick can be inserted over the round window niche and dexamethasone instilled for a week. It has been claimed up to 90% of patients can be controlled with this treatment (Bolas-Aguirre *et al.*, 2007) (most 'treatments' can claim a high success rate over the short term due to the fluctuating nature of the condition, so caution is required in quoting this to patients).

Intra-tympanic *gentamicin* therapy has proved much the most successful 'new' therapy for Ménière's disease in the last two decades. Instilled in a similar manner to the steroids, the most popular protocol involves a series of injections every 1 to 2 weeks up to an initial maximum of three or four. If hearing loss or dizziness occurs, the series is interrupted. Eighty per cent of patients have their vertigo abolished, and 96% find their vertigo much reduced. There is a risk of total hearing loss in the treated ear of 5%, but many patients have some loss before embarking on this treatment. This has proved a revolutionary treatment (Chia *et al.*, 2004). Caution is required if the hearing or balance is poor in the other ear, and in bilateral disease.

Endolymphatic sac decompression is a classic, if controversial, surgical procedure for Ménière's disease. The sac is approached via a cortical mastoidectomy. Total vertigo control is typically quoted at 50%, and good control at 80%. Paradoxically for a bigger operation, it is a more conservative approach than gentamicin and has much lower risks of hearing loss or post-treatment imbalance, so may be used for bilateral disease. It seems most successful in earlier disease.

For intractable Ménière's disease, a surgical labyrinthectomy may be employed, or vestibular nerve section performed via a neurosurgical approach.

Recurrent vestibular neuronitis (see also Vestibular neuronitis)

The presentation of recurrent vertigo seeming to last hours or days is common, but often nothing can be found on examination by the time the patient is seen. However, identifying the cause of recurrent vertigo in the absence of other neuro-otological symptoms can be very difficult. It has often been diagnosed as recurrent vestibular neuronitis. The theory is that latent neurotropic viruses, particularly the herpes simplex viruses, may reactivate in a similar way as is seen with cold sores or Bell's palsy, but on the vestibular nerve. It has led to trials of antiviral agents with

limited success. It may well be that many such cases represent recurrent BPPV, vestibular migraine, or a Ménière's disease variant.

Perilymph fistula

A perilymph fistula is an abnormal communication between the fluid-filled inner ear and the air-containing middle ear. Most commonly, the communication is via a defect in the oval or round window, although congenital abnormalities of the otic capsule can occur. Erosion of the lateral semicircular canal is also seen, usually resulting from cholesteatoma or, in past years, syphilis. 'Spontaneous' perilymph fistula is a controversial diagnosis. Trauma from surgery, especially stapedectomy, or implosive or explosive injuries is well described.

The clinical presentation is variable and hard to define. It usually includes a combination of hearing loss (which may be fluctuating, sudden or progressive), tinnitus, and dizziness. The dizziness is most commonly a mix of disequilibrium with intermittent vertiginous spells lasting seconds to hours. Classically, the vertigo will be induced by pressure change such as straining or air travel. There is no single diagnostic test. Nystagmus may be noted on VNG, while pressure change is induced through a tympanometer, and audiograms may vary. The differential diagnosis includes Ménière's disease and auto-immune inner ear disease.

Treatment in the acute phase is with head elevation and bed rest. Surgical plugging of the defect can be curative but it can be difficult to identify the site of the leak.

Superior semicircular canal dehiscence syndrome

Superior semicircular canal dehiscence syndrome (SSCD) was first described in 1998 and also presents with a variety of paroxysmal audiovestibular symptoms. It is likely to be increasingly commonly diagnosed as it becomes better recognised. It results from the bony covering between the superior border of the superior semicircular canal and the middle cranial fossa becoming deficient. Despite most likely representing a congenital thinning of the bone, it tends to present in middle age, or possibly after trauma.

Auditory symptoms include autophony and aural fullness, while audiometry often shows a low-frequency conductive hearing loss resulting from the mobile 'third window' into the middle fossa, which 'shunts' away sound energy. Vestibular symptoms are common but variable and not always present. Noise- and pressure-induced dizziness are sometimes seen. Both high-resolution computerised tomography (CT) scanning and vestibular evoked myogenic potentials (VEMPs) can aid diagnosis.

As treatment involves surgery, with a middle cranial fossa approach, many patients decide to live with the condition, but significant surgical series are developing around the world.

Auto-immune inner ear disease

Auto-immune inner ear disease (AIED) is usually associated with fluctuating bilateral sensorineural hearing loss that is responsive to immunosuppression. However, it may present with a Ménière's-type clustering of paroxysmal vertigo associated usually with hearing loss, which proves to be extremely responsive to steroids or indeed more potent immunosuppressants.

Fixed vestibular disorders

'Chronic vestibulopathy'

The most common presentation to a balance clinic is that of chronic dizziness resulting from permanent damage to the peripheral vestibular system affecting the eight nerve or the labyrinth. The symptoms are similar (Box 24.1), irrespective of the many causes discussed. They arise from inadequate central compensation to the vestibular injury. While most patients will be asymptomatic with this asymmetric input from the peripheral vestibular system, others will experience chronic disequilibrium and some motion-induced dizziness. The symptoms usually settle when the patient remains still. It is common for patients to experience relapses of symptoms under both physiological stress (for example

other illnesses or sleeplessness), or psychological stress, often over many years.

Clinical findings may include abnormal head thrust tests and Unterberger's marching test (the patient usually turns to the affected ear), indicating vestibular asymmetry. There is almost always an associated stress reaction from the patient with chronic disease.

Investigations include ENG or VNG, which may help distinguish peripheral from central causes and indicate which side is affected (nystagmus beats away from the affected ear). Computerised dynamic posturography (Figure 24.2) may be particularly helpful in difficult cases in defining the way in which the balance system has tried to compensate for the vestibular injury. 'Visual preference' is a common finding. In this condition, the eyes try to compensate for the lost vestibular function, so balance is more reliant on visual stimuli. However, in complex visual environments (such as supermarkets, scrolling down a computer screen, or walking on patterned carpets), the visual stimuli cannot be processed centrally in a form that is adequate for balance – the conflicting sensory stimuli result in dizziness.

Establishing the diagnosis is of great importance to most patients, many of whom have drifted without a clear understanding of their condition, and is the first step to recovery. Many will also have been taking vestibular sedatives over long periods, preventing recovery. These should be stopped. A simple analogy may help your patients:

> Imagine you are the pilot of an airplane which loses one of its two engines. You have three options. If nothing is done you will spin out of control. If you shut down both engines you will glide, which seems good in the short term – this is the same as taking vestibular sedatives – but the underlying damage will never be fixed. Alternatively, wrestle with the controls to stabilise the plane to its new situation – this is what physiotherapy aims to do.

An individually tailored programme of vestibular rehabilitation physiotherapy, targeting particularly the VOR, with the support of a specialist vestibular physiotherapist, can lead to a successful outcome in 85% of patients with chronic symptoms.

Vestibular neuronitis

Vestibular neuronitis is the most common cause of chronic vestibulopathy presenting to the balance clinic. Its acute phase is seen more commonly in general practice. It has many synonyms. Vestibular neuritis, viral labyrinthitis (it isn't, as it is the nerve that is affected, and the cochlea, which is part of the labyrinth, is spared), epidemic vertigo (as it is sometimes seen to cluster in communities, presumably due to a viral aetiology), and acute vestibulopathy.

Aetiology

It is believed to result most commonly from virally induced inflammation of the superior division of the vestibular nerve. This may result from reactivation of a latent herpes simplex virus in the vestibular ganglion, or may be a new infection from a neurotropic virus, as is seen occasionally in the 'epidemics' of vestibular neuronitis. A vascular event could also cause similar consequences. Inflammation of the nerve leads to an acute reduction in vestibular function and subsequent degeneration to chronic vestibular hypofunction. Since neither the vestibular labyrinth nor the cochlear nerve are affected, hearing is not lost.

Diagnosis

A rapid onset of severe vertigo associated with nausea and vomiting which settles over days, in the absence of any auditory or neurological symptoms or signs, is the typical presentation. The vertigo improves over days or weeks. Over subsequent weeks, months or even years, dizziness may persist because of the resulting chronic vestibulopathy. It is not uncommon for BPPV to develop later as a result of the degeneration in the labyrinth.

Treatment

In the acute phase, anti-emetics are the mainstay of treatment, along with reassurance. Antiviral medicines have been tried without great success. Corticosteroids have been shown to improve recovery in one well-conducted trial but are not yet widely used (Strupp *et al.*, 2004).

Other causes of vestibular hypofunction

Anything that can cause damage to the peripheral vestibular system may induce a chronic vestibulopathy that may not compensate and so leads to chronic symptoms. Common causes are trauma, middle ear surgery, and advanced Ménière's disease. Vertigo is an uncommon complaint with acoustic neuromas, but disequilibrium is common with larger tumours.

Ototoxicity from drug therapy can be devastating as it can induce bilateral vestibular failure. This induces the unpleasant symptom of oscillopsia. The horizon is seen to bob up and down as one walks. It is more difficult to treat than unilateral vestibular loss. Rather than the *adaptation* strategies described above, *substitution* strategies are employed using visual and postural cues. Much the most commonly implicated drug is the aminoglycoside antibiotic gentamicin, which is selectively vestibulotoxic, sparing cochlear function. Total dosage seems the most important risk factor, although a small proportion of the population is exquisitely sensitive to it, a factor coded for in their mitochondria due to genetic mutation. Other important ototoxic drugs include vancomycin, loop diuretics, and the chemotherapeutic drug cisplatin.

Multisystem balance disorders

So far we have been discussing relatively isolated vestibular events. In many patients there is a reason for their failure to recover from a vestibular insult and this should be sought with a thorough neuro-otological examination in the clinic. In elderly patients a multitude of medical and social problems may co-exist to prevent recovery. All three of the key areas of balance assessment outlined in the introduction are important: sensory inputs, central processing, and musculoskeletal responses. Nowhere is the multidisciplinary nature of balance medicine better seen than in the management of such patients. Many centres have developed 'falls clinics' run by physicians specialising in the care of the elderly, with support from physiotherapists, occupational health teams, audiologists, and community services. These clinics may run in parallel to more specialist balance clinics, cardiovascular and neurological services.

Ageing alone will slow recovery, as neuronal plasticity in the brain reduces, along with muscle bulk, and mobility. Diabetes or medications for hypertension may predispose to postural hypotension. Diabetes may also lead to peripheral neuropathy and poor vision. Parkinsonian symptoms may be seen in patients on long-term medication, particularly prochlorperazine, and Parkinson's disease is frequently diagnosed in the balance clinic.

Arthritis is more common and the elderly patient may find their additional vestibular disorder is the last straw, preventing them from self-caring. It is common to develop a 'fear of falling' at this stage. However, a team approach can not only greatly improve the quality of life of those affected, but also reduce the risks of fractures from falls.

Central balance disorders

Migraine and psychological disorder are extremely common causes of dizziness and must be clearly understood by anyone assessing dizziness. Tumours, multiple sclerosis, and rarer neurological disorders are very uncommon causes, although important and often a patient's first fear.

Migraine

Migraine is now widely recognised as one of the commonest causes of vertigo. Some claim it to be the second commonest cause after BPPV. It seems very likely that patients who might previously have been labelled with 'recurrent vestibular neuronitis' were in fact suffering from migraine. The annual prevalence of migrainous vertigo approaches 1% of the population (Neuhauser,

2007). The vertigo and dizziness may last seconds, minutes, hours, or even days. Headaches occur with the vertigo in only 25–50% of cases. To establish a diagnosis, a personal or family history of migraine is helpful. A migraine aura is diagnostic, and patients often report visual changes such as flashing lights or zigzag lines if prompted. Balance is usually good between attacks, although patients may be predisposed to motion sickness. There is a female predominance. Physical examination is usually normal, while ENG changes are noted in 10%. Treatment is with the lifestyle changes (stress reduction and sleep), dietary modifications, and range of migraine prophylactic medications that are used already for migraine management. Treatment can be very successful.

Psychological

Every patient with a chronic balance disorder has a psychological reaction to it, whether this is an anxiety or depressive reaction. In approximately 20% of patients, this reaction becomes the predominant disorder. Most of the time, by successfully treating the underlying balance disorder the psychological reaction will melt away. If possible, it is better to avoid medication, especially early in treatment. The support of a psychologist or psychiatrist can be very helpful, even alongside vestibular rehabilitation therapy.

A number of psychological disorders prove to be the primary cause of the dizziness. The commonest is panic disorder, often associated with hyperventilation. Peri-oral paraesthesia is often experienced, along with tingling in the fingers and toes during attacks. Hyperventilation tests in clinic can suggest the diagnosis but have been found to have a low specificity.

Antidepressant and sedative drugs are also common causes of chronic dizziness, and patients should be asked about these.

Tumours

Tumours are a surprisingly uncommon cause of dizziness and rarely cause vertigo. Audiometric asymmetry raises the possibility of an associated acoustic neuroma. The greatest risk is in those patients with progressive imbalance. Posterior fossa lesions are the most commonly seen. Fundoscopy should be performed to exclude papill-oedema, as raised intracranial pressure may require urgent neurosurgical referral.

Other central disorders

Many balance centres run joint clinics with neurologists. Given the huge range of possible associated neurological disorders, this can be a valuable educational and diagnostic set up. Only a selection of the more commonly considered conditions are explored in this section.

One common referral is for exclusion of *vertebrobasilar insufficiency* (VBI). This has often been described as presenting as acute dizziness on neck extension. Almost all cases turn out to be BPPV. True VBI is a transient ischaemic attack affecting the posterior brain circulation, culminating, if prolonged, in infarction. Hence true VBI is both rare and associated usually with visual dysfunction, and often drop attacks, inco-ordination, and confusion. When assessing for this condition, consider also *Arnold–Chiari malformation* which results from prolapse of the cerebellar tonsils into the foramen magnum. Downbeat nystagmus is often seen on neck extension, for example on Dix–Hallpike's test.

Neck injury, particularly whiplash injuries, may be associated with non-specific dizziness. This can be a difficult diagnosis as most patients with vestibular disorders have neck pain too. The resulting *cervical vertigo* is often a diagnosis of exclusion. Similarly, head injury can produce a *post-concussion* syndrome characterised by chronic non-specific dizziness.

Multiple sclerosis presents with an initial disturbance of balance in 20% of patients. There are, however, usually other neurological symptoms and signs – and indeed they are required to establish a diagnosis.

Assessment of the chronically dizzy patient does require careful assessment of cerebellar function. Cerebellar degeneration and atrophy are frequently seen in the balance clinic. Symp-

toms are often slowly progressive and constant. Walking on uneven surfaces becomes especially difficult. The integration of the sensory input to balance becomes deranged, and difficulties arise from both postural control and the VOR. The examination may reveal a broad-based ataxic gait, and tandem gait testing becomes difficult. Slow ocular pursuit and saccades will be abnormal. Brain imaging will be required. Vestibular rehabilitation therapy becomes more challenging but may be considered as part of a wider care package.

Summary

Balance disorders and dizziness are common and draw on many different specialties in a truly multidisciplinary approach. The establishment of increasing numbers of balance centres, and growing recognition of the disorders, will lead to significant improvements in patient care in the years ahead.

References

Bolas-Aguirre MS, Lin FR, Della Santina CC, Minor LB, Carey JP (2007) Longitudinal results with intratympanic dexamethasone in the treatment of Ménière's disease. *Otology and Neurotology* 29:33–38.

Brandt T, Daroff RB (1980) Physical therapy for benign paroxysmal positional vertigo. *Archives of Otolaryngology* 106:484–485.

Chia SH, Gamst AC, Anderson JP, Harris JP (2004) Intratympanic gentamicin therapy for Ménière's disease: a meta-analysis. *Otology and Neurotology* 25:544–552.

Epley JM (1992) The canalith repositioning procedure: for treatment of benign paroxysmal positional vertigo. *Otolaryngology – Head and Neck Surgery* 107:399–404.

Merchant SN, Adams JC, Nadol JB (2005) Pathophysiology of Ménière's syndrome: are symptoms caused by endolymphatic hydrops? *Otology and Neurotology* 26:74–81.

Nazareth I, Yardley L, Owens N, Luxon L (1999) Outcome of symptoms of dizziness in a general practice community sample. *Family Practice* 16:616–619.

Neuhauser HK (2007) Epidemiology of vertigo. *Current Opinion in Neurology* 20:40–46.

Neuhauser HK, von Brevern M, Radtke A *et al.* (2005) Epidemiology of vestibular vertigo. A neurotologic survey of the general population. *Neurology* 65:898–904.

Strupp M, Zingler V, Arbusow V *et al.* (2004) Methylprednisolone, valacyclovir or the combination for vestibular neuritis. *New England Journal of Medicine* 351:354–361.

Index

Note: page numbers in *italics* refer to figures, those in **bold** refer to tables